Veterinary Public Health & Epidemiology

Krishna Gopal Narayan •
Dharmendra Kumar Sinha •
Dhirendra Kumar Singh

Veterinary Public Health & Epidemiology

Veterinary Public Health- Epidemiology-Zoonosis-One Health

Springer

Krishna Gopal Narayan
Veterinary Public Health & Epidemiology
Ranchi Veterinary College
Ranchi, Jharkhand, India

Dharmendra Kumar Sinha
Division of Epidemiology
ICAR-Indian Veterinary Research Institute
Izatnagar, Uttar Pradesh, India

Dhirendra Kumar Singh
Division of Veterinary Public Health
ICAR-Indian Veterinary Research Institute
Izatnagar, Uttar Pradesh, India

ISBN 978-981-19-7799-2 ISBN 978-981-19-7800-5 (eBook)
https://doi.org/10.1007/978-981-19-7800-5

This Springer imprint is published by the registered company Springer Nature Singapore Pte Ltd.
The registered company address is: 152 Beach Road, #21-01/04 Gateway East, Singapore 189721, Singapore

Preface

We have covered four areas Veterinary Public Health, One Health, Epidemiology, and Zoonoses. While zoonoses are the problems the rest are the paths to control and prevent zoonoses. [*Our first book Veterinary Public Health and Epidemiology (Veterinary Public Health, Epidemiology, Zoonoses, One Health) deals with the basics.*]

Veterinary Public Health (VPH) is the sum of all contributions to the complete physical, mental, and social well-being of humans through an understanding and application of veterinary medical science. VPH impacts on human health by reducing exposure to hazards arising from animals (including wildlife), animal products, and their environment. One Health is defined as a collaborative, international, cross-sectoral, multidisciplinary mechanism to address threats and reduce risks of detrimental infectious diseases at the animal-human-ecosystem interface.

Zoonoses management requires knowledge of zoonotic pathogen, epidemiology, diagnosis, treatment, and prevention. We have organised the knowledge, data, and information on most of the zoonotic agents in this structure.

Epidemiology is basic to the understanding of disease in herd or population and comprises studies dedicated to the diseases (a) in single host species or to a single target species (classical epidemiology) and those (b) caused by multi-host pathogens (ecology of diseases). Understanding of this complex multi-host system (ecology of disease) is a prerequisite to designing measures to prevent zoonoses in the target hosts, i.e. human population.

Pathogens, insect vectors, and hosts (reservoir, bridge, and target) are influenced by climate and ecology. The vector population, development, activity, and spread are dependent upon environmental temperature, rainfall, humidity, soil, type of terrain, and vegetation around. Understanding the transmission of infectious agents between maintenance hosts, bridge hosts, and target hosts requires integration of ecological and epidemiological approaches.

The zoonotic pathogen-host interaction is an interesting and developing area. Understanding virulence factors, mechanism of invasion of host cells, and evasion of host immune system offers opportunities to search for antigens to prepare monoclonal antibodies (for specific detection and prevention of further invasion of host's cell) and therapeutic molecules.

Diagnostic methods and safety requirement of laboratory have been described.

Approaches to prevention like surveillance, active, passive, sentinel etc., and specific methods like vaccination are detailed. The role of state sectors like health and veterinary services, World Organization for Animal Health (WOAH) and World Health Organization, and specific recommendations have been described.

Zoonotic pandemics and serious outbreaks like bird flu, severe acute respiratory syndrome (SARS-1, SARS-2), Ebola, Rift Valley fever, West Nile fever, and the most recent monkeypox virus have been dealt with including details of some WHO managed outbreaks.

Managing events preceding the precipitation of clinical zoonotic illness/disease in population is dealt with in the first section. Diverse wildlife with a pool of variety of pathogens is in a state of equilibrium evolved through dynamic natural ecological processes. Interaction of human ecosystem is also dynamic but imperceptible till the balance (equilibrium) is altered. The wildlife and human share the same space at the interface. Pathogens spill over from the natural niche in the forest to cause pandemics. Understanding of what is happening or predicting the changes at the interfaces and ecotones is necessary in averting pandemics. Surveillance is a tool. Health system uses this with intervention methods to prevent infection progressing through sporadic, outbreak, and epidemic to pandemic.

Finally, available measures of averting zoonoses have been elucidated. Averting zoonotic pandemics is a matter of global concern.

Ranchi, Jharkhand, India — Krishna Gopal Narayan
Izatnagar, Uttar Pradesh, India — Dharmendra Kumar Sinha
Izatnagar, Uttar Pradesh, India — Dhirendra Kumar Singh

Contents

About the Authors

Krishna Gopal Narayan remained engaged actively for 39 years in veterinary education and research in various capacities and is continuing his academic interest. He has been a rank officer—beginning as House surgeon-cum-Demonstrator in Bihar Veterinary College, Patna, in 1959, kept on changing positions through selection, as Assistant professor in Panjab Agricultural University and Associate Professor in Haryana Agricultural University. He moved on to Rajendra Agricultural University as Professor of Veterinary Public Health and Epidemiology and became Dean, Faculty of Veterinary Sciences and Animal Husbandry in Birsa Agricultural University. He retired in 1998.

He continues his interest in Veterinary Public Health and Epidemiology right from the time earning his specialization degree (C. Sc., Budapest) in 1966 even after retirement. He is a recipient of the prestigious Fakhruddin Ali Ahmed Award for Outstanding Research in Tribal Farming Systems of ICAR (precisely for research on rabies). He was a member of the Veterinary Council of India. The Indian Association of Veterinary Public Health Specialists (IAVPHS) conferred him with Life Time Achievement Award for his outstanding contributions to the veterinary profession in general and Veterinary Public Health and Epidemiology in particular.

He has more than 70 research publications in peer-reviewed national and international journals besides many chapters in books. He has also authored a book and has been a member of the editorial commitee for various journals. He has chaired many scientific sessions at different conferences.

Dharmendra Kumar Sinha, Principal Scientist, is a senior faculty of Veterinary Public Health and Epidemiology at ICAR-Indian Veterinary Research Institute, Izatnagar, India. His fields of research are monitoring and surveillance, seroepidemiology, investigation of animal disease outbreak, meta-analysis, and economics losses due to animal diseases. He has handled several institutional projects as Principal Investigator (PI) and Co-PI of ICAR-funded projects. Dr Sinha has served as referee for a number of journals. He has 25 years of postgraduate teaching experience of epidemiology.

He has published more than 60 research papers in peer-reviewed national and international journals. He has authored one book on epidemiology besides many chapters. He is a member of several scientific societies, including Indian Association of Veterinary Microbiology, Immunology and Infectious Diseases; Indian

Association of Immunology and Immunopathology; and Indian Association of Veterinary Public Health Specialists.

Dhirendra Kumar Singh is a Principal Scientist (Retd. April 2022) in the Division of Veterinary Public Health at ICAR-Indian Veterinary Research Institute, Izatnagar, India. His research interests have been foodborne infections and intoxications and zoonoses particularly diagnosis and epidemiology. He has worked extensively in the field of brucellosis. Dr Singh has served as referee for numerous national and international journals which included *Indian Journal of Comparative Microbiology, Immunology and Infectious Diseases*; *Journal of Applied Animal Research*; *Tropical Animal Health and production*; and *Comparative Immunology, Microbiology and Infectious Diseases*. He was a member of many expert committees in the ICAR and Department of Animal Husbandry Dairying & Fisheries (DADF) under the Government of India. He has varied teaching experience of more than 28 years and taught veterinary public health; zoonoses; foodborne infections and intoxications; fish hygiene; environmental hygiene and epidemiology to undergraduate students and postgraduate scholars as faculty at the Division of Veterinary Public Health.

He has to his credit more than 50 research publications in peer-reviewed national and international journals. He has also authored many chapters in books. He is a member of many scientific societies like Indian Association of Veterinary Microbiology, Immunology and Infectious Diseases; Indian Society of Veterinary Immunologists and Biotechnologists; Indian Association for Advancement of Veterinary Research; and Indian Public Health Association.

Abbreviations

AAD	Antibiotic-associated diarrhoea
ACDP	Advisory Committee on Dangerous Pathogens
AF	Attributable fraction
AGPT	Agar gel precipitation test
AIDS	Acquired immunodeficiency syndrome
AM	Ante meridiem; Ante-mortem
AMP	Adenosine monophosphate
AMR	Antimicrobial resistance
AMUL	Anand Milk Union Limited, Gujarat
Anti-ABE	Anti-ABE trivalent antitoxin
AR	Attributable risk
AR	Attack rate
aW	Water activity
B/C ratio	Benefit cost ratio
BASE	Bovine amyloidotic spongiform encephalopathy
BEC	Binary enterotoxin of *C. perfringens*
Bfv	Blanched frozen vegetable
BoNTs	Botulinum neurotoxins
BSE	Bovine spongiform encephalitis
BTB	Bovine tuberculosis
C. botulinum	*Clostridium botulinum*
C. perfringens	*Clostridium perfringens*
CBPP	Contagious bovine pleuropneumonia
CCP	Critical control point
CDC	Centers for Disease Control and Prevention
CDR	Crude death rate
CDS	Department of Communicable Diseases, WHO/SEARO
CFIA	Canadian Food Inspection Agency
CFR	Case fatality rate
CFT	Complement fixation test
CFU	Colony forming unit
cGMP	Cyclic guanosine monophosphate
CH_4	Methane
CI	Confidence interval

Cia	*Campylobacter* invasive antigen
CIEP	Counterimmunoelectrophoresis
CIR	Cumulative incidence rate
CJDnv	Creutzfeldt-Jakob disease new variant
Cl. botulinum	*Clostridium botulinum*
Cl. perfringens	*Clostridium perfringens*
cm	Centimetre
CMO	Chief Medical Officer
CNS	Central nervous system
COVID-19	Coronavirus disease (originated in 2019 in Wuhan, China)
CPE	*C. perfringens* enterotoxin
CPILE	*C. perfringens* iota like enterotoxin
CSF	Cerebrospinal fluid
CSR	Communicable disease surveillance, outbreak alert and response
CVO	Chief Veterinary Officer
CWD	Chronic Wasting Disease
CytK	Cytotoxin K
DAEC	Diffuse adherent *Escherichia coli*
DALYs	Disability Adjusted Life Years
DEC	Diarrhoeagenic *Escherichia coli*
DEFRA	Department of Environment, Food and Rural Affairs
DH	Department of Health
DNA	Deoxyribonucleic acid
DZC	Danish Zoonosis Centre
E. coli	*Escherichia coli*
e.g.	Example
EAEC	Enteroaggregative *Escherichia coli*
Ed.	Edition
EEA	European Economic Area
EFSA	European Food Safety Authority
EHEC	Enterohaemorrhagic *Escherichia coli*
EIA	Enzyme immuno assay
EIDs	Emerging infectious diseases
EIEC	Enteroinvasive *Escherichia coli*
EIN	Emerging Infectious disease Network
ELISA	Enzyme-linked immunosorbent assay
EMB agar	Eosin methylene blue agar
EMG	Electromyography
EMPRESS	Emergency Prevention System
EN	Enteritis necroticans
EPEC	Enteropathogenic *Escherichia coli*
epg	Eggs per gram
ERIC-PCR	Enterobacterial Repetitive Intergenic Consensus-Polymerase Chain Reaction
ESBL	Extended spectrum beta-lactamase

ESBL-KP	Extended spectrum beta-lactamase producing *Klebsiella pneumoniae*
ESKAPE	*Enterococcus faecium*, *Staphylococcus aureus*, *Klebsiella pneumoniae*, *Acinetobacter baumannii*, *Pseudomonas aeruginosa*, and *Enterobacter* spp.
etc.	Et cetera
ETEC	Enterotoxigenic *Escherichia coli*
ETs	Exfoliative toxins
EU	European Union
ExPEC	Extra-intestinal pathogenic *Escherichia coli*
FAO	Food and Agriculture Organization of the United Nations
FAT	Fluorescent antibody test
FBD	Foodborne disease
FC	Food Chain
FCC-ICU	Food Chain Crisis-Intelligence and Coordination Unit, FAO
FDA	U.S. Food and Drug Administration
FDCs	Follicular dendritic cells
FERG	Foodborne Disease Epidemiology Reference Group, WHO
Fig.	Figure
FMC	Fairfield Medical Centre
FMD	Foot and mouth disease
FMDV	Foot and mouth disease virus
FPE	Food processing environment
FSA	Food Safety Agency
GBS	Guillain-Barre syndrome
GEIS	Global Emerging Infection Surveillance and Response System
GHP	Good hygienic practice
GIS	Geographic information system
GLEWS	Global Early Warning System
GMP	Guanosine monophosphate
GN cake	Groundnut cake
GNI	Gross national income
GPHIN	Global Public Health Information Network
GPS	Global Positioning System
GSSS	Gerstmann-Straussler-Scheinker syndrome
HA	Haemagglutinin
HACCP	Hazard Analysis Critical Control Point
HAV	Hepatitis A virus
Hbl	Haemolysin B l
HEV	Hepatitis E virus
HIV	Human immunodeficiency virus
Hl	Haemolysin
HPA	Health Protection Agency
HPAI	Highly pathogenic avian influenza
HS	Health service

HTLV	Human-T-lymphotropic virus
HUS	Haemolytic uraemic syndrome
i.e.	id est (that is)
IBC	Intrabacterial Community
ICCU	Intensive critical care units
ICMR	Indian Council of Medical Research
IDs	Infectious diseases
IDU	Injecting drug users
IFAT	Indirect fluorescent antibody test
IFN-y	Interferon gamma
Ig	Immunoglobulin
IHR	International Health Regulations
IMViC	Indole, Methyl red, Voges-Proskauer, and Citrate
INFOSAN	International Food Safety Authorities Network (WHO/FAO)
iNTS	Invasive non-typhoidal *Salmonella*
IP	Incubation period
IPEC	Intestinal pathogenic *Escherichia coli*
IPT	Immunoperoxidase test
IR	Incidence rate
IRR	Internal rate of return
ISO	International Organization for Standardization
JEV	Japanese encephalitis virus
K	Kelvin
kDA	Kilo Dalton
KFD	Kyasanur Forest disease
kg	Kilogramme
KPC	*Klebsiella pneumonia* carbapenemase
LBM	Live bird market
LPS	Lipopolysaccharide
LT	Heat labile
MALD-TOFMS	Matrix-assisted laser desorption/ionisation time of flight mass spectrophotometry
MBM	Meat cum bone meal
MDR	Multidrug resistance
MHC-II	Histocompatibility complex class II
MLD_{50}	Median lethal dose
MLPI	Multilocus phylogenetic analysis
MLST	Multilocus sequence typing
MLVA	Multiple locus variable-number tandem analysis
MRSA	Methicillin-resistant *Staphylococcus aureus*
MSM	Man sex with man
MSSA	Methicillin-sensitive *Staphylococcus aureus*
MYP agar	Mannitol egg yolk polymyxin agar
N	Nitrogen

N_2O	Nitrous oxide
NA	Neuraminidase
NCU	Neonatal care units
NEPNEI	National Expert Panel on New and Emerging Infections
Nhe	Non-haemolytic enterotoxin
NHPs	Non-human primates
NoV	Noro virus
NPV	Net present value
NSW	New South Wales
NTNH	Non-toxic non-haemagglutinin
ODH	Ohio Department of Health
OIE	World Organisation for Animal Health (Office International des epizootics)
OR	Odds ratio
ORpop	Population odds ratio
OWOH	One World One Health
P	Phosphorus
PAF	Population attributable fraction
PAHO	Pan American Health Organization
PAR	Population attributable rate
PCR	Polymerase chain reaction
PDS	Participatory disease surveillance
PET	Paraffin-embedded tissue
PFGE	Pulsed-field gel electrophoresis
pH	Potential of hydrogen
PH	Public Health
PHEIC	Public Health Emergency of International Concern
PI-PLC	Phosphatidylinositol-phospholipase C
PM	Post meridiem; post-mortem
PPR	Peste des Petits Ruminants
PRNP	Prion protein
ProMED	Programme for Monitoring Emerging Diseases
PRP/A	Prerequisite programme and activities
PrP^{res}	Protease-resistant prion protein
PSR	Polymerase spiral reaction
PSWID	Person who inject drugs
PVL	Panton-Valentine leucocidin
Q fever	Query fever
QMRA	Quantitative microbiological risk assessment
R. prowazekii	*Rickettsia prowazekii*
R_0	Basic reproduction number/Basic reproductive rate
RAPD-PCR	Random amplification of polymorphic DNA-polymerase chain reaction
REP-PCR	Repetitive extragenic palindromes-polymerase chain reaction
RNA	Ribonucleic acid

ROC	Receiver-operator characteristic
RODS	Real-time Outbreak Diseases Surveillance
RP	Rinderpest
RR	Relative risk
RRpop	Population relative risk
RTE	Ready to eat
RT-PCR	Reverse transcription polymerase chain reaction
RV	Rotavirus
RVA	Rota virus A
SAgs	Superantigens
SARS	Severe acute respiratory syndrome
SARSV	Severe acute respiratory syndrome virus
SCV	*Salmonella* containing vacuole
SD	Standard deviation
SDS-PAGE	Sodium dodecyl sulphate-polyacrylamide gel electrophoresis
SEs	*Staphylococcus* Exo/endotoxins
SFP	*S. aureus* food poisoning
SFV	Simian foamy virus
SIV	Simian immunodeficiency virus
SMS	Short Message Service
SNARE	Soluble N-ethylmaleimide-sensitive-factor attachment protein receptor
SNOMED	Systematized Nomenclature of Medicine
SNOVET	Systemic Nomenclature of Veterinary Medicine
SNVDO	Standard Nomenclature of Veterinary Diseases and Operations
spp.	Species
SRM	Specified risk materials
SRSVs	Small rounded structured viruses
ssE	Spore structural protein gene
ssRNA	Single-stranded ribonucleic acid
ST	Heat stable/sequence typing
STEC	Shiga toxin-producing *Escherichia coli*
STSS	Streptococcal toxic shock syndrome
Stx	Shiga-like toxin
T. canis	*Toxocara canis*
t/T	Time and treatment
TB	Tuberculosis
TGE	Transmissible Gastroenteritis
TSE	Transmissible spongiform encephalitis
TSI	Triple sugar iron
TSST	Toxic shock syndrome exotoxin
TTSS	Specialised protein secretion machinery
TTX	Tetrodotoxin
UK	United Kingdom
UKZG	United Kingdom Zoonoses Group

UNICEF	United Nations Children's Fund
UNSIC	United Nations System Influenza Coordinator
UPEC	Uropathogenic *Escherichia coli*
USA	United States of America
UTIs	Urinary tract infections
VAP	Ventilator-associated pneumonia
VBDs	Vector-borne diseases
vCJD	Variant Creutzfeldt-Jakob disease
VLA	Veterinary Laboratory Agency
VP	Viral protein
VPH	Veterinary Public Health
VPHE	Veterinary Public Health and Epidemiology
VS	Veterinary Service
VTEC	Verotoxigenic *Escherichia coli*
WAHIS	World Animal Health Information System
WGS	Whole genome sequencing
WHO	World Health Organization
WTO	World Trade Organization
WWTP	Wastewater treatment plant
Y. pestis	*Yersinia pestis*
ZEBOV	Zaire Ebola virus
%	Per cent
μg/mL	Microgram per millilitre
^{0}C	Degree centigrade
5-HT3	5-hydroxytryptamine 3

Veterinary Public Health

1

Abstract

Preventing the spread of infectious diseases is a global public good (public good is a concept associated with economic policies. Over 60% of human infectious diseases are zoonoses). Veterinary service stands on a tripod of (a) animal production, (b) animal health, and (c) veterinary public health (VPH). Claude Bourgelat, the founder of veterinary services and education mentioned in his testament 'interrelatedness of animals and human (Comparative Pathology)'. In fact, veterinary public health was born when Rudolf Virchow coined the term zoonoses after realising that man and animals acted as co-determinants. William Osler (1849–1919) organised a significant study of parasites in pork supply, suspecting human infection. Ante-mortem and post-mortem meat inspections protected humans from trichinellosis and taeniasis, besides other meat-borne diseases. Organised slaughter house and meat inspection enabled detection of bovine-tuberculosis-infected herd through back tracing economically, established a method of 'reverse tracing' as an important tool in epidemiological investigation. Epidemiology and zoonoses are the most important components. The Veterinary Public Health Division at the Centers for Disease Control and Prevention (CDC) was founded by James H. Steele (1947), who strongly advocated that 'good animal health is important for good public health'.

This chapter deals with Veterinary Public Health, the way it integrates human and animal health, the organisation at the international and national levels, and how the World Health Organization (WHO) and Office International des Epizooties (OIE) are integrated into it. The horizon of its activities is wide; it covers rural and urban health alike and provides food safety from farm to fork. VPH has access to several health-related areas.

K. G. Narayan et al., *Veterinary Public Health & Epidemiology*,
https://doi.org/10.1007/978-981-19-7800-5_1

1.1 Definitions

Veterinary services (VSs) are defined as governmental and non-governmental organisations that implement animal health and welfare measures and other standards and recommendations contained in the 'Terrestrial Code and the OIE Aquatic Animal Health Code in the Territory' (OIE 2012). VS is essentially a 'preventive medicine', where epidemiology is basic and inbuilt. The critical domains of a well-governed VS are the surveillance of animal health, the early detection of disease outbreaks, rapid response to disease outbreaks, at-source eradication of animal diseases (if possible), the coordination and implementation of specific disease control programmes and vaccination campaigns, the enforcement of veterinary legislation, and the establishment of public-private partnerships for sustainable animal health systems.

Veterinary services were born to promote 'Livestock production, prevention and cure of diseases, grazing and training of farmers and public' in France, as desired by King Louis XV. In his testament, founder Claude Bourgelat wrote about the concept of 'Inter-relatedness', i.e. comparative pathology. Many VSs were created to combat the devastating outbreaks of rinderpest, for example in India. Later, the 'control and eradication (wherever possible) of animal diseases in general' was added. Many countries are concerned about (a) increasing the level of production of livestock and fish, (b) the elimination of certain risks that threaten these animals, and (c) assuring the quality and safety of food produced along the chain of production, processing, conservation, and marketing at the national and international levels. Such efforts require an 'integrated approach', for which sharing of information is essential.

1.1.1 Office International des Epizooties (World Organization for Animal Health)

The Office International des Epizooties (OIE) was established in 1924 with office in Paris and with three main objectives: (a) to disseminate information on animal health worldwide, (b) to coordinate international research on important animal diseases and their control, and (c) to harmonise trade regulations relating to animals and animal products. OIE is involved in veterinary public health (VPH) issues in the context of these three objectives, and its activities are primarily to (a) survey information on internationally important animal diseases, including zoonoses and exchange; (b) harmonise international efforts to prevent and control animal diseases; and (c) publish and disseminate scientific materials. OIE presents a synthesis of animal health information obtained from member and non-member countries. It provides a unique tool for all those involved in animal production, wildlife disease surveillance, international trade in animals and animal products, and the epidemiology and control of animal diseases, including zoonoses (http://www.oie.int/animal-health-in-the-world/world-animal-health/). OIE has access to many links of global agencies, such as the World Health Organization (WHO), Food and Agriculture Organization (FAO), Food Safety International Authorities Network (INFOSAN), FAO/WHO/

OIE Global Early Warning System for Major Animal Diseases including Zoonoses (GLEWS+), Emergency Prevention System for Food Safety (EMPRES Food Safety), etc. VS *guarantees programmed development of the World Food system and its stability. Good governance is required.*

1.1.2 World Health Organization (WHO): VPH

Veterinary Public Health (VPH) was established in 1948 by the World Health Organization (WHO) during the First World Health Assembly, where rabies and brucellosis were discussed and various actions were proposed. It was in response to a memo submitted by Dr. James Harlan Steele dated 7 May 1946. Dr. Martin M. Kaplan developed the VPH programme in the Communicable Disease division (Steele 2008).

At present, the Communicable Disease Surveillance and Control (CSR) Department of WHO (TRS 907) implements the activities of VPH in collaboration with its food safety programmes. It contributes to the global efforts of CSR in strengthening the surveillance of and response to all communicable diseases that are or may emerge as a threat to public health.

CSR collaborates with the regional offices of WHO to support the surveillance and containment of zoonoses and food-borne zoonoses in man and animals in member states, which are of importance to public health. This collaboration is also extended for the disease of animal having known or potential public health implication besides for surveillance and containment of resistance to anti-microbial agents in animals having implications to human health.

All WHO regional offices have focal points, with the largest VPH programme by WHO at the Americas/Pan American Health Organization. For a global public goods (International Task Force on Global Public Goods 2006, p. 14) *there is a need of* public- and animal-health systems compliant with the WHO International Health Regulations (WHO 2005a) and OIE International Standards, through the pursuit of long-term interventions, which is robust as well as well governed. VPH is essentially a 'public good', and, therefore, the government needs to ensure the provision of VPH to all sections of the population, even though countries have variations in their actual mechanism for delivery (WHO 2002).

The International Task Force on Global Public Goods (2006) recognise 'the prevention of the spread of infectious diseases' as a global **public good**.

'Public good' is a concept associated with economic policies (Eloit 2012). *It is inclusive, encompasses several issues like education, environment, fundamental rights like 'right to health and food'. VS help improving animal health and reducing production losses, thus contributing directly and indirectly to food security and safeguarding human health and economic resources.*

Health is a state of complete physical, mental, and social well-being and not merely the absence of disease or infirmity (WHO 2005b). Health may also be defined as the ability of an individual to adapt and manage physical, mental, and social challenges throughout life.

Public health is the science and art of preventing disease, prolonging life, and promoting health through the organised efforts and informed choices of society; organisations, public and private; communities; and individuals (Winslow 1920).

Personal health is individuals' health, but to remain healthy is demanding, and a combined effort of the individuals and social and environmental protection institutions is required. Factors or determinants that influence individuals' health are a healthy community (i.e. social, economic, and educational), physical environment, and the individuals' characteristics, such as lifestyle, social status, and spiritual status.

Health service (HS) is a health delivery institution consisting of, mainly, two aspects—clinical medicine, which targets the 'individual', and public health, which targets the 'community and population'. Public health addresses the overall health of a community—from small to large—and is based on the analysis of the population's health, outbreaks, epidemics, and pandemics. HS uses surveillance, epidemiology, and biostatistics to study and address community health problems related to behaviour, the environment (natural, built, and social), and occupation. Common interventions are education and awareness programmes, the promotion of individual and community healthy behaviour and environmental hygiene, and vaccination during outbreaks.

Veterinary service contributes to (a) animal production, (b) animal health, and (c) human health by ensuring foods of animal origin and through protection from zoonoses. The contribution of the animal sector is >40% of the global value of agricultural production. An analysis of information on veterinary services (VS) from 178 countries showed that VS (see definition) impacted the food system and food security through six fields of activities—(1) organisation, (2) surveillance, (3) disease prevention and control, (4) sanitary inspection, (5) traceability, and (6) food hygiene, supported by institutional, legislative, and technical assistance.

'Animal-human interfaces' are better understood and realised by veterinarians. The principal beneficiary is the human population.

Robert Virchow realised that man and animals act as co-determinants of each other's health, and he created the term zoonoses for shared infections and diseases. Calvin W. Schwabe observed: 'The final objective of veterinary medicine does not lie in animal species that the veterinarians commonly treat, it lies very definitely in man and above all humanity.' He proposed 'One Medicine'. Dr. James H. Steele understood the important role of animals in the epidemiology of zoonotic diseases. The term veterinary public health (VPH) was coined by him. In 1947, he founded the Veterinary Public Health Division at CDC.

In 1975, a FAO/WHO joint expert committee met, of which Schwabe, Steele, and Dr. C.M. Singh from India were members, among others (*Veterinary Contribution to Public Health Practice—Joint Report of Expert Committee on VPH, 1975*). Areas of VPH activities were identified.

Veterinary public health is the sum of all contributions to the complete physical, mental, and social well-being of humans through the understanding and application of veterinary medical science. It concerns all aspects of the food production chain, from animal production to controlling epidemics that may impact agriculture, from ensuring the safe and humane slaughter of food animals to informing the public of safe ways to store and cook. It focuses on the interface between humans and animals and positively influences the human-animal connection, not only with regard to relevant diseases but also concerning the quality of life, health benefits, and environmental health issues. To attain optimum human health in a country, a sustainable relationship between humans, animals, and the environment is needed. All activities are based on epidemiological principles, methods, and practices; hence, it would be appropriate to use the term veterinary public health and epidemiology (VPHE).

1.1.2.1 A Sustainable Relationship

Animals and their insect vectors are sentinels for zoonotic agents, and the VPHE professional is the security guard. This is an old functional relationship. Detecting diseases, like bovine tuberculosis, cysticercosis, or trichinellosis, in an animal or its carcass during an ante-mortem/post-mortem inspection protected consumers. The practice of tracing back the infected herds of bovine tuberculosis, *Trichinella*, or *Salmonella*-infected pigs is 'detection of hotspots'. Pigs and mosquitoes used as sentinels for Japanese encephalitis virus (JEV) are scanned for virus/genome/antibodies, and concerned authorities, such as the health sector, are informed for risk assessment and proactive action to prevent an outbreak.

The 1999 West Nile outbreak in America (11% case fatality rate (CFR)) was misdiagnosed as St. Louis encephalitis till 27 September 1999. The veterinary pathologist at the Bronx Zoo helped in converging the up-to-then separate investigations. Dr. Laura Kahn observed that 'physicians treating the initial patients in New York City in 1999 might have benefited if they knew that in the previous months and concurrently, veterinarians in the surrounding area had been seeing dozens of crows dying with neurologic symptoms similar to those of the affected humans' (World Bank 2010).

According to the ancient account and modern hypothesis, death of the Alexander the Great in 323 BC in Babylon was due to encephalitis by West Nile virus with an extensive reservoir in wild birds. The death of flocks of ravens at the feet of Alexander showing unusual behaviour as he entered Babylon was reported by Marr and Calisher (Shanko et al. 2015).

1.1.3 Veterinary Public Health Functions

VPH is multi-sectoral. The core ministries to integrate, the sectors for liaison, and VPH functions are summed up below in Fig. 1.1 (from FAO/WHO 1975).

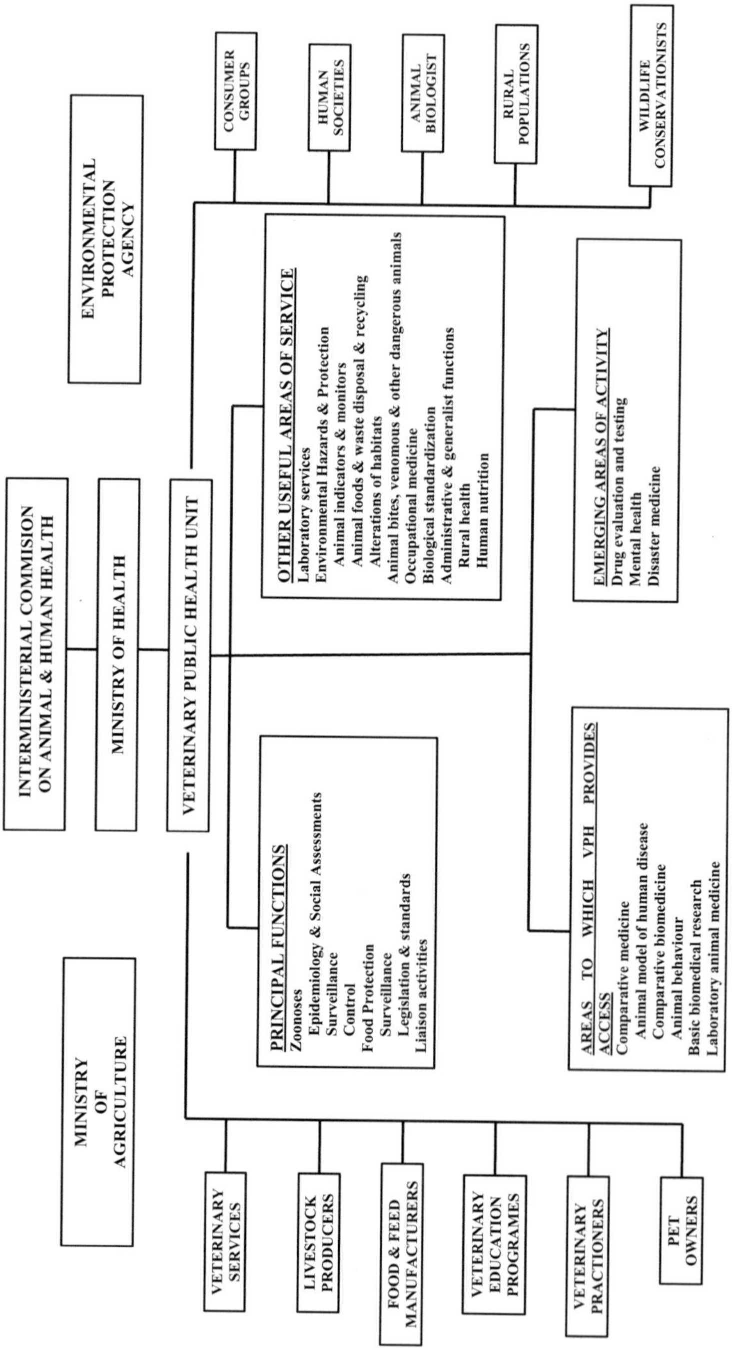

Fig. 1.1 Function and liaison relationships of a veterinary public health unit

1.1.4 Areas of Activities

The four areas of VPH activities—(1) principal function, (2) other areas of usual services, (3) areas to which VPH provides access, and (4) emerging areas—were identified, as shown in Fig. 1.1 (WHO 1975). These were redefined (WHO technical report series 907).

Food animals were reservoirs of zoonoses and agents like *Salmonella*, *Campylobacter*, *Escherichia coli*, and others responsible for food-borne infections. VPH leadership is essential to respond, especially for development of sustainable, integrated measures of safety to reduce risks to health along the entire food chain, from the point of primary production to the consumer (i.e. the 'farm-to-table' approach).

The core domains the diagnosis, surveillance, epidemiology, control, prevention, and elimination of zoonoses; food protection; health management of laboratory animal facilities and diagnostic laboratories; biomedical research; health education and extension; and the production and control of biological products and medical devices.

1.1.5 Other VPH Core Domains

- Management of domestic and wild animals and public health emergencies and the protection of drinking water and the environment
- Social, behavioural, and mental aspects of human-animal relationships (includes animal-assisted therapy and the development of standards for animal welfare)
- Leadership, management, and administration of agencies related to public health and the environment, covering government institutions, private sector organisations, and academic institutions
- Risk analysis (assessment, management, and communication), health economics, cost-benefit analysis, cost analysis, effectiveness analysis, and other methods for evaluating health service delivery and public health programmes
- Movement—trade and travel
- Farming methods, the food production chain, and Hazard Analysis Critical Control Points (HACCP)

An enhanced VPH curriculum for competent manpower to take up the above responsibilities was recommended.

1.1.6 VPH: Newer Areas of Activities

1. *Climate change and environmental hygiene*
   Global warming: global warming is causing the thawing of permafrost in the Arctic and Antarctic regions. It is postulated that once the frozen soil melts,

ancient viral strains and bacterial spores might be revived and cause outbreaks. A heat wave in 2016 in the Yamal Peninsula in the Arctic Circle caused the outbreak of anthrax. Anthrax-infected carcasses of reindeer buried in the permafrost released bacteria after thaw and caused epizootic infecting 2000 reindeer consequential transmission to infect humans after 75 years (Guarino 2016).

Anthrax hotspots can be located by examining specimens of soil for anthrax spores. Preventive vaccination can be done accordingly.

Intensive livestock production and trade: this demanded land use changes that contributed to environmental degradation and the emergence and spread of new animal and zoonotic diseases. Cattle ranching in Latin Americas, Brazil produced 40 million cattle/year. Brazil became an international feed bowl through large-scale deforestation and soya bean cultivation. The former released sequestrated carbon, and the latter added to CO_2 emission.

According to Gowri and Darrielle (2008), the industrial production system of livestock grew at double the rate of the mixed farming system and over six times the rate of production based on grazing. Playing with or switcing from dependence on natural resources led to a chain of demands: like energy and N-rich animal feed, soyabean, and corn; so cultivable land; so deforestation and so increased production of N-based fertiliser and also added to burden of tons of animal wastes—source of CH_4, N_2O and runoff of P, N, and other pollutants.

It is believed that industrial farming led to diseases—*E. coli*, campylobacteriosis, salmonellosis, and methicillin-resistant *Staphylococcus aureus* (MRSA)—the problem of anti-microbial resistance, bovine spongiform encephalopathy (BSE), and obesity.

Agriculture and animal farming are linked. A VPHE professional understands the human health consequences of intensive farming. Innovative mitigating changes in farming systems are most likely to come from him.

2. *Animal welfare* as well as social aspects, including service animals and human-animal bonding—e.g. animal therapy for depression cases.
3. *Laboratory services.*
4. *Nutrition and health education.*
5. *Laboratory animal medicine.*
6. *Invertebrate diseases and biological control.*
7. *Comparative pathology and microbiology*: monitor habitat change/migration/mortality due to environmental pollution and experimental surgery and medicine.
8. *Biomedical engineering.*
9. *Biotechnology.*
10. *Primate biology*: monkeys have been used as a model for studies in medical science. However, several important and often lethal infections originated from monkeys—monkeypox, Herpes virus simiae encephalomyelitis, infectious hepatitis A, simian immunodeficiency virus infection, dengue, and yellow fever.
11. *Wildlife diseases:* animals in natural habitats (forests) and captivity (zoos and recreational parks); zoonoses like severe acute respiratory syndrome (SARS), H5N1, and Ebola originated from wildlife and have pandemic potential.

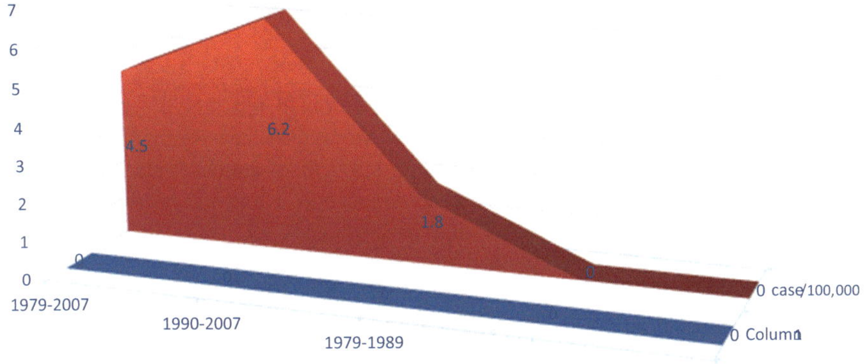

Fig. 1.2 Human trichinellosis in Romania (Neghina et al. 2010)

12. *Fish production and hygiene*: aquaculture has become both a necessity and a livelihood. Fish-borne diseases pose a threat. In Vietnam, zoonotic trematodes of fish origin have been reported to infect ≈1 million (Phan et al. 2010).
13. *Genetically engineered animals* for increasing production and raising biologicals (bio-farming): xenotransplantation is considered associated with the risk of emerging zoonoses. The emergence of anti-microbial drug resistance is associated with commercial farming.
14. *Disaster management.*
15. *Animals in the police and army.*

There is a breakdown of public health services during disasters. The capacity of public health services falls short of the requirement. Here are examples.

1.1.6.1 *Political Upheaval* and *Trichinellosis*

Romania recorded the first case of trichinosis in man and pigs in 1968. The incidence increased from 0.1 to 4.1 per lakh during 1963–1989 and increased to 2–15.9 during 1990–2007 (Fig. 1.2). A disaster caused by the Romanian Revolution, which overthrew the Communist regime in 1989, is ascribed. The upheaval caused the transportation of animals in improper conditions, the closure of large well-equipped national abattoirs, the slaughter of pigs in large numbers in private households and small ghost abattoirs with poor rules for hygiene, the trading of non-verified pork in illegal markets, and the lack of appropriate information either to consumers or pig breeders.

1.1.6.2 *Natural Disasters* and *Plagues*

A plague occurred between mid-August and the first week of October 1994. There were 234 deaths. Epidemiological investigations in Mamla, Beed district, Maharashtra, linked this epidemic to the 1993 earthquake in Latur. This village had the first warning—'rat fall' in mid-August. The survivors of the earthquake in September 1993 had converted the old damaged homes into granaries. The rodent and flea population grew exponentially; the intensity of flea infestation was 1.8 between October 1993 and July 1994 (Saxena and Verghese 1996).

1.1.6.3 Bioterrorism

WHO discussed anthrax letter bioterrorism and considered that the confirmatory detection of a deliberately caused outbreak is to strengthen the systems used to detect and respond to natural outbreaks. Besides anthrax, there are other zoonotic agents that can be used as a bioweapon. The epidemiological and laboratory principles being fundamentally the same, VPH must be kept ready.

1.2 Selected Areas of VPHE (Recommended in 1975 and 1999)

Pathogens are free; know no political and geographical boundaries; and infect trans-species of animals, birds, and vectors. Therefore, intelligence and combat tactics should be equally matched. The speed of action has to be faster than the speed of the spread of infection. This requires disease intelligence and information, combating and research, erasing the boundaries of disciplines, and creating bridges. VPHE has a direct responsibility when it comes to diseases at the 'domestic/pet animal-human interface'. It begins with 'Epidemiology'.

1.2.1 Epidemiology

It includes activities such as surveillance and disease mapping; screening against common infections—e.g. tuberculosis, brucellosis, etc.; epidemiological investigations of outbreaks and epidemics; the collection and dissemination of information on morbidity and mortality; the development of screening tools and testing; intervention studies—the testing of vaccines and other prophylactic measures; extending epidemiological and laboratory diagnostic services; connecting with local, state, and central vet services and Animal Disease Monitoring and Surveillance (ADMAS); and training and advisory services on the prevention, control, and eradication of animal diseases.

Zoonoses and food-borne infections are its principal focus (Fig. 1.1), and it covers most human health problems.

1.2.2 Zoonoses

The following are the functions of VPH: intelligence (diagnosis), surveillance, monitoring, risk assessment, search for natural *nidii* and determinants; search for animals as sentinels of zoonoses (e.g. pigs for JEV); dissemination of information; education and awareness of stakeholders and health administrators; prevention; and control.

Controlling zoonosis at the level of 'animal-source' is the best and most economical approach. Zoonotic infections that manifest clinically in animals, such as

Table 1.1 Sectors to integrate in the action plan

S. No.	Illness	Example	Sectors
1	Serious in man and animals	Rabies	VS + HS
2	Serious economic loss in animals	Anthrax, brucellosis, Q fever	VS + HS
3	No apparent illness in animals	Japanese encephalitis	HS + VS
4	Mild to inapparent in animals, wildlife as a source	Bovine TB (*M. bovis*)	VS + HS + Wildlife
5	Serious illness in man with wildlife as a source	SARS, Ebola	HS + Wildlife

Table 1.2 Cost-benefit ratio of the control of some zoonoses

Zoonoses	Cost:benefit	Country
Salmonellosis	19.8 for eggs, 5.4 for meat	Finland
Rabies	3.4–13.1	USA
Echinococcosis	3.0	Tibet
Bovine tuberculosis	1.71	England
Brucellosis	(6.5–21.7 in Cyprus) 3.88	Average of six countries

brucellosis, rift valley fever, and Q fever, are directly in the domain of VPH. VS controlled the Q fever epidemic in the Netherlands. Clinical human cases, such as of Q fever, JE, SARS, and Ebola, are handled best by health personnel. Important is intervention at the level of animals to prevent the appearance of such infections and human suffering, e.g. through rapid identification and communication between VPH and HS. For example, the control of the Q fever epidemic in the Netherlands (2007–2009) faltered because communication between the Ministries of Agriculture and Health was delayed (http://news.sciencemag.org/scienceinsider/2010/11/dutch-government-faulted.html#more).

Epidemiology of zoonoses suggests, delineates, and identifies the responsible sectors to come into action, with a specific action plan (Table 1.1).

The cost-benefit ratio of the control of zoonoses is always encouraging (Grace 2014); see Table 1.2.

In 1999, the WHO VPH study group deliberated on 'health for all in the twenty-first century' and the 'problems posed by emerging and re-emerging zoonoses'. At least half of the 1700 agents known to infect humans have a reservoir in animal or insect vectors, and a number of emerging infections are zoonoses or appear to be zoonoses (Table 1.3).

1.2.3 Food Hygiene

The following are the activities of VPH (see the core domain above):

- Farming methods, food chain, inspection and quality control of foods of animal origin and fish—*fluid milk, ante-mortem and post-mortem meat inspection, eggs,*

Table 1.3 Important host categories for human and emerging zoonoses (Cleaveland et al. 2001)[a]

Important host category	No. of zoonotic disease ($n = 800$)	No. of emerging zoonotic disease ($n = 125$)
Ungulate	315 (39.3%)	72 (57.6%)
Carnivore	344 (43.0%)	64 (51.2%)
Primate	103 (12.9%)	31 (24.8%)
Rodent	180 (22.5%)	43 (34.4%)
Marine mammal	41 (5.1%)	6 (4.8%)
Bat	15 (1.9%)	6 (4.8%)
Non-mammalian host (birds included)	109 (13.6%)	30 (24.0%)
Birds	82 (10.3%)	23 (18.4%)

[a] The host range shown represents minimums since the complete host range of many pathogens may not be known. Diseases with completely unknown animal hosts were not included ($n = 72$ diseases and eight emerging diseases)

etc.: greenstock, fresh/raw produce, value added products; inspection of production processes, product processing plants—slaughterhouses, dairies, restaurants, transportation, HACCP (farm to fork).

- Connecting and educating local, state, and central health agencies; manufacturers; traders; and consumer groups.
- Inspection and control of other non-edibles of animal origin, such as hide, endocrines and hormones, animal feeds, etc.; connecting manufacturers and traders.
- Analytical methods and quality standards.
- Use of slaughterhouse data by the National Animal Disease Control Centre (see Fig. 1.5 on food safety).
- Epidemiological investigation of food-borne infections and intoxication (figure-harmonised indicator) and educational programmes in the areas of food safety.
- The regulation (on elimination) of trade in trapped wildlife may help control transmission to market and farm animals, thereby to humans, besides eliminating infection in the farmed wildlife population. Ongoing monitoring might control transmission within this group and, thus, to wildlife markets and humans. This applies to *Trichinella spiralis*, which was very recently identified in wildlife in India.

1.2.3.1 Healthy Food Animals and Safe Produce

Agricultural production to the tune of 40% of the global value is contributed by livestock. This sector provides employment to 1.3 billion populations, besides supporting the livelihood and food security of one billion of the poor of the world, mostly living in the rural areas of Africa and Asia. About two third (2/3) of the world's population practices the 'mixed farming' system. This system accounts for 50% of the world's cereal production, generates 75% of milk, and is responsible for 60% of meat production in the developing world, providing millions of jobs simultaneously. Livestock and fish provide food security, which is, however, threatened by animal diseases.

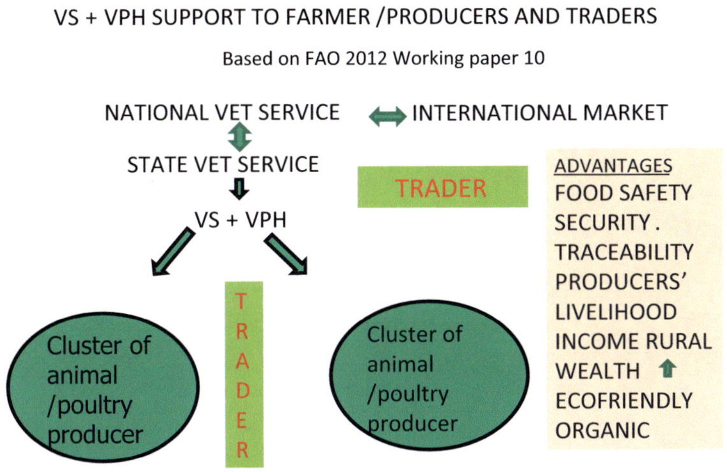

Fig. 1.3 Primary producers

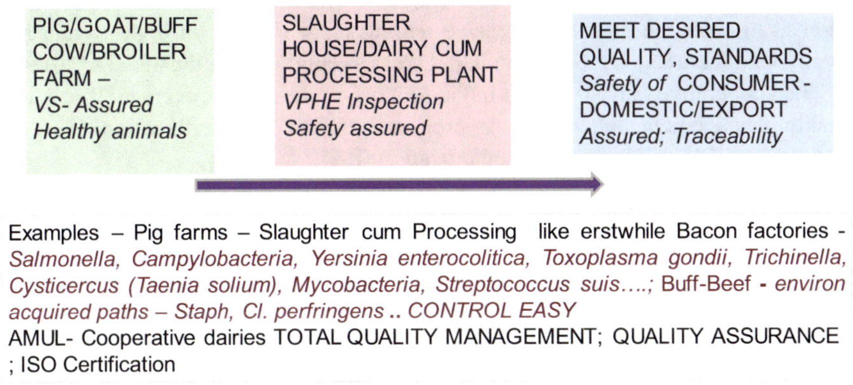

Fig. 1.4 Production, inspection, and safety

Linking 'primary producers forward to market/processing plant/slaughter house' assures income (Fig. 1.3). Food production systems were described (Narayan 2008). Backward integration of 160,000 farmers from 7200 villages in six districts of Uttar Pradesh (UP) raising >0.5 million buffaloes with forward linkages to the (plant) market resulted in (a) augmenting the income of farmers, (b) promoting male buffalo farming, (c) increasing buffalo beef lot, and (d) improving buffalo meat production and export. The entire system had a veterinary professional coverage of about 4 months per lot. It produced a 250 kg live weight buffalo calf yielding around 150 kg carcass (dressing % 60–65) and buffalo beef of excellent quality—lean, tender, juicy. Identification, certification of origin, and traceability were assured. Additional supervision and the inspection of slaughter and processing activities produce beef of exportable quality (Fig. 1.4). This began with the care of weaned

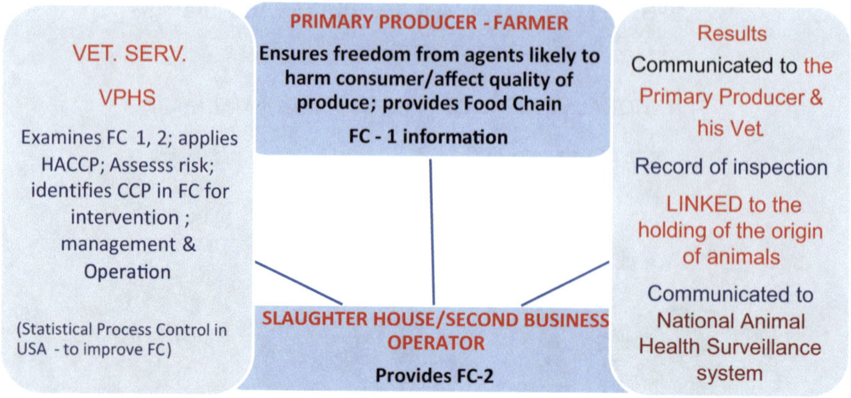

Fig. 1.5 Food safety

male buff calves (approximate age of 8–10 months purchased from farmers) kept under quarantine for a fortnight. Following deworming and vaccination, they were allowed to enter the farm for intensive rearing for 4 months on high protein and energy feed (courtesy Dr. S.K. Ranjhan, Director, Hind Agro Industries Ltd., 2007).

The cooperative dairy Amul in India, too, has professional coverage. It has total quality management and assurance programmes and also certification from the International Organization for Standardization (ISO).

Reverse tracing is inherent in these production systems. This facilitates rapid detection, intervention, and even the holding of contaminated consignments to save consumers from food poisoning.

Products of assured safety fetch a good price, augment farmers' income and creditability, and, finally, increase rural wealth. Production and connecting local markets with external markets increase employment.

Consumers feel secure when production is supervised and products are inspected (Fig. 1.4 on production and inspection). Composite system of pig and pork production has advantage of combining green stalk with processing at slaughterhouse. Veterinary supervision of pig farm can assure the freedom of pigs from pathogens like *Salmonella*, *Campylobacter*, *Streptococcus suis*, *Trichinella*, *Cysticercosis*, and *Toxoplasma*. Transport is nearly eliminated, and so muscle glycogen utilisation is minimised, resulting in good quality pork and minimising endogenous contamination with enteric microorganisms. Ante-mortem examination becomes ritual, and the escape of pathogens is detected during post-mortem meat inspection.

Food safety (Fig. 1.5) assurance connects primary producers to processors in the 'food chain (FC)'. Hazard Analysis Critical Control Point (HACCP) is used to find critical control points (CCPs) in the chain; risk is assessed for intervention. This is an additional step in food security after the healthy state of animals/birds is assured by primary producers/veterinarians.

The management of data concerning slaughterhouses, especially the findings of inspections, and the opening of a communication channel are important. In the case

HARMONISED EPIDEMIOLOGICALINDICATORS FOR SALMONELLA

PIG FARMS	TRANSPORT	SLAUGHTER HOUSE
HEI-1 BREEDING HEI-2 FATTENING POOLED FEED & FEACAL SAMPLE- CULTURE - DETERMINE PREVALENCE OF SEROTYPE HEI-3* HOUSING	HEI-4* TRANSPORT & LAIRAGE *AUDITING – TIME OF MIXING OF BATCHES, REUSE OF PENS IN LAIRAGE	HEI-5 CULTURE OF ILEAL CONTENT, LYMPH GLAND HEI-6 CULTURE OF CARCASS- SWAB HEI-7 CULTURE CARCASS SWAB POST CHILLING
INDICATOR OF FARM HYGIENE & FARMING	INDICATOR OF SL - BATCH RISK	INDICATOR OF SLAUGHTER LEVEL RISK

Note-Study at Ranchi Veterinary College– Salmonella spread in slaughter house of bacon factory – ileal content and carcass swab before chilling were positive. See HEI-5 and 6 above. HEI -1 to 7 apply to most of the food borne infections. Same may be extended to restaurants or fast food restaurants.

Fig. 1.6 Harmonised indicator

of a composite system (discussed above), it is just one step. The exchange of data improves the quality of both the farm and the processing unit.

Establishing a channel of communication with the national surveillance system for animal diseases and zoonoses contributes to the national database on endemic diseases and zoonoses and alerts for emerging ones. Then tracing back to the hotspot becomes easy.

Investigation into food poisoning is one of the most common and important activities.

A comprehensive investigation covers almost all activities in animal farming (harmonised indicators for *Salmonella*), shown in Fig. 1.6. The results reveal the site in the production line where contamination occurred, and thus corrective measures are taken (EFSA Scientific Report 2011).

1.2.3.2 Effects of Climate Change and Global Warming

Pathogens are more sensitive to climate change. Climate sensitivity has been observed in >50% of pathogens, including those associated with food- and water-borne diseases in Europe. It is implied that extreme weather conditions (e.g. El Niño), high temperatures, drought, and rains are likely to alter the distribution of pathogens, the routes of transmission by vectors and vehicles (soil, foods, and water), and incidence. There might also be a change in the severity and number of infection cycles per season (McIntyre et al. 2017).

Increased monthly temperatures and episodes of food-borne diarrhoeal were related, as was observed in the Pacific Islands (Singh et al. 2001). 'Changes in precipitation' affect enteric pathogens. *Salmonella* spp., *E. coli*, and norovirus are internalised by plants through their roots. These cannot be removed by post-harvest washing. If consumed uncooked or undercooked, which is more likely in the case of leafy vegetables and salads, they may cause infection. Internalisation increased under water stress (drought) and also excess water (excessive rainfall) (Ge et al. 2012). Water treatment and management plants unable to handle excessive rainfall will be supplying compromised quality of water. Low infective dose pathogens, like enteric viruses, enterohaemorrhagic *E. coli*, *E. coli* 0157:H7, and Shiga-toxin-producing *E. coli*, survive under high temperatures. *Salmonella* replicates rapidly. Animals shed enteric pathogens under heat stress (Venegas-Vargas et al. 2016). Changes in air temperatures and precipitation (relative humidity) positively influenced food-borne outbreaks caused by *E. coli*, *Vibrio parahaemolyticus*, *Campylobacter jejuni*, *Salmonella* spp., and *Bacillus cereus* in the Republic of Korea (Kim et al. 2015; Park et al. 2018).

In 2010, 600 million people were affected with >420,000 deaths by food-borne illnesses (WHO 2015). It is estimated that 33 million disability-adjusted life years (DALYs) were lost the world over. These were attributed to infectious agents causing diarrhoeal diseases, mainly involving norovirus, *Campylobacter* spp., *Vibrio cholerae*, *Shigella* spp., enteropathogenic *E. coli*, and enterohaemorrhagic *E. coli*. Fungal-contaminated crops are a source of aflatoxins, a major food-borne hazard associated with zinc and vitamin A deficiencies and stunted growth among children.

The emergence and re-emergence of food-borne pathogens, public health costs, loss to the food production sector due to removal from shelves, payment of damages, lawsuits, etc. are matters of concern.

Farming systems that do not use any agricultural chemicals and anti-microbials, say organic farming and innovative fine-tuning, are desired to mitigate the effects of global warming.

1.2.4 Rural Health

Leadership, management, and administration of public health qualities of VPHE professional (see Other VPH Core Domains above) are used for 'People centric approach' for making the livelihoods of farmers and small traders secured. The primary objectives are helping them to augment production and sale, the control of disease, emergency responses that reduce damage to poor people's livelihoods and dignity, the capacity building of agricultural and animal husbandry units in rural areas, and preparing rural people for 'Participatory Epidemiology'.

The rural posting of veterinarians and para-veterinarians and the nature of their jobs make them the nearest available professionals for villagers. The glue or connectivity is also better. They could share certain select public health activities, too.

Important areas contributing to the improvement of rural health include surveillance, the identification of human health problems, and offering of services; epidemiological investigation into occupational health hazards of farmers, livestock owners, attendants, and those engaged in handling animal produce and also hazards caused by the use of agrichemicals, pesticides, etc. and the resulting migration and habitat change of birds, etc.; accidents and bites; investigation on the effect of animal waste recycling; the health education of farmers and animal owners; and connecting with primary health centres.

1.3 VPHE Organization and Evolution

It was envisaged that the Ministries of Health and Animal Husbandry will have an Inter-ministerial Commission of Animal and Human Health. The VPH unit was placed in the Ministry of Health as it was contributing to human health. The horizontal linkages were identified as the Ministry of Agriculture and Environmental Protection Agency. Eleven sectors were identified for liaison. All governments in the Western Pacific Region agreed that VPH services protected against zoonoses and assured safe food (Wilks and Madie 1991). The organisation of VPH by the 'National government in Japan' appeared to be in line with the recommendations of FAO/WHO (1975). At a meeting in 1999 (WHO 2002), VPH activities and functions were defined to face the challenges of the twenty-first century. In most of the developing world, including India, VPH has not been organised. Ghatak and Singh (2015) reviewed the development of VPHE activities in India and summed up the strengths upon which a formal organisation can be shaped. Advocacy by academia and professional leaders supported by a strong and sustained political commitment is necessary.

VPH does not fit as a single organisational template. The functions, activities, and resources of VPH are dispersed throughout various agencies and sectors, like agriculture, health, and the environment. The programme of VPH may be a focal point having liaison functions, extensive operational responsibilities to provide technical cooperation to national programmes. Horizontal coordination between the three ministries and vertically down to the regional and local levels is essential for the delivery of VPH services. Vertical and horizontal channels of communication among different tiers of government and non-governmental organisations, including the private sector, are needed to ensure that community-level programmes are adjusted as needed.

1.3.1 An Example (Based on the Experience of Investigating the Japanese Encephalitis Epidemic in Champaran in 1980)

Tracing back a JE patient who discharged from hospital and reached his home. The house was constructed under the government's programme to help people like him. He received training in backyard horticulture and poultry and pig keeping. Being a diligent person, he adopted these and had in his house ducks, pigs, and a vegetable garden. The mini-ecosystem was favourable for a mosquito-JEV cycle introduced by birds in their natural habitat around water bodies near his house, which was without nets on its windows and doors. He was reconciled with mosquito menace and bites.

At the local level, each of the government departments is represented as 'vertical sectors'. VPH activities need to be horizontally dispersed through these. The provision of VPH knowledge/activities in these sectors is essential to protect people from zoonoses (JE in this case) and ensure the success of the programmes of these departments to augment the livelihood of and promote a comfortable life for the beneficiaries. In this case, the three service delivery departments and the recipient beneficiaries were required to be educated and made aware of the VPH activities. Understanding VPH like this promotes its application.

The evolution of VPHE varied based on the economic conditions of countries. It has evolved in countries that have highly organised systems for agricultural production and industrial meat and milk production, e.g. the USA. The VPH unit in the Centers for Disease Control and Prevention, USA, was founded by James H. Steele. It added to the 'Disease Intelligence capability'. During the COVID-19 pandemic, laboratories and scientists from ICAR-Indian Veterinary Research Institute and its research centres and veterinary universities were engaged in diagnostic services in India. They agree with the expression 'VPHE is route to One Health' (Narayan 2011). Chronologically, One Health came later. VPHE is evolving in India and is visible in areas of education and research.

Domestic and pet animal-associated zoonoses can be controlled and transmission blocked at the level of animals with strong veterinary efforts but generally fall outside the priority. Strengthening the veterinary sector, expanding areas of activities to include zoonoses, and enhancing capacity are required. The control of zoonoses like canine (dog) rabies, brucellosis, etc. is entirely under the veterinary sector. The burden of human illness due to domestic and pet-linked zoonoses would be eliminated only through veterinary efforts. As an example of expanding the veterinary sector to include VPHE activities, the Danish Zoonosis Centre (DZC) may be cited (World Bank 2010). In 1994, it was established as a separate unit within the Danish Veterinary Institute under the Ministry of Food, Agriculture, and Fisheries (now the National Food Institute, Technical University of Denmark) in compliance with the Zoonosis Directive of EU (92/117/92), and it is government funded. Reported pork-related zoonosis incidences in humans were increasing, and awareness was required. DZC was created to function as a coordinating body to integrate all data on the occurrence of zoonoses in animals, food, and humans in one place. A zoonosis epidemiological research unit was established. Its main functions include the creation of zoonosis-related database/statistics, surveillance (e.g. of antibiotic-resistant bacteria), tracking the routes of transmission and tracing the source of outbreaks, epidemiological research and the dissemination of information, and coordination between institutions and authorities. DZC guides on control and prevention of food-borne zoonotic diseases in Denmark pooling data from the Danish Veterinary Institute (food and animal data) and Statens Serum Institut (human data), makes scientific assessment and advice to the risk-managing institutions such as the Danish Veterinary and Food Administration. DZC has no power to make risk-management decisions.

There is scope and need to expand VPH activities to wildlife-domestic animals and human interface and environmental health. In most regions, wildlife falls under the ministry of environment, and areas are limited, with neglect of wildlife diseases. Inclusive VPH activities (wildlife-domestic animal-human interface) would be rewarding in the form of reduction of the burden of zoonoses.

References

Cleaveland S, Laurenson MK, Taylor LH (2001) Diseases of humans and their domestic mammals: pathogen characteristics, host range and the risk of emergence. Philos Trans R Soc Lond B 356: 991–999

EFSA (2011) Scientific report 2011. Technical specifications on harmonised epidemiological indicators for public health hazards to be covered by meat inspection of swine. EFSA J 9(10): 2371. 1–125

Eloit M (2012) The global public good concept: a means of promoting good veterinary governance. Rev Sci Tech 31(2):585–590

FAO/WHO (1975) Report of a Joint FAO/WHO Expert Committee on veterinary Public Health. The Veterinary Contribution to Public Health Practice. WHO Technical report series no. 573; FAO Agricultural studies no. 96. WHO, Geneva

Ge C, Lee C, Lee J (2012) The impact of extreme weather events on *Salmonella* internalization in lettuce and green onion. Food Res Int 45(2):1118–1122

Ghatak S, Singh BB (2015) Veterinary Public Health in India: current status and future needs. Rev Sci Tech 34(3):713–727

Gowri K, Darrielle N (2008) Global farm animal production and global warming: impacting and mitigating climate change. Environ Health Perspect 116(5):578–582

Grace D (2014) The business case for one health. Onderstepoort J Vet Res 81(2):725. 6 pages

Guarino B (2016) Anthrax sickens 13 in western Siberia, and a thawed-out reindeer corpse may be to blame. Wash Post

International Task Force on Global Public Goods (2006) Meeting global challenges: international cooperation in the national interest. Final report. International Task Force on Global Public Goods, Stockholm

Kim YS, Park KH, Chun HS, Choi C, Bahk GJ (2015) Correlations between climatic conditions and foodborne disease. Food Res Int 68:24–30

McIntyre KM, Setzkorn C, Hepworth PJ, Morand S, Morse AP, Baylis M (2017) Systematic assessment of the climate sensitivity of important human and domestic animals pathogens in Europe. Sci Rep 7(1):7134

Narayan KG (2008) Food production systems, safety and education. In: Singh SP, Julie Funk SC (eds) Food safety, quality assurance and global trade: concerns and strategies. Tripathi and Nanda Joshi' International Book Distributing Co. (Publishing Division.), Lucknow, pp 1–11

Narayan KG (2011) Veterinary Public Health – a route to 'One Health'. Dr. M. R. Dhanda oration. In: 9th All India Conference of Association of Public Health Veterinarians and National Symposium on "Challenges and strategies for Veterinary Public Health in India" February 18–19, 2011

Neghina R, Neghina AM, Marincu I, Moldovan R, Iacobiciu I (2010) Epidemiology and epizootiology of trichinellosis in Romania 1868–2007. Vect Borne Zoonot Dis 10(4):323–328

OIE. Office International Des Epizooties (2012) Terrestrial Animal Health Code, 21st edn. OIE, Paris. http://www.oie.int/en/international-standard-setting/terrestrialcode/

Park MS, Park KH, Bahk GJ (2018) Interrelationships between multiple climatic factors and incidence of foodborne diseases. Int J Environ Res Public Health 15(11):2482

Phan VT, Ersbøll AK, Nguyen TT et al (2010) Freshwater aquaculture nurseries and infection of fish with zoonotic trematodes, Vietnam. Emerg Infect Dis 16(12):1905–1909

Ranjhan SK (2007) Buffalo as a social animal for humanity. Asian Buffalo Magazine 3:22–31

Saxena VK, Verghese T (1996) Ecology of flea transmitted zoonotic infection in village Mamla, district Beed. Curr Sci 71:800–802

Shanko K, Kemal J, Kenea D (2015) A review on confronting zoonoses: the role of veterinarian and physician. J Veterinar Sci Technol 6:221

Singh RB, Hales S, de Wet N, Raj R, Hearnden M et al (2001) The influence of climate variation and change on diarrhoeal disease in the Pacific Islands. Environ Health Perspect 109(2): 155–159

Steele JH (2008) Veterinary public health: past success, new opportunities. Prev Med 86(3): 224–243

Venegas-Vargas C, Henderson S, Khare A, Mosci RE, Lehnert JD et al (2016) Factors associated with Shiga toxin-producing *Escherichia coli* shedding by dairy and beef cattle. Appl Environ Microbiol 82(16):5049–5056

WHO (2005a) International health regulations. WHO, Geneva. Second edition January 1, 2008. https://www.who.int/publications/i/item/9789241580410

WHO (2005b) Constitution of the World Health Organization. Organization: basic documents, 45th edn. World Health Organization, Geneva

WHO (2015) WHO estimates of the global burden of foodborne diseases. Foodborne disease burden epidemiology reference group 2007–2015. WHO, Geneva. https://apps.who.int/iris/bitstream/handle/10665/199350/9789241565165_eng.pdf?sequence=1

WHO. WHO Study Group on Future Trends in Veterinary Public Health (1999): Teramo (2002) Future trends in veterinary public health: report of a WHO study group (WHO technical report series 907). WHO Study Group on Future Trends in Veterinary Public Health, Geneva

Wilks CR, Madie P (1991) Organisation of veterinary public health in the Western Pacific region. Rev Sci Tech 10(4):1131–1158

Winslow CE (*1920*) The untilled fields of public health. *Science 51*(*1306*)*:23–33*

World Bank (2010) People, pathogens and our planet. Vol. 1: Towards a one health approach for controlling zoonotic diseases. Report No. 50833-GLB. The World Bank, Agriculture and Rural Development Health, Nutrition and Population, Washington, DC

2 Zoonoses

Abstract

Animals are an integral part of human life. Human interacts with animals in their daily life, in either urban or rural settings, during travel, while visiting animal exhibits, or while enjoying outdoor activities. Animals provide food, fibre, livelihood, travel, sport, and companionship to people. However, animals harbour harmful germs, like viruses, bacteria, fungi, and parasites that can spread to people, causing mild to serious illness and even death—these are known as zoonotic diseases or zoonoses, which are very common. It is estimated that >6 of ten known infectious diseases of man can be transmitted from animals, and three out of four new or emerging infectious diseases in man originate from animals. However, there are certain diseases (tuberculosis, COVID-19) that spill over from humans to animals, too.

Zoonoses are no longer a national problem, but due to the increased and fast international movement of humans, animals, and animal products, these diseases spread across the world by transcending natural boundaries, causing a bad impact not only on human health but also on the global economy. Therefore, for the control of zoonoses, global monitoring and surveillance are mandatory. The control of zoonoses retains its prominent place among the actions of international agencies, like the World Health Organization (WHO), World Organisation for Animal Health (WOAH), and Food and Agriculture Organization (FAO).

The history of civilisation has been shaped by many infectious diseases, and zoonoses have played a major role. Zoonotic diseases have shaped the life of human beings for centuries. About 25% of the total annual human death worldwide is caused by zoonotic diseases. It is estimated that of the 1415 infectious diseases pathogenic to man, 868 (61%) are zoonotic. Among these 217 are viral, 538 are

K. G. Narayan et al., *Veterinary Public Health & Epidemiology*,
https://doi.org/10.1007/978-981-19-7800-5_2

bacterial and rickettsial, 307 are fungal, 66 are protozoal, and 287 are helminthic (Taylor et al. 2001). Of the 175 emerging infections, 132 (75%) are zoonotic.

2.1 Definition

Zoonoses are diseases and infections, the agents of which are naturally transmitted between other vertebrate animals and man. Coined by Rudolf Virchow, it consists of two Greek words—zoon (animals) and noses (disease).

Infectious diseases originating in man and transmitted to animals are referred to as reverse zoonoses—also referred to as zooanthroponosis and/or anthroponosis (Greek: zoon—'animal', anthropos—'man', nosos—'disease').

The causative agents of animal diseases get adapted to animals and exist in these through uninterrupted chains of infection. The adaptation may be restricted to a single or more than one species of animal. Some such disease agents may infect man, too. Most of the time, man is almost always an accidental host. Once the disease is transmitted to man from animals, its epidemiologic course is halted and man often acts as a dead-end host.

2.2 Classification of Zoonoses

Zoonoses are classified in many ways, which are described below.

2.2.1 Based on the Maintenance Cycle of the Infectious Agent

This classification is the most useful when it comes to formulating a control programme:

1. Direct zoonoses (*orthozoonoses*): the agent is transmitted from an infected host to a susceptible host by direct contact—through fomites or a mechanical vector (Fig. 2.1). It is maintained in the nature through transmission between single vertebrate host e.g., rabies, brucellosis.
2. *Cyclozoonoses*: the infectious agents require more than one vertebrate host for maintenance in nature (Fig. 2.2). No invertebrates are involved. Examples are taeniasis and pentastomiasis, but a majority of the cyclozoonoses are cestodiasis.

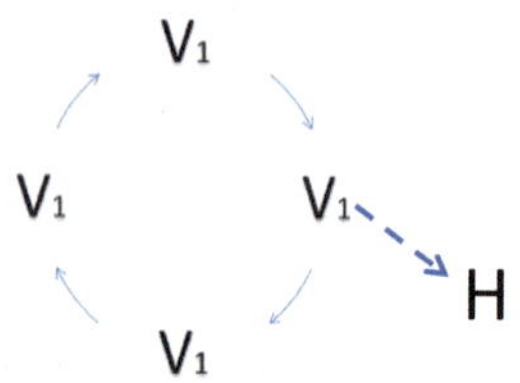

Fig. 2.1 Direct Zoonosis

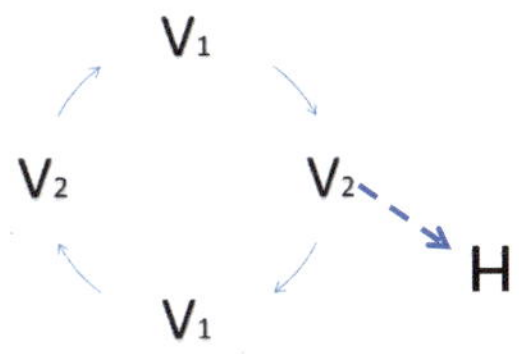

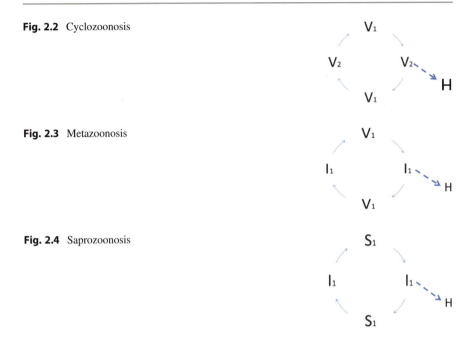

Fig. 2.2 Cyclozoonosis

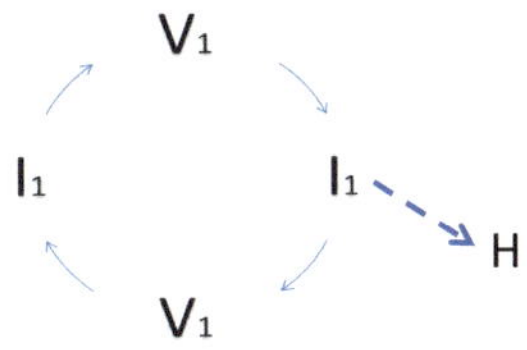

Fig. 2.3 Metazoonosis

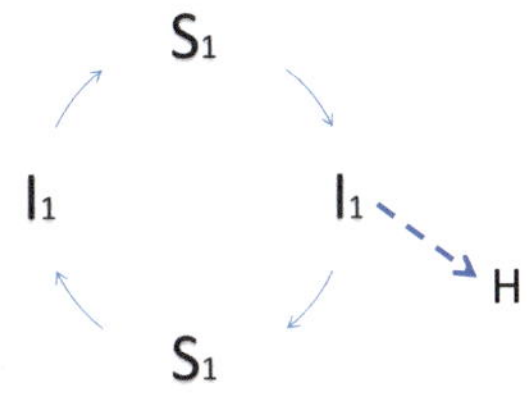

Fig. 2.4 Saprozoonosis

3. Metazoonoses (*pherozoonoses*): this class of zoonoses needs vertebrate as well as invertebrate hosts for its maintenance in nature. An extrinsic incubation period is required inside the invertebrate host for transmission to take place (Fig. 2.3). The infectious agent either undergoes multiplication (called propagative transmission) or development (i.e. developmental transmission) in the invertebrate host, e.g. plague.
4. *Saprozoonoses*: a vertebrate host as well as an inanimate object are involved in the maintenance and transmission of the agent, e.g. histoplasmosis. Here, direct transmission of the agent is rarely observed or is absent altogether. The agent develops or multiplies on an inanimate object, like an organic matter, which may be food or soil (Fig. 2.4).

2.2.2 Based on the Direction of the Transmission of the Agent (Fig. 2.5)

1. Anthropozoonoses: disease-causing agents adapted to human beings in the course of evolution and exist in them through uninterrupted chains of transmission, e.g. cholera and smallpox.
2. Zooanthropozoonoses: human infectious agents able to infect animals (transmission from man to animals), e.g. *Corynebacterium diphtheria.*
3. Amphixenoses: disease-causing agents transmitted equally from animals to human beings and from human beings to animals; the agents are usually

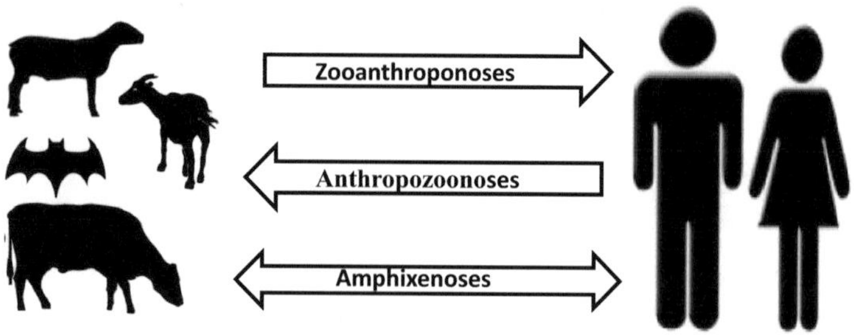

Fig. 2.5 Classification of zoonosis according to transmission

ubiquitous, and man and animals are equally suitable reservoir hosts, e.g. *Staphylococcal* infection.

2.2.3 Based on the Nature of the Causative Agent

1. Bacterial zoonoses: brucellosis, leptospirosis
2. Viral zoonoses: rabies, Japanese encephalitis
3. Parasitic zoonoses: hydatidosis, trichinellosis
4. Fungal zoonoses: histoplasmosis, cryptococcosis
5. Rickettsial zoonoses: coxiellosis

2.2.4 Based on Likely History (Hart et al. 1999)

1. *Old zoonoses*: epidemic and endemic human-specific infections with a temporally distant non-human source, e.g. measles
2. *Recent zoonoses*: human epidemic or endemic diseases—new or emerging with a recent non-human source, e.g. human immunodeficiency virus (HIV)
3. *Established zoonoses*: infectious diseases occasionally transmitted to man with a non-human reservoir, e.g. monkeypox
4. *New and emerging zoonoses*: infectious diseases that have only recently been detected found to spread to humans having a non-human reservoir host, e.g. hantaviruses and Ebola virus
5. *Parazoonoses*: epidemic or endemic diseases of man, infectious agent(s) of which undergo periodic changes in their virulence by acquiring genes from non-human pathogens, e.g. re-assortment of genes in influenza A

Man may be incidentally trapped in the chain of infection of certain zoonoses like hydatidoses and trichinellosis, and the agents meet a dead end. A contrasting situation happens when man-to-man transmission occurs—as in Ebola, Marburg, and pneumonic plague.

2.2.5 Other Classification of Zoonoses

Zoonoses can be (1) **emerging** or (2) **re-emerging**.

Zoonotic diseases that appear and affect a population for the first time or have existed previously but are increasing rapidly in terms of the number of new cases within a population or their spread to new geographical areas are known as emerging zoonoses.

Zoonoses affecting a given area in the past, which declined or were controlled, but are again being reported in increasing numbers are known as re-emerging zoonoses. At times, a new clinical form of an old disease appears with high severity or fatality, e.g. chikungunya in India.

2.2.6 Mechanism of Emergence of Disease

Two distinct mechanisms of the emergence of zoonoses are recognised. Some pathogens jump from animals to humans, become adapted to transmission from human to human, and evolve predominantly or exclusively as human infections ($Ro > 1$ in humans), e.g. measles originating from closely related morbilliviruses of cattle (rinderpest) or smallpox from poxviruses of either camel or cattle. Other zoonoses with $Ro < 1$ in humans require continuous reintroduction from animal reservoirs (obligate zoonoses).

Logical speculation of the 'origin of zoonoses' is traced to man's forebears. Microorganisms were carried vertically from man's forebears to the present race of man, as suggested by the antigenic similarity between certain viruses (cytomegalovirus) of anthropoid apes. Communicable diseases are often density dependent. The likelihood of transmission depends on the increase in the number of susceptible and infectious individuals.

Pathogen transmission from a vertebrate animal to a human has been identified as a global public health issue. This zoonotic spillover is largely poorly understood. Such zoonotic spillover is an outcome of several factors, which include climatic, ecological, epidemiological, and behavioural determinants of pathogens (e.g. infectivity, pathogenicity, virulence, drug resistance, etc.) and human factors (e.g. susceptibility to infection, nutritional factors, comorbidities, cultural factors, socio-economic factors, etc.).

2.2.6.1 Environmental Changes

Global warming and its consequential effects on hosts, vectors, and agents are subtle but are going on, leading to habitat change, migration, and the extension or creation of new *nidii* of infection. Because of this, identification of new infection in an area earlier known to be free from it, expansion or shrinkage or change in vector borne zoonoses and other vector borne anthroponotic infection may be seen. Global warming might change the migratory route of birds, which has relevance to the spread of bird flu.

Another important difficulty posed to public health veterinarians is that the *pathogenicity of agents that cross species barriers is unpredictable*; for example, hantaviruses of rodents as well as the Ebola, Lassa, and Marburg viruses cause serious diseases in man.

The breakdown of public health services during political upheaval and natural calamities like floods and earthquakes may also result in the spread and outbreak of zoonotic diseases such as cholera, cryptosporidiosis, and plague.

Revelation of new agents/reservoirs/intermediate hosts/vectors: these might have existed and are not new, e.g. lyssavirus in bats in Australia, *Brucella* spp. in marine animals, black rats in synanthropic nidus as reservoir of *Fasciola* infection in absence of domestic animals and discovered now. Such animals are as capable reservoirs as domestic animals and are responsible for human infection.

Immunosuppression: environmental pollution with pesticides and mycotoxins, infection with HIV in man/simian immunodeficiency virus (SIV) in monkeys/ Gumboro in birds, immunosuppressive drugs in the treatment of cancer, and transplant surgery have resulted in a sizeable susceptible population for relatively innocuous microbes, besides the known pathogens. Acquired immunodeficiency syndrome (AIDS) patients have provided an opportunity to understand the possible response of immunocompromised hosts. There is increased (a) frequency of infection, (b) infection with opportunistic pathogens, (c) severity of disease, (d) shedding of infectious agents, and (d) difficulty in diagnosis leading to delayed appropriate intervention. *Immunocompromised hosts thus would be playing a significant role in evolution (opportunistic to pathogens) and in increasing the density of pathogens per unit of susceptible hosts.*

Persistence of infection: sometimes infection is symptomless or persists after clinical recovery. The persisting infecting agent may cause a relapse, e.g. Brill Zinsser's (rickettsiosis) and tuberculosis. Such 'silent patients' pose a danger to others, infecting them. The infecting agent may undergo antigenic changes in them, as happens in trypanosomiasis and HIV patients. Genetic swapping in viruses may occur in the case of co-infection, resulting in the emergence of a new pathogen. 'Re-emergence' may also result in the case of latent infection/long incubation period (for example, trichina larvae may remain viable and infective for 12 years in pigs and 31 years in man; long incubation period may occur in the case of slow-growing viruses and prion, such as bovine spongiform encephalopathy (BSE) and related conditions). A recent estimate of incubation period for kuru is 12 years with a range of 5–56 years. A gene variant responsible for resistance to prion diseases was probably responsible for the long incubation period. Rabies virus hides itself in the subscapular fats of bats. The transmission of rabies through corneal transplant and recently through organ transplant raises similar issues of the persistence of this agent in humans and its baffling appearance in the recipients.

2.2.6.2 Emergence and Re-emergence

The term 'emerging' was defined in 1981 by Krause and Lederberg. Emerging diseases are those 'that have recently increased in incidence, impact, geographic distribution or host range (e.g. Lyme disease, Nipah virus), that are caused by pathogens that have recently evolved (e.g. new strains of influenza virus, drug resistant strains of malaria), that are newly discovered (e.g. Hendra virus) or diseases that have recently changed their clinical presentation (e.g. Hantavirus pulmonary syndrome)'. The time span for the term 'recent' may vary, but to address this ambiguity, a time frame of 2–3 decades has been agreed upon. Re-emerging diseases form a sub-class of emerging diseases historically prevalent at a significant level but became significantly less with only a recent increase in incidence (Daszak and Cunningham 2003; Yale et al. 2013).

The majority of emerging infectious diseases (EIDs) or events are zoonoses (60.3% of EIDs): a majority (71.8%) originate in wildlife (e.g., SARS, Ebola), and 54.3% of EIDs are caused by bacteria or rickettsia, primarily drug-resistant microbes. The origins of EID show a significant correlation with socio-economic, environmental, and ecological factors. This provides a basis for identifying regions where new EIDs are most likely to originate ('hotspots' of emerging disease); at lower latitudes where reporting effort is poor and have substantial risk of originating wildlife zoonotic and vector-borne EIDs and therefore global resources need to be diverted to these (Jones et al. 2008).

The distance between various species of animals and human beings is reducing. This is driving species towards extinction, disrupting ecosystems, introducing pathogens, and increasing opportunities for zoonoses.

2.2.7 Anthropogenic Factors/Determinants of Zoonoses

1. Intensive agriculture and production: water logging (e.g. JE and leptospirosis); deforestation, forcing fruit bats to change their habitat (e.g. Nipah) or expand habitat—the Kyasanur Forest disease (KFD) epidemic in 1983 is linked to deforestation for cashew plantation.
2. Intensive animal farming led to the abuse of antibiotics in the form of sub-therapeutic, meta-therapeutic, and prophylactic antibiotics in animal farming, causing the emergence of anti-microbial resistance.
3. Changing food preference/habit: sushi, a Japanese fish food item, causes fish-borne parasitic infection; trichinellosis and Ebola are associated with the consumption of bushmeat.
4. Wildlife meat demanded as delicacies: civet cats were identified as a source of SARS, which first emerged in a trader in November 2003 in a small industrial town—Foshan in the southern Chinese province of Guangdong. Four health workers who were attending to him also fell critically ill. *Wildlife restaurants in Guangdong are known to serve a range of exotic and sometimes endangered species.*
5. Wildlife farming: the introduction of ostrich farming and slaughter resulted in the emergence of Congo-Crimean haemorrhagic fever in slaughterhouses specialising in ostrich slaughter in South Africa
6. Change in feed processing: BSE (CJDnv), not known until 1986 (1986–1996, approximately 160,000 cases were reported in the UK)—during 1981–1982,

rendering temperature for preparing cattle feed was reduced; by May 1996, BSE was reported from areas outside the UK and ten countries.

7. Change in storage technique: ice preservation of marine mammals and fishes on harvest caused the larvae of nematode *Anisakis* spp. to migrate from the intestine to the muscles, infecting consumers. Thus, in 1955, the first human case of a serious intestinal granulomatous disease caused by larvae was diagnosed in the Netherlands.
8. Trade and transport: the shipment of goods to and from India, African islands, and Nigeria resulted in the entry of chikungunya to India, causing an epidemic (March 2005–2009) affecting over 1.35 million people. Transportation vehicles acted as mechanical vectors for the entry and dispersal of *Aedes albopictus*.
9. Water reservoirs and dams constructed in eastern India resulted in a significance in visceral leishmaniasis in Bangladesh and West Bengal since water bodies served as a habitat for the multiplication of sand flies (Bern and Chowdhury 2006).
10. Travel/tourism: African tick bite fever, caused by *Rickettsia africae* and transmitted in rural sub-Saharan Africa by ungulate ticks of the *Amblyomma* genus, infects man mostly during wild game safaris and bush walks.
11. Recreational activities/sites: giardiasis, cryptococcosis, and schistosomiasis are linked to swimming in water bodies, especially during summer.
12. Trade in wildlife and exotic pets: *Lagos bat lyssavirus* infection in 120 persons resulted from exposure to infected Egyptian rousette bats (*Rousettus aegyptiacus*) that had been imported from Belgium and sold in a pet shop in South West France. Tarantulas are growing in popularity in the exotic pet trade. Others are horned toads, Partridge Cochin, prairie dogs, big cats, wolves, and bears—examples of zoonoses they may cause are *prairie-dog-associated plague, bird-associated psittacosis and ornithosis, and other wildlife-associated zoonoses.*
13. Xenozoonoses
    (a) Allograft is another means of the spread of zoonoses, e.g. rabies through corneal and other organ transplants and West Nile through infected blood transfusion.
    (b) Xenograft: the transplantation of animal cells, tissues, or organs to humans is likely to spread zoonoses. Organs and tissues are grown in pigs raised specifically for this. Once the species barrier is breached, new infection in the recipient may be established and may spread subsequently to others in the population.
    (c) Transgenic products (products of human genes raised in animals): here, again, the risks involved are the same as above. Weiss et al. (2000) cited examples of agents jumping over the species barrier—HIV-1 jumping from chimpanzees, HIV-2 from sooty mangabey, and BSE from bovine.
14. Bioterrorism: many zoonotic agents have bioweapon potentiality, e.g. *Bacillus anthracis*.

2.2.8 Management of Zoonoses

The control of zoonoses contributes significantly to ensuring food security and public health. The control and prevention of zoonoses could be achieved through different approaches, as discussed below, depending upon the situation.

2.2.8.1 Conventional Approach (Veterinary Service-Veterinary Public Health)

Referring to the classification of zoonoses (Hart et al. 1999) above, most of the 'established' and obligate zoonoses (with domestic and pet animals as hosts) can be controlled by veterinary service (VS). These zoonoses are very important, and some of them have pandemic potential, like bird flu and swine flu.

These are common among economically weak farmers and occur in rural areas.

Lembo et al. (2010) presented a comparison of estimated deaths (Table 2.1) from rabies and other neglected zoonoses in comparison with pandemic-potential zoonoses, such as influenza, SARS, Ebola, and others. Rabies and other neglected 'established zoonoses' cause huge losses in terms of death and disability-adjusted life years (DALYs). DALY burden for rabies is higher than most other neglected zoonotic diseases. Interestingly, all these are controllable and preventable with a functional veterinary public health service provided by the veterinary sector.

2.2.8.2 Multi-sectoral Approach (One Health)

Some zoonoses, like SARS, H5N1 avian influenza in Asia, BSE in the UK, West Nile and monkeypox viruses in North America, and H7N7 avian influenza in the Netherlands, caused great suffering, loss of life, and huge economic loss. Fruit bats have been identified as reservoirs of important emerging zoonoses—Hendra, Nipah, and SARS. Serious combined thinking by international organisations revealed other threats also, like bioterrorism, anti-microbial resistance, xenotransplantation, environmental pollution, and climate change.

Table 2.1 Data from Figure 1 of Lembo et al. (2010)

Zoonoses	Estimated number of deaths	Method of control
Rabies	55,000	VPH (for obligate/established zoonoses)
Leishmaniasis	46,862	
Human African trypanosomiasis	52,342	
Chagas disease	11,367	
Japanese encephalitis	10,988	
Rift Valley fever	537	
SARS	774	One Health (for pandemic-potential zoonoses; human-human transmission)
Influenza A H5N1	79	
Nipah	105	

The experience and methods of eliminating smallpox and polio by the health sector (HS) and rinderpest and vesicular exanthema through VS were inadequate to tackle these because zoonotic agents have many escape routes in the form of more than one host and/or vector and routes of spread. The determinants of zoonoses and issues like bioterrorism and anti-microbial resistance fall under the administrative areas of many sectors, and so efforts need to be multi-sectoral. Success demands the participation of all, including those who suffer and are likely to suffer. "Success in controlling the disease requires sensible, strict vigil of animals, control on their movement and elimination of infected ones. These efforts will fail without the participation of willing and an educated public".

In Malta, failure to control rogue flocks and small flocks kept for family-use led to an epidemic caused by the sale of cheeselets (small cheeses). It took nearly 100 years for Malta to attain freedom from brucellosis (Wyatt 2013).

Of the three criteria for disease eradication programmes—(1) biological and technical feasibility, (2) costs and benefits, and (3) societal and political (Aylward et al. 2000)—the last one is critical.

One health approach considers and integrates these. The core sectors work out the first two, but without societal acceptance and political will, it is not possible to achieve the goal.

Experience with the control of dengue is illustrative. Blood-feeding mosquitoes—*Aedes aegypti*, *Ae. albopictus*, and *Ae. polynesiensis*, besides several species of the *Ae. scutellaris* complex—are the key to the maintenance of the virus and its transmission. Mosquito eggs survive long periods of desiccation. Infection in mosquitoes persists throughout their life, which may run for days or weeks (CDC, 2010. http://www.cdc.gov/dengue/epidemiology/index.html). There is vertical transmission of virus—transovarian—in mosquitoes. Both female and male progenies may carry the virus. Female mosquitoes may get infected by males venereally; the genital tract may also be infected. There is also horizontal transmission among mosquitoes (De Siva et al. 1999). Most human cases cluster in mosquito-breeding sites and within their flight range, which is 100–200 m. Water-filled habitats, such as water containers, tanks of coolers, and potted plants in and around human dwellings, are preferred sites where immature stages develop into adults.

The recommended five elements of integrated mosquito control (WHO 2009) are as follows:

1. Advocacy, social mobilisation, and legislation to strengthen public health bodies and communities
2. Collaboration between the health and other sectors (both public and private)
3. An integrated approach to disease control to maximise the use of resources
4. Evidence-based decision-making to ensure the appropriate implementation of any interventions
5. Capacity building to ensure an adequate response to the local situation

Epidemiological surveillance consists of the identification of locations where the dengue virus is active, through (a) the detection of viraemic human cases in sentinel hospitals in strategic locations and (b) the detection of infected mosquitoes and eggs from houses. Entomological surveillance was considered sensitive for the *detection of circulating virus even before the occurrence of human cases and was thus useful for initiating early intervention.*

The term 'zoonosis' was coined in the late nineteenth century by Rudolf Virchow (1821–1902), a German physician and pathologist, while studying a roundworm, *Trichinella spiralis*, in swine. He said: '... between animal and human medicine there are no dividing lines—nor should there be'. The Canadian physician William Osler (1849–1919), father of modern medicine and internal medicine, had a deep interest in the linkages between human and veterinary medicine and published 'The Relation of Animals to Man' (see Box-Birth of One Health). Calvin W. Schwabe (1927–2006), in his book 'Veterinary Medicine and Human Health', explained the relationship between general medicine and zoology. He coined the term *One Medicine*—the two complimentary sectors being human medicine and veterinary medicine—and called for a unified approach against zoonoses. Veterinary medicine stands on a tripod—animal production, animal health, and veterinary public health. The last one has direct access to human health. VPH is a route to One Medicine.

Today, 'One Medicine/One World One Medicine' is usually referred to as 'One Health' worldwide (birth of One Health). The core components are HS and VS. This terminology change occurred during the first decade of the twenty-first century. One Health recognises humans as part of a larger living ecosystem, that they do not exist in isolation, and that the activities of each member affect the others. Therefore, One Health considers 'health' in a holistic manner—humans, animals, and the environment they exist in.

The 12 Manhattan Principles was published by the Wildlife Conservation Society on 29 September 2004. The Society brought together a group of human and animal health experts for a symposium, 'Building Interdisciplinary Bridges to Health in a "Globalized World"', at Rockefeller University in New York City to discuss the movement of diseases among humans, domestic animals, and wildlife. To combat health threats to human and animal health, 12 priorities were set, known as the 'Manhattan Principles'. They formed the basis of 'One Health, One World' and called for an international, interdisciplinary approach to prevent diseases.

The One Health approach is currently the best in the management of zoonoses. One Health is a '"Unifying concept" i.e. an interdisciplinary and cross-sectoral approach, which strives to promote and develop a better understanding of the "drivers" and "causes" surrounding the emergence and spread of infectious diseases' (www.oneworldhealth.org). It is based on the identification of service delivery sectors/stakeholders/target or suffering groups and unifying them into a 'working group/team'.

2.2.8.3 Drivers of Diseases—One Health Team

The theory of natural nidality of infectious agents states that a vector-borne pathogen has a natural nidus, wherein it maintains itself through a spiral transmission between a reservoir and a vector in natural habitat (i.e., the environment) in a balanced relationship (of host-agent-environment). The One Health concept attempts to identify the 'drivers' that challenge the 'balanced ecosystem/landscape' and create bridges between pathogens and susceptible populations. Planning suitable control measures becomes easy. Drivers are of a diverse nature, falling into different administrative domains or sectors. Hence, 'inter-sectoral' collaboration is essential.

2.2.8.4 One Health Is Economical

According to Grace (2013), in developing countries, an estimated 14% of livestock are infected with one or more zoonotic diseases annually, accounting for a 10% reduction in their productivity. Grace (2013) used the FAOSTAT 2012 value of livestock production (US $639 billion/year) in these countries and estimated the productivity losses related to zoonoses to be around US $9.26 billion/year (assuming that current values of losses are 1.4% and that, without these, production would be US $648 billion).

The benefits of the application of the 'One Health' approach are in terms of averting pandemics (estimated US $30.0 billion expenditure (see Table 2.1), improving the timelines of responses to outbreaks (estimated US $6.0 billion expenditure per year), saved DALYs, and the reduction of the spillover of zoonoses to wildlife, thus conserving the ecosystem. This is against an estimated expenditure of US $3.4 billion on strengthening VS to deliver. The One Health concept benefits greatest the low- and middle-income countries where extensive veterinary health and food safety frameworks are not developed.

References

Aylward B, Hennessey KA, Zagaria N, Olivé J-M, Cochi S (2000) When is a disease eradicable? 100 years of lesson learned. Am J Public Health 90:1515–1520

Bern C, Chowdhury R (2006) The epidemiology of visceral leishmaniasis in Bangladesh: prospects for improved control. Indian J Med Res 123:275–288

Daszak P, Cunningham AA (2003) Anthropogenic change, biodiversity loss, and a new agenda for emerging diseases. J Parasitol 89(Suppl):37–41

De Siva AM, Dittus WPJ, Ersinghe PH, Amersingh FP (1999) Serologic evidence for an epizootic dengue virus infecting Toque macaques (*Macacasinica*) at Polonnaruwa, Sri Lanka. Am J Trop Med Hyg 60(2):300–306

Grace D (2013) One health approach makes sense in the changing socio-economic landscape of developing countries. Presented at the 27th Annual Joint Scientific Conference and 2nd One Health Conference in Africa, 16–19 April 2013, Snow Crest Hotel, Arusha, Tanzania

Hart CA, Bennet M, Begon ME (1999) Zoonoses. J Epidemiol Community Health 53:514–515

Jones KE, Patel NG, Levy MA, Storeygard A, Balk D et al (2008) Global trends in emerging infectious diseases. Nature 451(7181):990–993

Lembo T, Hampson K, Kaare MT, Ernest E, Knobel D et al (2010) The feasibility of canine rabies elimination in Africa: dispelling doubts with data. PLoS Negl Trop Dis 4(2):e626

Taylor LH, Latham SM, Woolhouse ME (2001) Risk factors for human disease emergence. Philos Trans R Soc Lond Ser B Biol Sci 356(1411):983–989

Weiss RA, Magre S, Takeuchi Y (2000) Infection hazards of Xenotransplantation (a review article). J Infect 40:21–25

WHO (2009) Dengue and dengue haemorrhagic fever fact sheet No. 117. WHO, Geneva. http://www.who.int/mediacentre/factsheets/fs117/en/

Wyatt HV (2013) Lessons from the history of brucellosis. Rev Sci Tech 32(1):17–25

Yale G, Bhanurekha V, Ganesan PI (2013) Anthropogenic factors responsible for emerging and re-emerging infectious diseases. Curr Sci 105(7):940–946

3 Epidemiology

Abstract

Man's experience of epidemics dates back to prehistoric times. Epidemics have taken a heavy toll on human and animal life from time to time and have often changed the course of history. The science of epidemiology has taken birth from human curiosity to learn more and more about epidemics. Epidemiology has varied applications and is an important discipline, which forms the very core of all investigational studies. Its interest extends beyond the boundaries of the epidemic/outbreak. Epidemiological investigation does not end with the epidemic but only starts with it, to extend and continue through the inter-epidemic period, when interactions between various factors take place that culminate in an epidemic. The basic difference of epidemiology from other diagnostic disciplines is its ability to search for population/herd/flock-based indicators of disease based on observation, comparison, and, in some cases, experimentation. To detect the presence of indicators of disease(s) in a population, there are two epidemiological approaches: (a) qualitative (landscape, serological, and molecular epidemiology) and (b) quantitative (survey, surveillance, analytical and mathematical epidemiology, economics-related methods, and information systems). These two approaches are applied in an integrated manner during the course of an investigation. Therefore, epidemiology is rightly called the basic/mother science of preventive medicine and public health.

Epidemiology is concerned with the mass phenomenon of disease and can be defined as the study of the frequency, distribution, and determinants of disease in a population, with the primary objective of developing suitable prevention and control measures as well as providing a scientific basis for planning public/animal health programmes.

The complex and dynamic relationship between the host, agent, and environment is involved in an unstable and delicate balance of health; therefore, all areas of veterinary/medical education are fundamental to epidemiology. These

K. G. Narayan et al., *Veterinary Public Health & Epidemiology*,
https://doi.org/10.1007/978-981-19-7800-5_3

relationships include (1) the infectivity and pathogenicity of the causative organism; (2) host susceptibility, resistance, and/or immunity; and (3) the physical, biological, and socio-economic factors of the environment. Epidemiology encompasses not only the diseased population but also the population at risk. Thus, epidemiology is an orderly scientific approach to the study of the conditions/situations and diseases affecting the health and welfare of man and animals.

3.1 Introduction

Human history has witnessed disease outbreaks at different points in time. The outbreaks can be best tackled through the investigation of disease in a population, affected and at risk rather than individual. This requires the study of the natural history of the disease in relation to its distribution in the population, the nature of the infective agent, and the environmental attributes affecting the causative agent as well as the host, reservoir, and vectors. Such study in relation to the population in question forms the basis of epidemiology.

Epidemiology is a study (*logy* = science) on (= *epi*) a population (= *demos*). The term epizootiology is more inclusive (study on a population of animals, including *Homo sapiens*). However, epidemiology is the term most commonly used to denote studies on both human and animal populations, unless specifically mentioned. The study of this subject is basic to population/herd medicine, which is essentially 'preventive medicine'. It is the study of disease in its natural habitat and the medical aspect of ecology. It investigates the connection between the populations of infectious agents or other causative factors, the host population, and their environment, which is referred to as the epidemiological triad (Fig. 3.1) of a multifactorial system for causing epidemics. It is equally applicable to infectious and non-infectious diseases. It aims to protect, promote, and restore the health of the population. The study of the natural history of disease in a nation can be used as an index to assess its progress. The same applied on a global level can indicate 'human progress, e.g., global eradication of smallpox from human being and rinderpest from cattle'.

Epidemiology includes the investigation of the connection between the population of infectious agent(s) or other causative factor(s), the host population, and their environment, which can lead to a multifactorial system for causing epidemics. It is

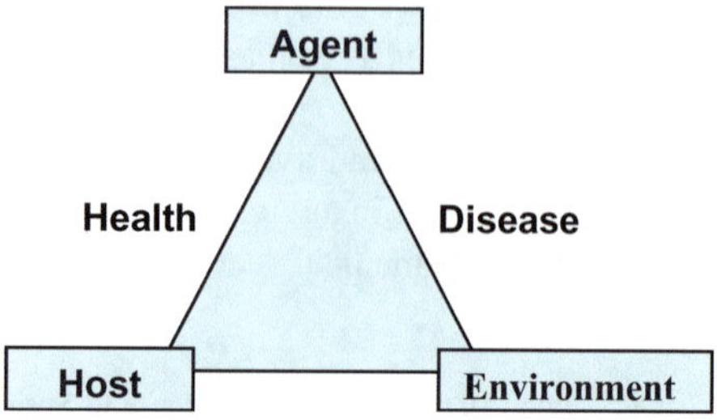

Fig. 3.1 Epidemiological triad

equally applicable to infectious and non-infectious diseases. Epidemiology is the study of disease in nature. The study of the natural history of disease in a nation can be used as an index to assess its progress. The same applied on a global level can indicate 'human progress, e.g., global eradication of smallpox'.

The purpose of epidemiology is searching the cause of an epidemic and the revelation of the cause-effect relationship. It is often known as shoe-leather epidemiology. Investigations on two cholera epidemics—around Broad Street Lamp, London, 1854, and the Ferrara City Council, Italy, 1855—shed light on the evolution of epidemiology. In London, John Snow used simple forms of comparisons and frequency measures. In the Ferrara City Council, Italy data were collected in such a way that comparing groups on specific exposure could not shed light on the possible causal association. John Snow (anaesthesiologist) and William Farr (statistician, Registrar General) knew that a 'controlled experiment' was needed to demonstrate the causal effect of polluted water. This team of two—medicine and public health surveillance—discovered the mode of transmission of cholera years before the causative agent was discovered. Farr had created a unique and innovative system of standardised procedures for the collection, classification, analysis, and reporting of the causes of deaths. Snow's horse sense grouped the households according to water suppliers. This comparison of death rate per 1000 households supplied by Southwark and Vauxhall Company vs. Lambeth Company—30 vs. 4 and 6/1000 in other districts of London demonstrated that the polluted water caused cholera. Group comparison became a strategy or method. This grand experiment or a natural experiment on the rate of deaths among the exposed vs. the non-exposed is cited in most books on epidemiology (Morabia 2004).

The epidemiologic study designs evolved from intuitive group comparisons, and there has been a progressive refinement of principles, concepts, and methods. Epidemiology has rightly been said to be an open-end discipline that derives information from a variety of established disciplines, such as microbiology, biotechnology, statistics-biostatistics, environment, forestry, wildlife and ecology, economics, social science-anthropology, etc. An epidemiologist is the captain and possesses sixth or horse sense. He collects information on the 'epidemic' under investigation as per the plan drawn through his 'vision', collates data, tabulates to draw conclusions that enable to formulate hypothesis(es), revisits the data if needed, and revises the plan.

The actual trajectory of the disease is not only the mathematics of virus progression but also the behaviour of the community, society, and the people at large. For example, in case of SARS-CoV-2, referred to as 2019-nCoV shows—the complexity of 'the problem of containment of epidemic' and maze of factors, stakeholders, requirement of a team of widely diverse nature of professionals. Epidemiology is basic and essential to the implementation of the One Health concept.

3.2 Objectives and Application of Epidemiology

Epidemiology provides an answer to all relevant questions pertaining to the disease in a population, such as who, what, when, where, why, and how. It

1. Enables the identification of aetiology and transmission pathways
2. Provides information on the health status of the population in an area
3. Helps in health administration, e.g. planning for medical/veterinary facilities, preventive inoculation, special care to a specific occupation group (e.g. all pregnant and lactating cows), etc.
4. Provides knowledge about local disease patterns in animals and also searches for human linkages
5. Provides information/data that can be combined with information from areas/ disciplines like genetics, biochemistry, microbiology, etc. to elucidate disease causation and also planning for integrated multidisciplinary disease management programmes
6. Provides the opportunity to examine if the epidemiological data are consistent with epidemiological hypotheses developed either clinically or experimentally in the laboratory
7. Provides a basis for the development of preventive and intervention measures, public health, and other useful disease management practices
8. Provides opportunities for the evaluation of disease management tactics, prophylactic vaccination, and chemoprophylactic drenching programmes.
9. Enables the estimation of economic loss due to the disease as well as gains resulting from intervention measures
10. Provides a basis for devising the means to optimise productivity and minimise disease in the animal population

3.3 Types of Epidemiology

There is no systematic classification. The various types of epidemiology have been described in the literature. Most types or classes are indicative of the uses of epidemiology.

3.3.1 Based on the Fundamentals/Basics

1. **General epidemiology** deals with the fundamental aspects of the multifactorial causation of epidemics—the epidemic or epizootic process involving the agent; the hosts—reservoir and the susceptibles; the transmission process and the environment—social, ethnological, ecological, etc.; and temporal factors.
2. **Landscape epidemiology** is the study of disease in relation to the ecosystem in which the disease is found. It can be used to analyse both risk patterns and environmental risk factors.

3. **Descriptive epidemiology** aims to describe the distribution of diseases and determinants. It provides a way of organising and analysing these data to describe the variations in disease frequency among populations by geographical areas and over time (i.e. person, place, and time).
4. **Analytic epidemiology** is concerned with the search for causes and effects—or the why and how. It is used to quantify the association between exposures and outcomes and to test hypotheses about causal relationships.
5. **Experimental epidemiology** is a type of investigation where an experimental model is used to confirm a causal relationship. It studies the relationships of various factors to determine the frequency and distribution of diseases in a population.

3.3.2 Based on Diagnostic Methods and the Diagnosis of Infection/Disease

1. **Clinical epidemiology**: the clinical manifestation and pathology of the disease constitute the basis of description, but the biological and sociological trends are also included to understand the epidemic process. Thus, the knowledge of clinicians, pathologists, and epidemiologists is combined to understand the epidemic process in order to find out a control strategy. Akin to clinical epidemiology are sub-clinical epidemiology and serological epidemiology, which deal with such cases where the disease is not manifested clinically and serological testing is required to establish its prevalence/incidence.
2. **Sub-clinical epidemiology**: it involves the study of an illness that is staying below the surface of clinical detection. A sub-clinical disease has no recognisable clinical findings. It is distinct from a clinical disease, which has signs and symptoms that can be recognised.
3. **Serological epidemiology**: it is the study of disease on the basis of variables (antibodies, minerals, hormones, enzymes, etc.) present in the serum or body fluid.
4. **Molecular epidemiology**: Kilbourne (1973) was the first to use the word molecular epidemiology in a study of the influenza virus. It involves the use of molecular (ribonucleic acid (RNA), deoxyribonucleic acid (DNA)) techniques to identify and differentiate causative organisms in order to understand the origin and relatedness of outbreaks.

In the study of epidemics, it is essential to establish the identity of the infectious agent. Molecular epidemiology utilises genetic markers. Once the causative agent is identified, tracing out its source to the reservoir and the circuitous routes through a vehicle or vector becomes easy with the marker. Molecular biology has made tremendous development, and various methods have become handy. Some of these are chromosomal DNA analysis, chromosomal DNA banding, plasmid DNA analysis, DNA and RNA homology, etc. In the study of infectious diseases, particularly viral diseases, molecular tools are especially useful as the time required for virus isolation and characterisation by conventional methods is eliminated. Molecular biology has enabled the understanding of the mechanism of disease causation, resistance, latency, and persistence and also the emergence of new strains. Host susceptibility and resistance are also better understood.

3.3.3 Based on Attributes in the Study Population

1. **Occupational epidemiology**: each occupation has associated health hazards. The application of the knowledge of both occupational hazard and epidemiology in the management of the health of the occupational groups is dealt with in occupational epidemiology, e.g. pneumoconiosis among miners and zoonoses among animal owners.
2. **Disaster epidemiology**: disaster epidemiology is the use of epidemiology to assess the short- and long-term adverse health effects of disasters and to predict the consequences of future disasters.
3. **Genetic epidemiology**: clusters of cases in the families of human beings and certain breeds of animals point to genetic factors. The study of genetically inherited diseases is dealt with in 'genetic epidemiology'. The genetic nature of a disease is indicated in the following circumstances: (a) the incidence of the disease is more among the relatives of cases than among the relatives of controls, (b) the relatives of cases from a defined population have a higher frequency of risk of the condition than the population from which the cases were selected, (c) a higher proportion of cases than of controls has a relative with the disease condition, (d) a higher proportion of the cohort of healthy individuals with a family history of the disease condition develops the condition over a period of time than of otherwise comparable individuals without a family history of the disease, and (e) the correlation of the values of the trait between pairs of related individuals is significantly greater than 0.
4. **Nutritional epidemiology**: an exciting branch of epidemiology, it is the study of nutritional determinants of disease in a population, which gives insights into the potential causes and prevention of many health conditions.

3.3.4 Based on Application

1. **Applied epidemiology**: it describes how best to apply traditional epidemiological methods for determining disease aetiology to 'real-life' problems in public health and health service research.
2. **Special epidemiology**: it is the theory of the development, control, and prophylaxis of special epidemic or epizootic diseases, e.g. acquired immunodeficiency syndrome and bovine spongiform encephalitis.
3. **Practical epidemiology**: it deals with the application of the results of epidemiological studies in collaboration with many specialists, like practicing veterinarians/physicians, microbiologists, pathologists, public animal health

specialists, etc., for the control, eradication, and prevention of epidemics. This is essentially applied epidemiology with a multidisciplinary approach.

4. **Theoretical epidemiology**: in this type of epidemiology, models are designed to simulate epidemics so as to examine the factors associated with or responsible for the occurrence of epidemics and work out a strategy to control ongoing epidemics as well as prevent their occurrence in future. The relationship between the suspected causal factors (attribute) and the disease is quantified, and mathematical models are developed, e.g. the Reed and Frost model for measles. An agent, a susceptible host, and an environment that brings the host and agent together constitute an epidemiological triad or triangle, the simplest model for an infectious disease (Fig. 3.1).
5. **Predictive epidemiology**: the occurrence and trends of a disease can be predicted once the determinants have been identified and their fluctuation has been quantified. Then parameters of various determinants are used in a model to predict the possible occurrence of an epidemic of the disease so as to make preparatory arrangements for prevention and control. For example, knowledge about the amount of rainfall has been possible to predict the trend of liver fluke morbidity since the population of vectors and the intermediate hosts of parasites are dependent upon environmental factors, such as rainfall, humidity, and temperature.
6. **Participatory epidemiology**: it is the application of participatory methods to epidemiological research and disease surveillance, which overcomes the limitations of conventional epidemiological methods. The Global Rinderpest Eradication Program adopted participatory epidemiology as a surveillance tool for controlling rinderpest. This approach was subsequently used in both rural and urban settings in Africa and Asia for foot and mouth disease (FMD), *peste des petits ruminants* (PPR), and highly pathogenic avian influenza.
7. **Computational epidemiology**: it involves the application of computer science to epidemiological studies. Its use particularly in theoretical epidemiology is very important, basically in the development of mathematical models and the use of expert systems (disease diagnosis).

References

Kilbourne ED (1973) The molecular epidemiology of influenza. J Infect Dis 127(4):478–487. https://doi.org/10.1093/infdis/127.4.478

Morabia A (2004) A history of epidemiologic methods and concepts. Springer, Basel

Ecological Concept

4

The word 'ecology' comes from the Greek root 'oikos', meaning 'home'. Ecology may, thus, be defined as the science of the 'home relations of organisms (biotic components), their interaction with each other and environment'. It includes biological diversity. Ecology defines relationships between organisms and their environment. The environment of any organism consists of everything external to that particular organism. There are two major components of the environment: biotic (living organisms) and abiotic or physical forces, including the wind, sunlight, and soil, as well as man-made infrastructure. In a given unit, ecosystem brings these factors together—a dynamic complex of plant, animal, and microorganism communities and their non-living environment interacting as a functional unit. For example, Rift Valley fever virus transmission involves stages of drought and rainfall, soil conditions, particular vector species, susceptible host species, and their interactions among other determinants. Biotic and abiotic conditions may affect the potential for persistence and/or the dissemination of contaminants (whether pathogens, chemicals, etc.).

Soil, water, air and other non-living objects constitute the abiotic environment. Besides, there are forces like solar radiation, gravity, nuclear energy, etc. that are also in the environment surrounding an organism. The biotic components of the environment consist of animals, plants, microbes, and all other living organisms. The inter-species and intra-species relationships of the biota are dynamic. While creating a place for its existence, an organism has to struggle against various competitive fauna and environmental factors. It creates a 'niche' for itself. Numbers of organisms settle down after such struggle in a defined place. The binders among the biotic community are ethnology (behaviour), food chain, shelter, reproduction/propagation, and other necessities of life of the organisms sharing an ecosystem. Any organism, like the others, is related to and influenced by the environment. The relationship may be both friendly and hostile. The ecological environment may be considered as the sum total of all the external influences and conditions that affect the life process.

K. G. Narayan et al., *Veterinary Public Health & Epidemiology*,
https://doi.org/10.1007/978-981-19-7800-5_4

The habitat and the micro- and macro-organisms (including plants and animals) are all considered one interacting unit—the ecosystem. An ecosystem, which provides uniform conditions of life, is called a 'biotope' (the address), and the biotic community sharing the 'biotope' is called 'biocoenosis'. The 'niche' of an organism in the biotope is its special position, something like the profession with which it is identified. 'Biome' is a well-differentiated and climatically uniform geographical region, such as tundra, grassland, savannah, tropical forest, and desert.

The biotic community in any ecosystem is the result of the interaction of all living agents affecting the biotic communities and the soil, water, air, physical forces, chemical forces, plants, and animals—all interacting with each other and affecting other's behaviour. In other words, the biotic community appears to be in a dynamic equilibrium. This organisation is held intact because the agencies involved approximately balance each other. If the potency of one is changed, the composition of the biota in the community will continue to change until a new balance is reached. Such changes are known as 'succession'. When the equilibrium is reached, in which the main biotic components are not overthrown by new invaders, a stage is reached, called 'climax'. In this stage, a slow evolution may lead to a better adaptation of the species to fit each other and the habitat. However, no two species have the same requirement, nor do they behave similarly. In the competition between different species for a place in the community, those that can obtain the necessities of life have a better chance of survival than those that cannot. In the resulting organisation, each species tends to find a particular part of the habitat, in which it can hold an advantage over its competitive species in obtaining the necessities of life. Such part of the habitat in any community occupied by a species is called a 'niche'. Individuals, families, or colonies of a given species are in direct competition with each other in the same niche, which exacerbates during critical periods, such as overpopulation, drought, or shortage of food or shelter. It usually results in the selective elimination of some and the selective survival of those best suited to stand the competition. This natural selection contributes to the evolution of a species as well as to the reorganisation of a biotic community. During the process of competition in response to stimuli of the environment, an organism may develop a particular morphological form, a physiological response, or a behavioural pattern. Such a response is considered an adjustment, which may remain fixed under given stimuli (dauermodification) or may become fixed in heredity (adaptation). A biotic community is an outcome of an age-old struggle to reconcile its constitutional organisation with the exigencies of the environment. The dynamics of ecology involve fluctuating physical environments, active living organisms, changing populations, and the passing of time and have a direct bearing on the behaviour of organisms, their survival, their distribution in space or time, and evolution.

The emergence and re-emergence of infectious agents, including zoonoses, can be considered a logical consequence of their ecology and evolution as microbes exploit new niches and adapt to new hosts. Human activities like land use, the extraction of natural resources, animal production systems and the use of antimicrobials, global trade, etc. create or provide access to these new niches. The ecological niche for the arthropod vectors is shaped by environmental and anthropogenic determinants.

The reservoir, insect vectors, and pathogens constitute the components of a biocenosis. The reservoir becomes the donor of infection, with the insect vector a recipient, which in turn becomes the donor to donate the infectious agent to another susceptible vertebrate (another individual of the reservoir species). This cycle of transmission maintains the infectious agent in the biotope, which becomes the 'natural nidus' of infection. The agent-vector-reservoir host being in a balanced state, the infection remains confined to this nidus, as explained in Pavlovsky's theory of natural nidality of diseases. Once this balance is disturbed, the agent is likely to spill over to cause an epidemic.

Disease or departure from health is the result of an interaction among both animate and inanimate disease causing agents, man/animals, and the total environment, including its physical, economic, social, and biological aspects. Ecological relationships that lead to the causation of a particular disturbance are called 'epidemosis'.

Each disorder represents a complex epidemiological unit that constitutes only a segment of the total ecology. Human/animal ecology is his mutual relationships, his organic and inorganic environment, his adaptations, the struggle for his existence, his parasites, etc.

The study of the natural history of disease requires knowledge of (a) the surrounding outer world, (b) the organic and inorganic conditions of existence, (c) the so-called economy of nature, (d) the correlation between all organisms living together in one and the same locality, (e) their adaptation to the surroundings, (f) their modifications, (g) their struggle for existence, etc.

There are a number of natural nidii of infection, like the following:

1. Conjugate nidus harbouring causative agents of two or more diseases.
2. Poly-hostal nidus has more than one species of reservoir host with regard to the disease-producing agent.
3. Poly-vector nidus harbouring more than one species of vectors with regard to the disease-producing agent.

A nidus is called 'elementary' if there is a continuous circulation of the agent of a transmissible disease. The extent of a nidus may be narrow, like a rodent burrow or a hollow in the branch of a tree. It may be diffuse, as wide as a deciduous forest.

Autochthonous nidus is a natural nidus that has not been influenced or altered by human activities. It is a virgin landscape containing a nidus of infection.

Anthropurgic nidus refers to a natural nidus that appeared in a cultivated landscape where the virgin structure of biocoenosis was changed as a result of cultivation. The nidii of many helminthiasis were created like this.

Synanthropic nidus refers to a nidus of infection that is shared by human beings (Syn = together, anthropos = man). Synanthropes are domestic animals, birds, reptiles, etc. that may act as a link between anthropurgic nidii and the human dwelling or his farms. There may be independent synanthropic nidii in a populated area. The agent's environment in a synanthropic nidus is extremely mobile and wholly under the influence of human activity. Usually, agents have a wide range of adaptations and a wide host range, e.g. *Salmonella* and *Toxoplasma*.

Soil nidus certain fungi are common in soil enriched with organic matter. For example, *Histoplasma capsulatum* is especially found in soil enriched with bird faeces. *Cryptococcus neoformans* is found common in soil enriched with pigeon droppings.

Water nidii some of the trematodes have natural water nidii (hydrobiocoenosis), e.g. liver fluke and amphistomes.

4.1 Persistence of a Natural Nidus of Infection

Disturbances may affect the structure and composition of a biotic community, influencing the circulation of the infectious agent. The circulation may decline, yet the nidus continues and persists. For example, the tick *Ornithodoros* may maintain spirochaetes for 20 years. Reservoir host-vector-agent interaction is complex and maintains the perpetuation of the agent, at times even thwarting directed actions, e.g. the transovarial transmission of infection in ixodid ticks, e.g. *Babesia bigemina.* The maintenance of Japanese encephalitis virus by some species of birds without any harm/manifestation of signs and symptoms, rabies virus in the subscapular fats of bats, and masked/occult swine influenza virus in earthworms are examples of such mechanisms.

Activity in a nidus is determined by a variety of factors, such as vector density, reservoirs' density, vectors' efficiency, and the infectivity and pathogenicity of agents. Most of these are influenced by environmental conditions. The extent of activity is determined by the flight range of the host (birds, bats) and vectors and the availability of susceptible hosts within that range.

4.2 Escape of an Agent and the Formation of a New Nidus

An agent may escape from its nidii to establish a new nidus to spread the infection through various ways, as detailed hereunder:

1. Introduction of a new host species into an ecosystem, of which the infectious agent is a part, e.g. blue tongue in Africa—local breeds of sheep may have no mortality, but in imported breeds, it may be up to 90%.

2. Introduction of an infected host species into a new ecosystem; e.g., the introduction of a single sheep suffering from peste des petits ruminants (PPR) to a new flock of sheep may cause 90% infection and 30–70% mortality.
3. Changes in the population dynamics of a usual host, a potentially new host, or an intermediary transport host, e.g. measles in newborns (turnover of the population).
4. Ecological changes that bring two previously separated ecosystems in contact, e.g. cholera in floods and plague during an earthquake.
5. Changes in the habits of a host, including its food habits, e.g. food-borne trematodiasis (*Clonorchis sinensis*, *Paragonimus* spp., *Fasciola* spp., and *Opisthorchis* spp.), are emerging public health problems in Southeast Asia and Western Pacific regions because of attraction to local dishes, like raw crab soaked in soya sauce, drunken crabs, raw grass carp, raw fish, which are considered delicacies by tourists.
6. Technological changes brought about by man, e.g. anisakiasis.
7. Mutation or genetic recombination of an agent, e.g. influenza virus.

4.3 Landscape Epidemiology

The study of landscape epidemiology provides insight into the mechanism of a disease's process, its maintenance in nature, and the possible points of attack. The identification of weak links enables one to design a strategy for the control of diseases. The ecological aspect of certain diseases is better explained by 'landscape epidemiology'. Certain diseases, like liver fluke, amphistomiasis, and Kayasanur forest disease, tend to restrict themselves to geographical areas possessing some ecological characteristics. The infectious agent, the vector, and the intermediate host are members of the biotic community, which share the same biotope to constitute the natural nidus or focus of infection. The infection/epidemic process is initiated from this primary source. The infectious agent perpetuates here. This niche of the infectious agent gets established after a lot of struggles and adjustments with the fauna and environmental factors. Any disturbance affecting the essential components of the biotic community that maintains the infectious agent results in serious consequences. For example, a flood or an earthquake affecting a 'plague nidus' may lead to the spillover of the infectious agent from the natural nidus to rodents in the synanthropic nidus (a nidus where man is also a component of the biotic community), initiating an 'epidemic plague'. Pavlovsky's theory of 'natural nidality of transmissible diseases' states that 'the infectious agent is maintained in nature by a wild life reservoir and a vector in an enzootic state' (Pavlovsky et al. 1966). There is a successive transit of the agent from the body of the animal reservoir (donor) to the vector (the recipient). The infected vector becomes the 'donor', in turn, and the agent is transferred to an animal recipient. The agent is, thus, maintained in the nidus through a spiral-chain-like transmission (Fig. 4.1). The natural nidus is said to be an aggregate of epizootic foci. The epizootic focus may be considered the abode of the source of infection (the reservoir host) and the adjacent area through which the agent

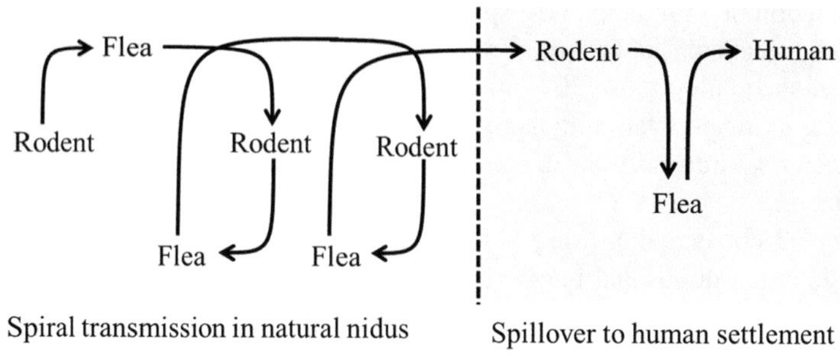

Fig. 4.1 Spiral transmission of *Yersinia pestis*

can be disseminated. A medico-geographical map of such ‘natural-focal’ diseases can be made.

Reference

Pavlovsky EN, Plous FK, Levine ND (1966) Natural nidality of transmissible diseases. Am J Med Sci 252:161

Causation of Disease 5

5.1 Different Hypothesis of Disease Causation

It is difficult to define disease. Health, opposite to disease, has been defined, for human beings, as 'a state of physical, mental and social wellbeing and not merely the absence of disease or infirmity'. In the case of animals, a working definition has been proposed by Thaplyal and Misra (1996): 'animal health is a state of physical, physiological and behavioural wellbeing of animals, which lead to maximum possible levels of production, draught efficiency and economic benefit'. Any departure from this is then 'disease', which is a morbid state, affecting organs or systems of the host body and manifesting variously, such as a rise in body temperature, a loss of appetite, body aches, etc. It usually also results in the inability of an individual to perform normal physiological functions despite being in optimum nutritional and environmental conditions. Health is considered to be the result of a harmonious relationship of an individual with the environment. Any disturbance in this state of harmonious relationship brings about 'dis-harmony or dis-ease'.

This departure from a state of health may have many causes, the search for which and the explanation of diseased state has been going on. Many hypotheses have been proposed, and some of these are summed up below:

- **Superstitious belief**: disease is caused by the wrath of God or an evil spirit.
- **Environmental effect**: exposure to foul air (mal air) causes disease. Hippocrates explained disease causation in his 'Air, Waters, and Places'.
- **Humoral theory**: body fluids (*vat*, *pit*, *rakt*) are stable or balanced (homeostasis) in a state of health but not so in a diseased state.
- **Taoist (Chinese) theory**: there are opposite forces, called *yan* and *yin.* A balanced state is indicated when both are equal. The Chinese considered three 'Self'—'earth-self', 'heaven-self', and 'health-self'—to explain health and disease.

K. G. Narayan et al., *Veterinary Public Health & Epidemiology*,
https://doi.org/10.1007/978-981-19-7800-5_5

- **Germ theory**: each disease is caused by a specific etiological agent; e.g., *Mycobacterium tuberculosis* causes TB, and the foot and mouth disease virus causes FMD. Scurvy is a result of vitamin C deficiency, anaemia is caused by iron deficiency, and the excess of fluorine leads to fluorosis.

The above theories are deficient in one or the other way or emphasise 'one factor' as a cause. For example, 'environmental effect', the 'humoral theory', and the 'germ theory' emphasise only the 'environment', 'host', and 'agent', respectively.

When the germ theory of disease causation was propounded, it became necessary to convince people that a bacterium was causally associated with disease. Henle-Koch's postulates were put forward to demonstrate the causal association of *Bacillus anthracis* and *Mycobacterium tuberculosis.* In brief, an organism, to be accepted as a cause of disease, must (a) be isolated in pure culture from a diseased case and grown in artificial culture media, (b) be found in all cases and regularly, (c) reproduce the disease in experimental animals, and (d) be re-isolated from the experimental animal in pure culture.

These commonly known Koch postulates continued to be the guideline for many years till some diseases could not be adequately explained. Most of these diseases that are caused by exotoxins of bacteria could not satisfy the four postulates, e.g. *Corynebacterium diphtheriae* and *Vibrio cholera.* In addition, bacterial food poisoning caused by enterotoxins (*Staphylococcus aureus*, *Clostridium perfringens*); diseases caused by slow-growing viruses, fungi, and parasites; and genetic and immunological disorders could not be explained. The theory of 'multi-factorial causation of disease' brought forward evidence of an association of factors, other than the specific infectious agent, in disease causation. Evans' postulates (Evans 1976) considered these epidemiological evidence defining the 'causal association of a factor with disease'. They are as follows: (a) the incidence and prevalence of disease must be more in the exposed than in the control cohorts, (b) the cause is more common in the diseased, (c) exposure to the agent precedes the appearance of disease, (d) the elimination of the agent results in a decrease in the incidence of disease, (e) disease is experimentally produced, and (f) the prevention or modification of the host response decreases the expression of disease. The deficiencies of Henle-Koch's postulates were mostly made up. The causal association of factors in cases of most chronic and slowly developing diseases could be explained. Susser's criteria are worth considering when establishing causal association (Susser 1977). These are the following: (a) strength—a stronger statistical association denotes a greater possibility for one variable to positively affect the other; (b) consistency—the causal association is established on the basis of repeated tests, and the results are reproducible; (c) coherence—the association appears reasonable in biological terms; (d) specificity—the suspected characteristic relates favourably to the precision with which the occurrence of one variable predicts the other variable; (e) time order and logical structure—historically, the exposure to disease precedes its actual occurrence; and (f) dose-response—the intensity of disease occurrence is related to the dose of the causal agent.

Factors that contribute to disease causation may be classified as follows:

- *Predisposing* factors create a state of susceptibility, making the host vulnerable to the agent, e.g. genetics, age, sex, previous illness, etc.
- *Enabling* factors are those that assist in the development of the disease, e.g. poor nutrition, unhygienic housing, poor sanitation, inadequate medical care, etc.
- *Precipitating* factors are those that are associated with immediate exposure to the disease agent or the onset of the disease, e.g. exposure to a specific disease agent, like Ebola, while nursing; attending a funeral; drinking contaminated water; etc.
- *Reinforcing* factors are those that aggravate an already existing disease, e.g. repeated exposure, malnutrition, overwork/exhaustion, environmental conditions, etc.

Multiple causalities of disease is the theory that considers holistically the contribution of each of the three major factors—'environment', 'host', and 'agent'—to the causation of the disease. *A balanced state of the interaction of 'host-environment-agent' results in 'health', and any alteration or imbalance leads to disease* (Fig. 5.1).

The balanced state can be altered by any change in the constellation of the host, agent, and environment. The balanced state of the host is dependent upon age, sex, race, habits, customs, genetic factors, defence system, etc.; that of the agent is determined by the nature and characteristics of the agent in relation to the host and the environment; and that of the environment is the aggregate of all external conditions and influences affecting the agent (non-infectious) or the life of the agent, host, intermediate hosts, and vectors; behaviour/management; or animal husbandry practices.

This is best illustrated by 'smog death' events, which occurred in 1948, 1950, and 1952 in Pennsylvania, Poza Rica, and London (HMSO 1954), respectively. The chemical pollutants (agents) affected those who had a cardio-pulmonary weakness (hosts) when a thick smog (environment) prevented the clearance of harmful chemical pollutants. The meteorological conditions initiated the disturbance in the balance state, and the result was morbidity and mortality of both man and animals who had a cardio-pulmonary weakness. In the case of shipping fever (haemorrhagic septicaemia), a similar situation is observed. During the shipping of cattle, the ocean environment increases host's susceptibility to the agent, *Pasteurella multocida* present in the respiratory tract of the animals as a commensal—the relationship changes from commensalism to parasitism. Biotic and abiotic conditions may affect the potential for persistence and/or the dissemination of pathogens, chemicals, etc. The transmission of Rift Valley fever virus involves stages of drought and rainfall, particular vector species, susceptible host specie(s) and their interactions, and soil conditions, among other determinants.

The environment affects both the agents and the hosts. There are diseases where insect vectors and intermediate hosts are also involved. These are also affected by the environment. Thus, a number of interactive combinations of the host (H), agent (A), vector (V), intermediate host (IH), and environment (E)—A-H, A-V-H, A-IH-H, A-H-E, A-H-V-E, A-IH-H-E, V-H, H-E, etc.—influence the occurrence of a disease.

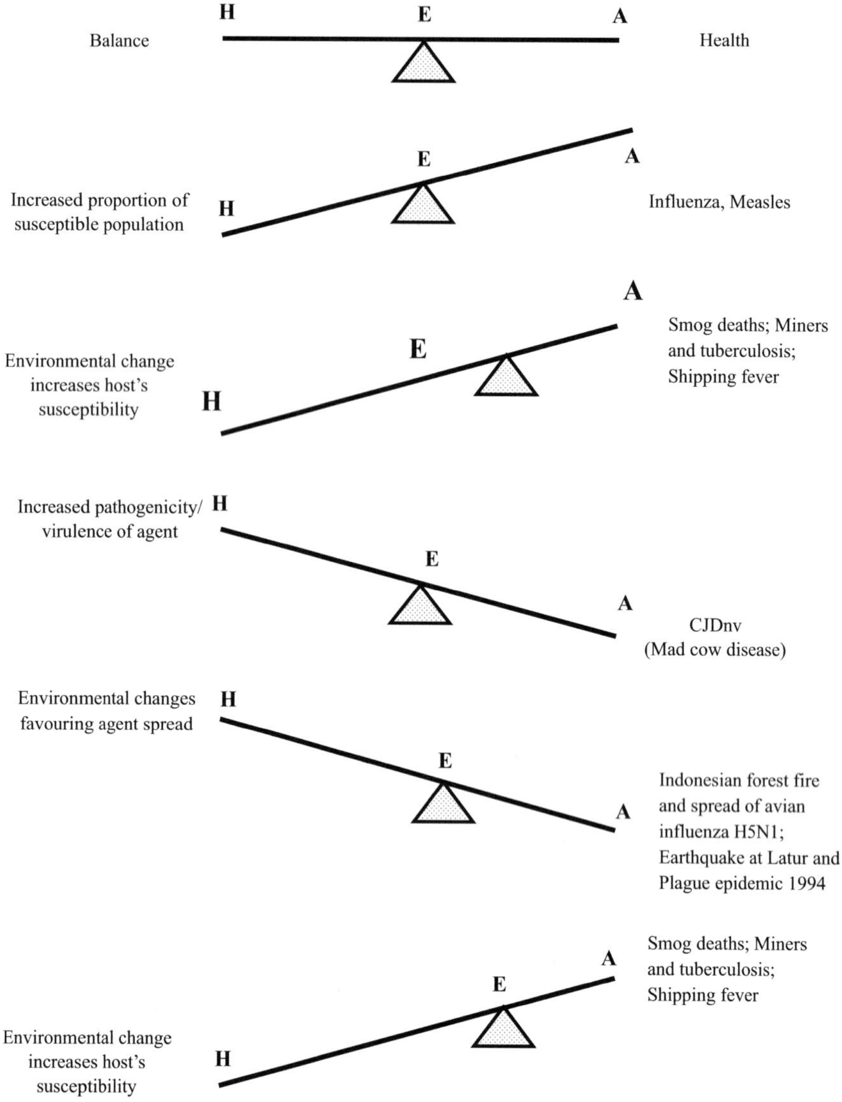

Fig. 5.1 Multiple causalities of disease

5.2 The Multiple Causality Hypothesis and Its Utility

- It is not essential to know the entire web of causation for controlling disease. The identification of one significant strand in the web is enough to control the disease. For example, the identification of the fact that 'cholera was caused by drinking sewage-contaminated water' was enough to control the outbreak in London even before *Vibrio cholera* was identified as the specific cause.

- Enormously increased opportunities are provided to prevent or control disease. This is particularly true in the case of parasitic diseases.
- Disease can be prevented in such cases also where it is not possible to manipulate the cause. Phenylketonuria is a genetic disorder. The clinical disease occurs when a diet contains phenylalanine. This knowledge enables one to exclude this amino acid or such food.
- This theory provides the use of alternatives to unacceptable measures of control. For example, smoking causes lung cancer, and if smoking cannot be prevented, filters can be used to keep out carcinogens.

5.3 Drivers of Disease in the Population

Pandemics, due to emerging and re-emerging infectious diseases, are experienced primarily because of the practices that fundamentally change the ecological dynamics and the environment, leading to increased contact between people and animals in unexplored areas. Such practices pose a host of other impacts on the ecosystems associated, which affect human health. The leading drivers of emerging diseases include land use change causing habitat loss (such as deforestation, land conversion for agriculture, and processes associated with the extraction of natural resources), human susceptibility to infection, agricultural industry changes, international travel and commerce, war, and famine (Loh et al. 2015).

References

Evans AS (1976) Causation and disease: the Henle-Koch postulates revisited. Yale J Biol Med 49(2):175–195

HMSO (1954) Mortality and morbidity during the London fog of December 1952. Reports on Public Health and Medical Subjects, No. 95. Her Majesty 's Stationary Office, London

Loh EH, Olival KJ, Zambrana-Torrelio C, Bogich TL, Johnson CK et al (2015) (2015). Targeting transmission pathways for emerging zoonotic disease surveillance and control. Vect Borne Zoonot Dis 15(7):432–437

Susser M (1977) Causal thinking in the health science: concepts and Strategies in epidemiology. Oxford University Press, New York, NY

Thaplyal DC, Misra DS (1996) Fundamentals of animal hygiene and epidemiology. International Book distributing Co., Lucknow

Agent, Host, and Environmental Factors 6

The interaction and interdependence of the agent, the host, the environment, and time are used to explain diseases and epidemics. The agent is the cause of disease; the host is an organism, usually a human or an animal, that harbours the disease; the environments are those surroundings and conditions external to the human or animal that cause or allow disease transmission; and time accounts for incubation periods, the life expectancy of the host or the pathogen, and the duration of the course of illness or condition.

6.1 The Agent

Diseases may be caused by the impact of a fall or accident, emotional breakdown, burn, excess or lack of certain chemicals, or microscopic and sub-microscopic agents, as explained below.

The agent causing disease may be physical, chemical, biological, or a variety of other factors whose presence or absence in the host's environment leads to ill health, i.e. disease:

- *Physical agents*: such as heat, electricity, radiation, fall, beating, drowning, etc.
- *Chemical agents*: such as toxic plants and feed, agrochemicals, chlorinated naphthalene used as additives in farm lubricants (causes bovine hyperkeratosis), and insecticides used for spray or dips; excess of certain chemicals (e.g. fluorine) and deficiency of other chemicals (e.g. iodine, vitamins) are also chemical causes of disease.
- *Biological agents*: the bites of venomous insects and reptiles, snakes, dogs, and microorganisms—bacteria, viruses, prions, fungi, parasites, etc.—are all biological agents of disease.

K. G. Narayan et al., *Veterinary Public Health & Epidemiology*,
https://doi.org/10.1007/978-981-19-7800-5_6

Three sets of properties of microorganisms are important for understanding infection, disease, and epidemic. These are (a) properties useful for identification; (b) properties useful for understanding the agent's interaction with the host's tissues and cells, even at the molecular level; and (c) host-related properties that explain the further spread of infection.

Properties useful for identification: These are the taxonomic and antigenic characteristics of a microorganism. The conventional laboratory tests in isolation and the characterisation of a microorganism are useful for identification on the basis of taxonomy, e.g. Gram's staining, morphology, certain differential biochemical tests, tissue culture and specific cytopathy, and antigens, like somatic, flagellar, etc., for serological tests. Specific antigens may be used to identify the exposure group in the population. A significant increase in the levels of a specific antibody indicates definite exposure (i.e. it is diagnostic).

The agent's ability to survive in the environment outside the host is important for the transmission of infection. For example, *Yersinia pestis* survived for 18 months in the dark in fleas' faeces. If protected from the ultraviolet (UV) rays of the sun, all viruses survive longer during winter than in summer. Over 90% of outbreaks of transmissible gastroenteritis (transmissible gastroenteritis virus (TGE)) occur during winter. The TGE virus survives at 5 °C for more than 3 weeks in contrast to 3 days in faeces. Swine pox and contagious pustular dermatitis viruses can survive for months in the premises and buildings to infect a fresh batch of young animals. The wine fever virus has a short survival time in sties although is resistant to phenol and cresol, and therefore, if susceptible pigs are kept in the sties vacated by diseased pigs even 2 days earlier, they may not be infected. Polio virus does not survive in a drying well but survives better in moist conditions, and possibly faecal transmission is thus facilitated. Spore-bearing bacteria survive for long outside the host (Murray et al. 2021).

The growth requirements of agents differ. Water does not provide nutrients for growth and as such acts as a mechanical vehicle. Waterborne infections therefore are caused by agents that are highly infective even in low doses, e.g. *Vibrio cholera.*

Vulnerability to chemotherapeutic agents does affect the transmission process as the period of infectivity is reduced in case an effective chemotherapeutic agent is administered to patients. The agent may be resistant to the drug, and so the control of disease becomes problematic, e.g. multiple drug resistance in *Mycobacterium tuberculosis.*

Antigenic changes in the agent present two problems. The diagnosis becomes difficult unless antiserum for the antigenically changed strain is available in the laboratory. The host naturally immune to the parent agent due to earlier exposure is susceptible to infection with the new antigen-bearing strain.

Properties useful for understanding the agent's interaction with the host's tissue, cells, and even cell molecules are various properties useful in invasion and initiating pathological changes in the hosts. Examples are the following:

- Lipopolysaccharides (LPSs) and lipoproteins which are present in the bacterial cell wall, particularly of Gram-negative bacteria (*Escherichia coli*); they are also called endotoxins, which cause fever.
- Means to evade phagocytosis like capsules, certain proteins (M protein of *Streptococcus*, protein A of *Staphylococcus*), the mycolic acid of *Mycobacterium tuberculosis*, etc.
- Bacterial adhesins, fimbria and flagella, or viral haemagglutinin used for adherence to specific cell enzymes, like coagulase, proteinase, lipase, neuraminidase, and nuclease.
- Exotoxins of specific activities, such as the neuroparalytic toxin of *Clostridium botulinum*; the exotoxin of *Corynebacterium diphtheriae* inhibiting protein synthesis of cells; the enterotoxins of *Vibrio cholera* and *E. coli* inhibiting the cyclic adenosine monophosphate (AMP) and cyclic guanosine monophosphate (GMP), respectively, of intestinal cells; and the cytotoxins of *Shigella dysenteriae*.

Parasites may bring about pathology through any or a combination of the following: mechanical injury, chemical changes, the digestion of mucosa, and using the host's nutrition, causing deficiencies, toxins, and neurotoxins, etc.

Host-related properties useful in explaining the spread of disease: infectivity, pathogenicity, and virulence. These terms are already defined. Suitable examples to differentiate these are the following: rabies virus has low infectivity but high pathogenicity and virulence; poliovirus has high infectivity, low pathogenicity, but high virulence; smallpox virus has high infectivity, pathogenicity, and virulence; measles virus has high infectivity and pathogenicity but low virulence; chickenpox virus has high infectivity, low pathogenicity, and very low virulence; leprosy bacilli have very low infectivity and pathogenicity but high virulence; and common cold virus has high infectivity and pathogenicity but low virulence.

6.2 Host

Host factors of concern are breed, race, ethnic group, occupation or uses, age, sex, husbandry practices, management conditons/socio-economic status, physiological state, previous and concurrent infection/disease history, herd immunity, behaviour and resistance, reservoirs, and host specificity of infection:

- *Heredity*: umbilical hernia in calves and imperforate anus in piglets.
- *Age*: lamb dysentery in young ones; coccidiosis and Johne's disease are more common and severe in young ones. Some diseases are more common or severe in older than in young ones, e.g. red water (calves up to 12 months are less susceptible) and brucellosis.

- *Sex*: abortion and mastitis are diseases of females, whereas fistulous wither is more common in males.
- *Occupation or use*: fracture of the long bone in race horses, fistulous wither in bullocks, mastitis in milch animals.
- *Nutrition*: a well-nourished animal is generally less susceptible to diseases. Exceptions are enterotoxaemia in sheep and black quarter in cattle.
- *Breed*: generally exotic breeds of cattle are the most, cross-breds are less, and the indigenous ones are the least susceptible to blood protozoan diseases in India. Boran cattle are less susceptible to piroplasmosis than Ayrshire cattle. Light-skinned breeds are more susceptible to photosensitisation than dark skinned. In humans, duodenal ulcer is more common in those having blood group O; stomach ulcers, pernicious anaemia, and diabetes mellitus are more prevalent in those having blood group A.

6.3 Environment

Environment is a general term but very inclusive. Important components are climate and weather, husbandry, open and closed population, management, housing, transport, etc. The climate and weather affect the agent, host, vector, and intermediate hosts and thus determine the geographic distribution of diseases.

Effect on the host fluctuating environmental temperature and humidity predispose pigs to pneumonia and calves to mortality. The onset of rains is associated with outbreaks of haemorrhagic septicaemia. Winter and frost lower the resistance in sheep so that they may suffer from braxy. Pendulous crops in turkey of Bronze breed found in the Central Valley of California are recognised as a disease with genetic as well as climatic determinants. A hot, dry environment of central valley of Californa causes turkey of Bronze breed with genetic host disposition to pendulous crop condition due to consumption of excessive amount of water leading usually to irreversible stretching of crop (Schwabe et al. 1977).

Effect on the agent climatic conditions affect the survival of the agent in the environment. *Bacillus anthracis* forms spores very slowly at temperature 21 °C or below. The vegetative forms are fragile and are destroyed easily in nature. Therefore, serious outbreaks of anthrax do not occur in places where atmospheric temperature is maintained below 21 °C. *Plasmodium* can multiply in mosquitoes' body at a temperature not less than 15–16 °C.

Effect on vectors insect vectors like mosquitoes, blow flies, and mites are more active during warm months. The occurrence of spring-summer encephalitis is indicative of the effect of season; this is because of the high tick density during these months. Eastern equine encephalitis in horses and human beings in Massachusetts and New Jersey is usually associated with heavy rains during autumn in the previous year and summer rains during the epidemic year, which favour the build-up of the vector mosquito *Culiseta melanura*. Vector distribution may exceed the range of infection but not the other way, e.g. *Aedes aegypti* widely distributed but not yellow fever. Environmental temperature affects the infected host and also influences vector transmission. Mosquitoes feeding upon yellow fever cases in humans can transmit to susceptibles and can produce disease in 4 days and 18 days at temperatures of 37 °C and 21 °C, respectively. At a temperature of 16 ° C, no fatal disease is caused but immunity is induced. The survival of *Yersinia pestis* in the body of fleas is again temperature dependent. The plague bacilli disappear from the body of infected fleas at 30–32 °C but survive for 3 weeks at 22–25 °C.

Effect on intermediate hosts snails are active during rains and near pools of water. The development of the intermediate stages of liver fluke and amphistomes is dependent upon the snails' physiology. During drought or in summer, snails stop feeding and become quiescent, and the development of immature flukes in snails also ceases. Cercaria will not be laid on the blades of grasses for infecting cattle.

Effect on disease distribution the effect on the distribution of diseases could be indirect through the effect on the host, agent, vector, and intermediate hosts. Besides, there may be a direct effect, too. The geo-climatic conditions determine the type of vegetation. The distribution of plant toxicities is, thus, dependent on the environment. Goitre and fluorosis are other examples. The landscape epidemiology defines natural nidii of infections. A few diseases are named after the location as their distribution is defined, East Coast fever, Eastern Equine encephalitis, Western equine encephalitis, Degnala disease.

6.4 Husbandry Practices

Open population a population in which there is no restriction upon the incoming and outgoing animals, i.e. the movement is unrestricted, is called open population.

Closed population in contrast, the movement of animals in the closed population is restricted. These are important. A bullock brought from an open population, say, a village or an animal fair, may be carrying FMD (incubatory carrier). Its introduction to a farm is likely to introduce FMD in the farm. This may lead to an outbreak. The farm population is an example of a closed population. Any newly brought animal should be kept under observation (quarantine) separately before allowing it to mix with the rest of the animals. Animals sent for 'shows', 'competition', or 'fair' should similarly be treated on return. Examples of a closed population in the case of human beings are jails, mental hospitals, hostels, etc.

Social distance it measures the distance between two human beings, e.g. the distance between two siblings, between husband and wife, or between parent and children. In epidemiology, it measures the physical distance, an opportunity of contact between two individuals, man or animals. The more intimate or close is the contact, the more is the possibility of transmission of infection.

Free-range system this system is associated more with gastrointestinal parasitic diseases. In contrast, animals kept in confinement have more chances of tuberculosis infection. Damp, ill-ventilated houses lead to respiratory problems in pigs and poultry. The infrequent removal of litter in a deep litter system is likely to create nidii of coccidiosis and ascaridiasis.

Feed vitamin-A-deficient feed increases susceptibility to diseases, particularly to colibacillosis and respiratory diseases. Mineral deficiency, phosphorus in particular, leads to pica (mud eating, bone licking). On the other hand, overfeeding or a sudden change over to good feed leads to enterotoxaemia. Feeding a large amount of cold milk or contaminated milk to calves causes scour.

Transport and other stress factors may lead to increased salmonellosis and sporadic pneumonia.

Altitude and latitude high altitude has a direct effect on the host, e.g. brisket disease in cattle (enlarged heart). Toxoplasmosis is more common in areas of low altitude; sunburn, photosensitivity, and skin cancer are more prevalent in areas near the equator, where sunshine is intense. Bronze turkey disease leads to death in poults when reared in a hot climate. This genetic disorder is not manifested in cold climates or cold places.

6.5 Time

Time is also a determinant of disease occurrence. An example is Monday morning or after a holiday (post-holiday sickness). Horses suffer from azoturia, particularly on Mondays. Overwork on weekend, followed by rest on Sunday, leads to azoturia or myoglobinuria on Monday morning. Photoperiodism may determine the biting time of a vector; e.g., *Culex tarsalis* feeds at sunset when birds roost, *Haemagogus* feeds in the daytime when animals rest, and vampire bat rabies is mostly transmitted at night. There are seasonal diseases, too, e.g. pollen allergy; most of the enteric diseases occur during summer and respiratory diseases during winter. Measles occurs in a cyclic pattern, every 3–4 years when the susceptible population increases (population turnover).

References

Murray PR, Rosenthal KS, Pfaller MA (2021) Chapter: Bacterial classification, structure, and replication. In: Medical microbiology, vol 12, 9th edn. Elsevier Inc., Amsterdam, pp 114–126.e1

Schwabe CW, Riemann HP, Franti CE (1977) Epidemiology in veterinary practice. Lea & Febiger, Philadelphia, PA

Disease Transmission 7

Disease is a departure from health and a manifestation of a morbid condition. It is a deviation from physiological condition in which the activities of an organ or more than one organ are affected, leading to a state of imbalance and altered homeostasis. Disease may be infectious or non-infectious. Infectious diseases are caused by infectious agents. Non-infectious diseases, on the other hand, may have a variety of causes, like metabolic disorder, e.g. ketosis and milk fever; hormonal causes, like breeding problems; immunological causes, like allergy; neoplastic disorder, like cancer; deficiency, like goitre; or excess of a certain chemical, like selenium toxicity.

7.1 Infection Process

Two important components of the infection process are a host and an infectious agent. The entry of an infectious agent into the host requires 'portals of entry'. After entry, the agent takes some time to establish in the host's tissues and then multiplies (Fig. 7.1), which is called the 'incubation period' (stage 1). This is followed by the appearance of symptoms of the disease (stage 2). This stage may be subdivided into the prodromal phase (stage A); classical symptoms, when the disease is at its peak form, or fastigium/most intense phase (stage B); and the phase of decline or defervescence (stage C). The host defence system fights, and antibodies are formed, resulting in specific immunity. This alone or therapeutic intervention results in the control of the disease and the cessation of clinical symptoms (stage 3). It takes some time for the patient to return to a healthy state (stage 4). The host's system is cleared of the infectious agent at the end of the convalescent stage, with some exceptions where the agent persists. Clinical disease may be classified as per-acute, acute, sub-acute, and chronic. Per-acute cases last only for a few hours, as in anthrax, when cases are generally found dead. Most acute diseases have a short course, e.g. foot and mouth disease (FMD) and rinderpest (RP). The course of sub-acute diseases lasts long, and these are mild, e.g. mastitis. When the diseases progress

K. G. Narayan et al., *Veterinary Public Health & Epidemiology*,
https://doi.org/10.1007/978-981-19-7800-5_7

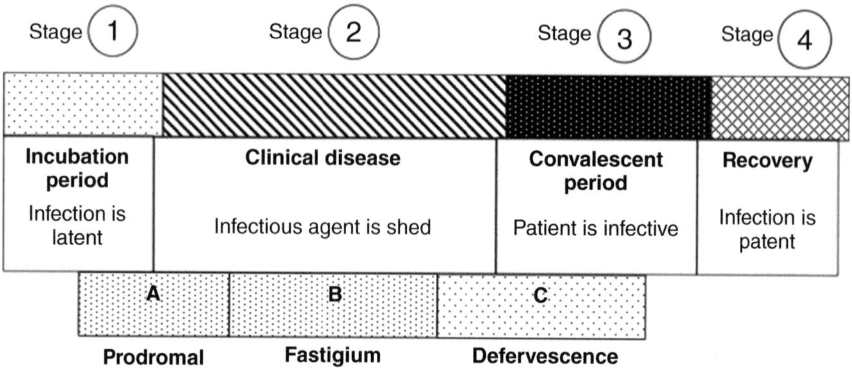

Fig. 7.1 Stages of infectious disease

slowly and last longer, say for months, these are called chronic, e.g. actinomycosis and Johne's disease. Some diseases may run a short, long, or longer course.

Epidemic is recognised by the appearance of a higher number of cases than expected. Obviously, the first case must have gotten the infection from some source/reservoir, of the same species or some other and sharing the same habitat or introduced from outside of the place of epidemic. Thus, two important components of the event need to be addressed: a reservoir/source and the modes of spread to the susceptible population.

In the study of an epidemic, the stages in the development of the disease are important. The activity of the infectious agent in a host (host-agent interaction) is observed, and it has a bearing on the understanding of the disease's spread/process in a population.

Infectiousness is the ability of an infectious agent to invade a new host. Generally, the diseases in which the infectious agents are shed for a short period tend to be highly infectious and spread quickly. FMD, hog cholera, and influenza are highly infectious. The time for an infective agent to find a susceptible host (i.e. the length of link) is short. On the other hand, diseases with a long incubation period and a long period of shedding spread slowly (an exception is the availability of favourable conditions, such as overcrowding of the susceptible population), and not all exposed become infected; examples are bovine/caprine contagious pleuropneumonia and tuberculosis.

7.1.1 *Latent and Patent* Infection

A latent (implying dormancy or having potential) infection may be defined as an inapparent infection having the potential to show/develop signs and symptoms of the disease. In an inapparent infection, the host carries an infection without disease and the host-parasite relationship may be commensal. During latent infection or the period of latency, the infective agent remains quiescent and is, thus, difficult to detect in the host. Nevertheless, the agent does have the potential to become active and to manifest the clinical disease. Once the infective agent becomes detectable in the host, maybe in secretions or excretions or recovered from or detected in the blood or tissues of the host, the infection is said to be patent. During the period of patency, the infection may be transmitted.

Periods of latency and patency influence the spread of infection. The infectious agent is quiescent or perhaps hidden in the host cell during latency. In the later part of the incubation period, the agent usually starts getting out of the host's system. This continues throughout the clinical disease and convalescence stages. The patient is infective to others, i.e. may act as a source of infection in the population, during the period of patency. The latent state is also important because such individuals who are latent carriers of infectious agents pose potential dangers to the susceptible population. In the case of chicken pox and epidemic typhus (*Rickettsia prowazekii*), latent infection can become patent after years. Herpes simplex and many adenovirus infections are intermittently patent over a long period of time.

Latency may be a mechanism adopted by an infectious agent to escape from threats or evade threats to its existence. The host's micro-environment and the availability or otherwise of certain chemicals either induce latency or cause reactivation. For example, *Brucella abortus* organisms hiding in the cells of cows' supramammary lymph gland get reactivated to cause infective abortion in the presence of erythritol, which is made available in cotyledon and chorion only during pregnancy. Some of the nematodes' larvae stop development (arrested larval development) during the pregnancy of the host and restart after parturition, when hormonal changes are favourable.

Carriers animals that harbour an infecting/disease agent, but displays no symptoms i.e inapparent infection. They may be shedders, non-shedders, or intermittent shedders. Temporary carriers include animals in incubative and convalescent stages. Chronic carriers remain carriers for a long period and are most important in the spread of infection. Healthy carriers are animals that have recovered from the disease but continue to harbour the infective agent. Animals that have become infected but the infective agent persists in them and there is no sign or symptom of the disease (inapparent infection) are also called healthy carriers. It may be an incubatory carrier where the host can transmit infection during the incubation period of infection before manifesting the clinical disease. On the other hand, a convalescent carrier is one that can transmit the infectious agent after the clinical recovery of the host, when the signs and symptoms of the disease disappeared. The carrier may be continuously infective (e.g. typhoid) or intermittently infective (e.g. herpes simplex virus). A persisting infection may be transmitted congenitally from generation to generation (e.g. lymphocytic choriomeningitis in mice).

A non-shedder may be considered a potential shedder. Intermittent shedders may constitute greater danger as they remain undetected compared to continuous

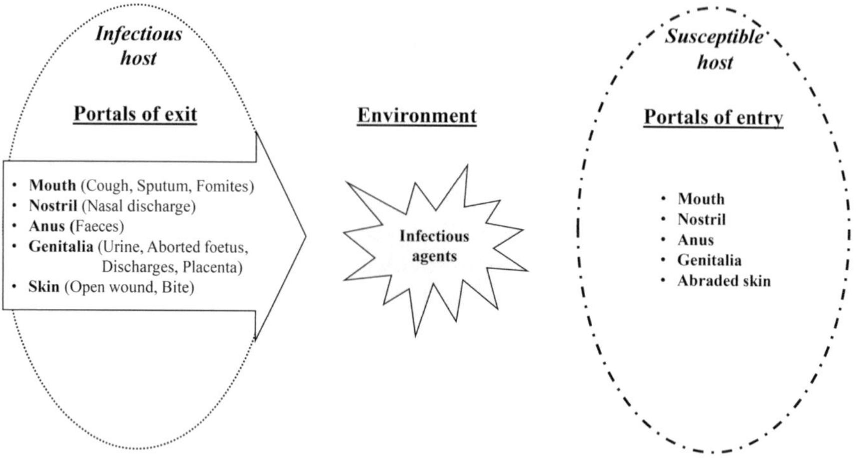

Fig. 7.2 Transmission and spread of infection/disease

shedders. Infective agents persist in carriers; e.g., canine infectious hepatitis persists and multiplies in the kidney and sheds in urine. Infectious laryngotracheitis virus persists for weeks (maximum 741 days) in the trachea of 1–10% of recovered birds.

A **reservoir** of infectious agents is one in which the infectious agent naturally lives and multiples. This may be a human, animal, insect, or inanimate object like soil, which remains a common source of infection to susceptible hosts. Diseases of human beings for which man is the natural reservoir are called anthroponotic diseases, e.g. rubella, smallpox, gonorrhoea, etc. Scientifically, zoonoses are diseases of animals and also include diseases of human beings for which animals are the reservoirs. Similarly, diseases for which soil and other inanimate objects (rich in organic) are the sources are called saprozoonoses, e.g. listeriosis, histoplasmosis, etc. Insect vectors also act as reservoirs. Some infections are passed vertically to the progeny of insects or horizontally to another metamorphic stage.

Source it is the immediate man, animal, object, or substance from which the infectious agent passes to a host. A contaminated feed/food, contaminated water supply, or infected man, animal, or insect could be a source of infection.

The infectious agents are shed from a case, starting from the late incubation period till the end of the convalescent stage or may be even later. The amount of infectious agent excreted by a case depends upon the stage of the disease and its acuteness. The infectious agent uses the natural portals of entry and exit in the hosts (Fig. 7.2).

Epidemic focus is the abode of a source of infection and the adjacent region throughout which the source of infection can disseminate the infective agent—the extent of an area depends upon the circumstances and the particular infection concerned. An epidemic process is a series of interrelated sequential epidemic foci.

7.2 Modes of Transmission

An infectious agent may adopt any of the following methods of transmission:

1. Contact
   (a) Direct
   (b) Indirect
2. Air
3. Vehicle
4. Vector

Contact-borne transmission includes infections transmitted by direct or indirect contact with the source of infection. Indirect-contact-borne infections, such as FMD, RP, and anthrax, are spread through contact with infective discharges from the diseased or dead animals. Direct-contact-borne infections require direct intimate contact with the infected, e.g. syphilis, gonorrhoea, acquired immunodeficiency syndrome (AIDS), dourine in animals, and fungal skin infections. The cases are found clustered in a close community and sporadic in nature.

Airborne infections are also sometimes classed as indirect-contact-borne infections. Infectious agents, like FMD virus and influenza virus, remain suspended in the air in droplet nuclei. Of the suspended particles in the air—dust, drops, and droplet nuclei—the last is the smallest (less than 10 μm) and can reach the lung alveoli directly to deposit the infectious agent. Overcrowding and inadequate ventilation facilitate transmission.

Infectious agents may ride over any non-living object, like a vehicle, to travel to the susceptible hosts, e.g. milk, meat, water, and soil. The vehicle-borne infections/diseases are seen distributed along the line of distribution of the common contaminated vehicle, e.g. *Salmonella*-contaminated sausage. The epidemic curve is explosive in nature, and cases are confined to the area of supply of the contaminated food.

Insects may also carry infectious agents as vectors. The distribution of cases is dependent upon vector density and is confined to the area of vector activity, depending on the climatic conditions. The disease, therefore, is seasonal in appearance with a gradual build-up of cases as the population of infected vectors increases.

Vehicle- and vector-borne infections can be mechanical and biological.

In mechanical transmission, the disease agent is transferred mechanically by the vehicle or vector (an arthropod) without undergoing multiplication. The transfer of *Vibrio cholerae* by water and the transport of *Shigella dysenteriae* by houseflies are examples of mechanical transmission.

When the infectious agent of disease undergoes multiplication or some developmental changes with or without multiplication, it is called biological transmission. It has been subdivided into three: (a) propagative transmission, where the infective agent undergoes multiplication only without any developmental changes, e.g. *Clostridium perfringens* type A in meat gravy and plague bacilli in rats; (b) cyclo-propagative transmission, where the infective agent undergoes cyclical changes as well as multiplication, e.g. malarial parasites in anopheles mosquitoes; and (c) cyclo-developmental transmission, where the infective agent undergoes cyclical (i.e. metamorphic) changes only without multiplication in the vector, e.g. filarial parasites in Culex mosquitoes and guinea worm in cyclops. There is also another group (developmento-propagative) that does both, increasing the number as well as changing the stage of the parasite (example: a single miracidium stage of the liver fluke *Fasciola hepatica* enters a *Lymnaea* snail vector, It then successively converts into the sporocyst, redia, and cercarial stages, with the latter two stages also multiplying in numbers. Eventually, numerous cercariae emerge from the snail).

The infectious agents take time to multiply or develop and multiply, which is called 'extrinsic' incubation period, to differentiate from the 'incubation' period, which is the time taken by the infectious agents to multiply in the vertebrate host. In the vectors, the infectious agents may pass from the mother to the progenies, called 'transovarial transmission', e.g. *Babesia bigemina.* In some cases, the infectious agents pass from one developmental stage to the next, which is known as 'transstadial' transmission.

Transmission from parents to offspring is called 'vertical transmission', e.g. *Salmonella gallinarum* infection in poultry. Most of the infections spread laterally to those sharing the exposure, which is called 'horizontal' spread. Alternate transmission from one type of host (say an animal) to another type of host (say invertebrate) is called zig-zag transmission.

The extent of transmission of infectious agents is dependent upon a number of factors:

1. The range of movement of the reservoir, vector, or vehicle
2. Survival of the agent outside of the host
3. The ability of the agent to multiply and increase in number in the vertebrate and invertebrate hosts and in inanimate objects
4. Its host range
5. Its infectivity, pathogenicity, virulence, etc.
6. The availability of susceptible hosts
7. Social distance

7.3 Mysterious Mechanisms of Transmission

Infecting agents in the arthropod vectors and in the intermediate hosts are carried through the developmental stages or the hibernation of these. The egress of the infecting agent from the vector may be active or passive. The egress related to the activity of the vector is called 'active egress', e.g. blood-sucking ticks or fleas, allowing simultaneous egress of the infecting agent. Blood sucking is the vector's activity. If the agent egresses through faeces, urine, tears, or secretions of surface lesions, it is called 'passive egress'. Passive egress is common in coprophagous insects, e.g. earthworms, molluscs, and crustaceans.

An adult infected vector hibernating over the winter harbours an infectious agent. This explains the appearance of disease after a long period of lull during the cold winter season. The infection/disease is called overwintering. This represents a long chain of transmission cycle. An adult infected female vector passes on the infectious agent to its progenies through the ovary (transovarial transmission). This seems to be a mechanism adopted by the infectious agent to escape the methods of control.

Histomonas meleagridis, a protozoon, infects birds. It hides itself in a nematode, *Heterakis gallinarum*. The ovary of the nematode is infected, and the protozoa escape in the eggs of this nematode. The egress is 'passive'. The protozoa then infect a subsequent vertebrate host.

Metastrongylus is the lungworm of swine. The nematode carries the swine fever virus through its entire developmental cycle. The lung tissue already damaged by the migrating larvae of the nematode prepares a fertile soil for the seed, i.e. the virus. The stress of the cold winter favours the reactivation of the masked virus. Earthworms are the intermediate host/vector of the nematode. The swine influenza virus can persist in the 'masked' form for 16 months in the third-stage larvae of the lungworm in their earthworm intermediate host. The virus has thus two systems through which to hide and meet the threats to its life. The lungworm is involved in providing the virus that would infect the *first case* of a swine fever outbreak. Subsequently, the transmission of the virus from swine to swine occurs.

Salmon poisoning is another interesting example. *Neorickettsia helminthoeca* is a rickettsia infecting dogs and wild carnivores. The dogs/wild carnivores are infected through the stomach fluke *Troglotrema salmincola*. The life cycle of the fluke requires a snail (*Goniobasis plicifera*) as an intermediate host and a salmonid fish (salmon or trout) as the other host. The fish spawns in fresh water. The dogs/wild carnivores get infected with the fluke by eating salmonid fish that carries metacercaria. The rickettsiae are carried through the entire worm cycle. This infection is carried out to sea by the salmon over 2–4 years before they return for spawning in fresh water. Viable rickettsia is present in the metacercaria observed in salmon fish tissues caught in the sea.

7.2 Modes of Transmission

An infectious agent may adopt any of the following methods of transmission:

1. Contact
   (a) Direct
   (b) Indirect
2. Air
3. Vehicle
4. Vector

Contact-borne transmission includes infections transmitted by direct or indirect contact with the source of infection. Indirect-contact-borne infections, such as FMD, RP, and anthrax, are spread through contact with infective discharges from the diseased or dead animals. Direct-contact-borne infections require direct intimate contact with the infected, e.g. syphilis, gonorrhoea, acquired immunodeficiency syndrome (AIDS), dourine in animals, and fungal skin infections. The cases are found clustered in a close community and sporadic in nature.

Airborne infections are also sometimes classed as indirect-contact-borne infections. Infectious agents, like FMD virus and influenza virus, remain suspended in the air in droplet nuclei. Of the suspended particles in the air—dust, drops, and droplet nuclei—the last is the smallest (less than 10 μm) and can reach the lung alveoli directly to deposit the infectious agent. Overcrowding and inadequate ventilation facilitate transmission.

Infectious agents may ride over any non-living object, like a vehicle, to travel to the susceptible hosts, e.g. milk, meat, water, and soil. The vehicle-borne infections/diseases are seen distributed along the line of distribution of the common contaminated vehicle, e.g. *Salmonella*-contaminated sausage. The epidemic curve is explosive in nature, and cases are confined to the area of supply of the contaminated food.

Insects may also carry infectious agents as vectors. The distribution of cases is dependent upon vector density and is confined to the area of vector activity, depending on the climatic conditions. The disease, therefore, is seasonal in appearance with a gradual build-up of cases as the population of infected vectors increases.

Vehicle- and vector-borne infections can be mechanical and biological.

In mechanical transmission, the disease agent is transferred mechanically by the vehicle or vector (an arthropod) without undergoing multiplication. The transfer of *Vibrio cholerae* by water and the transport of *Shigella dysenteriae* by houseflies are examples of mechanical transmission.

When the infectious agent of disease undergoes multiplication or some developmental changes with or without multiplication, it is called biological transmission. It has been subdivided into three: (a) propagative transmission, where the infective agent undergoes multiplication only without any developmental changes, e.g. *Clostridium perfringens* type A in meat gravy and plague bacilli in rats; (b) cyclo-propagative transmission, where the infective agent undergoes cyclical changes as well as multiplication, e.g. malarial parasites in anopheles mosquitoes; and (c) cyclo-developmental transmission, where the infective agent undergoes cyclical (i.e. metamorphic) changes only without multiplication in the vector, e.g. filarial parasites in Culex mosquitoes and guinea worm in cyclops. There is also another group (developmento-propagative) that does both, increasing the number as well as changing the stage of the parasite (example: a single miracidium stage of the liver fluke *Fasciola hepatica* enters a *Lymnaea* snail vector, It then successively converts into the sporocyst, redia, and cercarial stages, with the latter two stages also multiplying in numbers. Eventually, numerous cercariae emerge from the snail).

The infectious agents take time to multiply or develop and multiply, which is called 'extrinsic' incubation period, to differentiate from the 'incubation' period, which is the time taken by the infectious agents to multiply in the vertebrate host. In the vectors, the infectious agents may pass from the mother to the progenies, called 'transovarial transmission', e.g. *Babesia bigemina.* In some cases, the infectious agents pass from one developmental stage to the next, which is known as 'transstadial' transmission.

Transmission from parents to offspring is called 'vertical transmission', e.g. *Salmonella gallinarum* infection in poultry. Most of the infections spread laterally to those sharing the exposure, which is called 'horizontal' spread. Alternate transmission from one type of host (say an animal) to another type of host (say invertebrate) is called zig-zag transmission.

The extent of transmission of infectious agents is dependent upon a number of factors:

1. The range of movement of the reservoir, vector, or vehicle
2. Survival of the agent outside of the host
3. The ability of the agent to multiply and increase in number in the vertebrate and invertebrate hosts and in inanimate objects
4. Its host range
5. Its infectivity, pathogenicity, virulence, etc.
6. The availability of susceptible hosts
7. Social distance

7.3 Mysterious Mechanisms of Transmission

Infecting agents in the arthropod vectors and in the intermediate hosts are carried through the developmental stages or the hibernation of these. The egress of the infecting agent from the vector may be active or passive. The egress related to the activity of the vector is called 'active egress', e.g. blood-sucking ticks or fleas, allowing simultaneous egress of the infecting agent. Blood sucking is the vector's activity. If the agent egresses through faeces, urine, tears, or secretions of surface lesions, it is called 'passive egress'. Passive egress is common in coprophagous insects, e.g. earthworms, molluscs, and crustaceans.

8 Disease Distribution in Population

A case is presented to a veterinary physician. He observes signs and symptoms and arrives at a certain diagnosis. When disease appears in a herd/population, there are certain manifestations helpful to an epidemiologist in making a diagnosis. The first thing an epidemiologist does is to count the cases and study their distribution in time (temporal) and place (spatial). He then plots the incidence, consults past records, and compares. It becomes possible for him to describe the disease occurrence as sporadic, outbreak, epidemic, endemic, pandemic, exotic, emerging, or exotic. The definitions of these terms are already given. These are called attributes of herd disease.

8.1 Sporadic

The occurrence of cases in an uneven and scattered manner in time and space is indicated by the term sporadic. It is suggestive of the presence of a source of infection in the same species or any other species or an inanimate object located in the same area (the area of occurrence of disease) or outside. The infection is introduced from the source occasionally.

8.2 Outbreak, Epidemic, and Pandemic

These are indicative of the number of cases clearly in excess of the expected number (Figs. 8.1, 8.2, 8.3, 8.4, 8.5, and 8.6). The extent of spatial distribution is very small (local, such as students' hostel or a farm), called an outbreak; large (district, state, country), called an epidemic; and very large (a number of countries), known as a pandemic. The epidemiologist looks for the source of infection in the population affected in the area of occurrence and in other species of animals in the same area. The host-agent relationship is relatively new and unstable. Sometimes, the infection

K. G. Narayan et al., *Veterinary Public Health & Epidemiology*,
https://doi.org/10.1007/978-981-19-7800-5_8

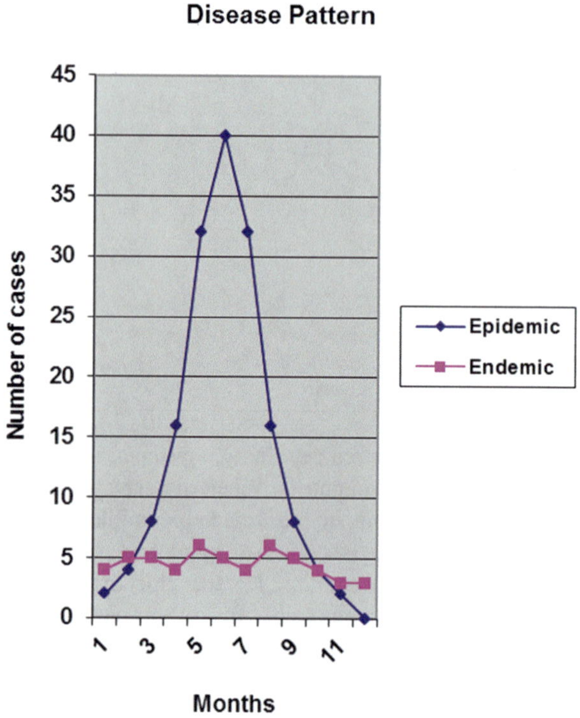

Fig. 8.1 Cases are clearly in excess of the expected number

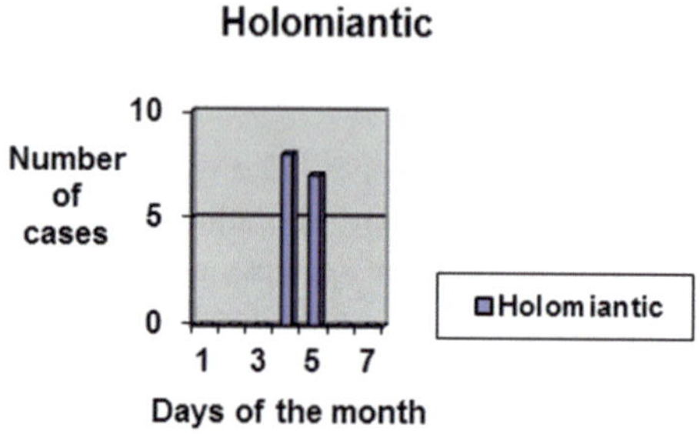

Fig. 8.2 In an explosive/point epidemic pattern, almost all cases cluster at almost a single point in time

may be imported also. In general, however, an imported infection usually occurs sporadically in the beginning before assuming an epidemic state. Certain *Salmonella* serotypes were first imported with contaminated animal feed, fishmeal in particular, in countries where these did not exist. *Salmonella menston*, for example, introduced in England like this, initially infected poultry sporadically. Increased isolations from poultry, eggs, and poultry meat/egg-associated human salmonellosis caught the attention of epidemiologists, who revealed the undelying facts. Epidemiologists may find that an endemic state has changed to an epidemic state and may also find out the reason. The factors which altered/changed the stable host-agent relationship of the endemic disease, such as turnover of susceptible population, altered

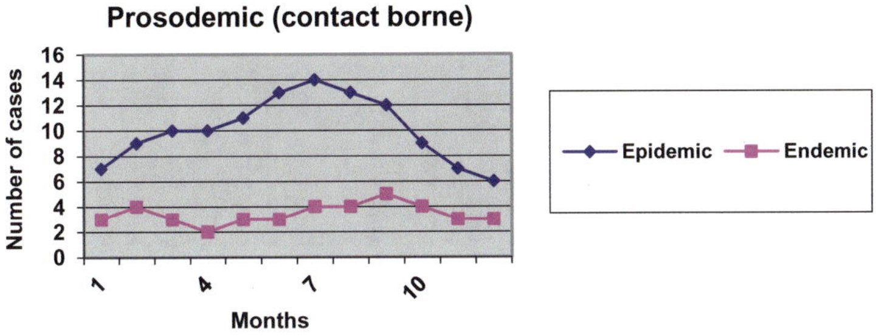

Fig. 8.3 Contact-borne infection, wherein the cases continue to appear

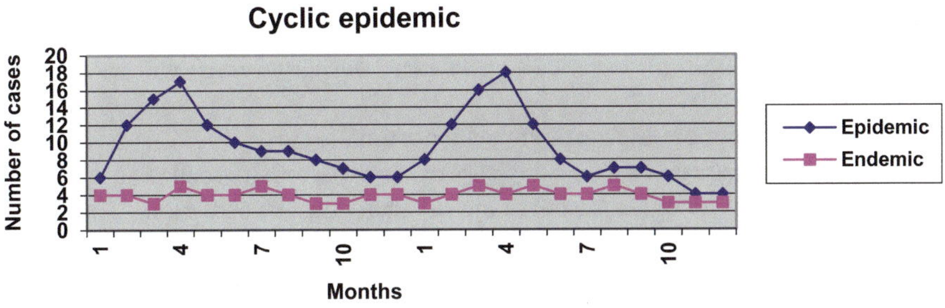

Fig. 8.4 Cyclic epidemic

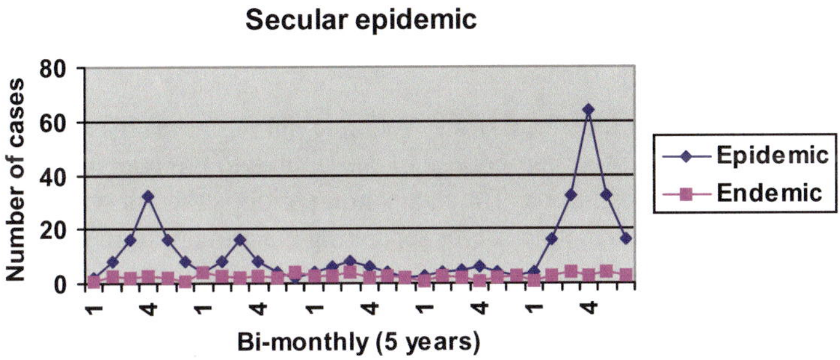

Fig. 8.5 Secular trend

pathogenicity of the agent or circumstances favouring increased exposure to the agent may also be revealed.

The *basic reproduction number* (R_0) denotes how many would be infected by one infected person if all contacts were non-immune and susceptible. For endemic infections, many contacts would be already immune, hence non-susceptible, so $R_0 = 1$ means that among all exposed contacts, at least one was susceptible and successfully infected. The *effective reproduction number*, R_0, should be 1 for a stable endemic infection. When $R_0 > 1$, an outbreak is expected. When $R_0 < 1$, there is a decline in infection. For endemic diseases like seasonal influenza, R_0 fluctuates

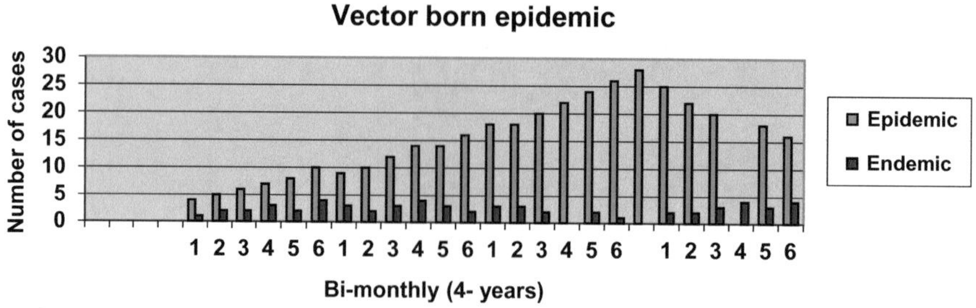

Fig. 8.6 Vector borne epidemic

between <1 (low season) and >1 (high season), but the average will be 1 over a period of time.

When the number of cases is plotted against time, a curve (Fig. 8.1) is obtained. When the number of cases is in clear excess of the expected, it is called an epidemic. The components of an epidemic curve are (a) accretion, (b) egression—consists of progression and regression, and (c) decrescence. As the infection proceeds, the number of cases rises. The initial rise touching the level of endemicity is the 'accretion' portion. The cases further increase in number. This 'progression' reaches a peak, following which a decline in the number of cases begins; this 'regression' touches the level of endemicity. When 'progression' and 'regression' are taken together, this is termed as 'egression'. A further decline in the number of cases touching zero is the grade called 'decrescence'. This is also called the 'gradation' of an epidemic.

The factors affecting the shape of an epidemic curve are (a) incubation period, (b) infectivity of the agent, (c) proportion of susceptible to immune in a population, and (d) density of the population. The incubation period is the interval between the peaks of two successive epidemic curves separating the primary from the subsequent or secondary epidemic peak.

The threshold level of a population density for an epidemic is the 'minimum density of susceptible required to allow a contact-transmitted epidemic to commence'. This is also called 'Kendall's threshold'. Examples are >1 fox/km^2 for fox rabies (Macdonald and Bacon 1980) and 12 dogs/km^2 for parvovirus (Wierup 1983).

Generally, 20–30% susceptibles in a population are required for a contact-borne epidemic to proceed. In other words, a reduction in the susceptible population below this rate should not allow the infection, i.e. the epidemic, to proceed.

An epidemic may be 'point epidemic', in which all or most of the cases cluster at a single point in time (Fig. 8.2). An example is 'food poisoning'. Almost all cases report at a single point in time as they were exposed to a common cause and at the same point in time, i.e. contaminated food served at a dinner. This also measures an 'event', such as a plane crash resulting in all deaths clustered at one point in time. An epidemic is also called 'explosive' in nature. Contrasting is 'propagative epidemic'.

Epidemiologists find cases gradually increasing year after year. The epidemic curve presents as if cases are propagating. This is indicative of a slowly increasing disease and points to a factor that is gradually building up. An example is spring-summer encephalitis. The vector tick population increases gradually. Each stage—larvae, nymph, and adult stages—is infective. The infection in vectors may be transovarial and transstadial. The ticks moult approximately in a year. Thus, a crop of first-stage larvae is added to the already existing second-stage larvae in the second year. By the third year, there will be first-, second-, and third-stage larvae available to infect the host (Fig. 8.6).

8.3 Endemic

Diseases indigenous to an area are called endemic or enzootic. The number of cases is maintained with less amount of variation. Occasionally, the endemic state may change to an epidemic state. The host-agent relationship is considered stable. In between endemic and epidemic, there is a range of terms like hypoendemic, mesoendemic, hyperendemic, and holoendemic. FMD and theileriasis are examples of endemic diseases.

8.4 Emerging Diseases

Investigations made into some uncommon, unusual disease reveal that the disease was either exotic (not reported earlier in the place/country of investigation) or emerging (a new disease or an endemic and not so significant). Bovine spongiform encephalitis or mad cow disease is an emerging disease caused by prions. Cryptosporidiosis, Lyme disease, yersiniosis, and campylobacteriosis are re-emerging.

8.5 Cyclic Epidemic Curve

The epidemic is observed every year (Fig. 8.4). As in the case of measles, most cases appear during spring (March–April) every year.

A regular, predictable cyclic fluctuation in incidence is called 'endemic pulsation'.

The possible reasons for the season-related cyclic trend are (a) host density, (b) management practices, (c) survival of the infectious agent, (d) vector dynamics, and (e) other ecological factors.

8.6 Secular Epidemic

Observe that epidemics appeared (Fig. 8.5) in the first 2 years, followed by almost an endemic state to a fresh epidemic in the fifth year. This is indicative of a change in the infecting agent, e.g. the influenza virus undergoing an antigenic 'shift' (major changes) or 'drift' (minor changes) and causing a pandemic almost every decade. The antigenic nature of a new variant of the infectious agent, e.g. influenza virus, is such that the population that suffered or was exposed earlier to the parent virus has antibodies specific to the parent virus but not to the new variant, and so they suffer. The new variant emerged during the time that elapsed between the two epidemics. Students may refer to the antigenic shift and antigenic drift observed in the influenza virus leading to changes in the haemagglutinin and neuraminidase antigens.

References

Macdonald DW, Bacon PJ (1980) To control rabies: vaccinate foxes. New Scient 87:640–645

Wierup M (1983) The Swedish canine parvovirus epidemic- an epidemiological study in a dog population of defined size. Prevent Veterin Med 1:273–288

Data in Epidemiology 9

Data are very important and are the backbone of epidemiology. Data (singular: datum) can be defined as 'Facts, especially numerical facts, collected together for reference or information' (Anonymous 1989). These data may relate to clinical signs, therapy, post-mortem and laboratory examinations, etc. A collection of data is called a *data set*. The initial measurements that form the basis of analysis are called *raw data*.

The body weight, milk yield, and number of cases of a disease and the number of animals are numerical facts that can vary from animal to animal and disease to disease and are, therefore, called *variables*, which may be either continuous (e.g. body weight, milk yield, etc.) or discrete (e.g. number of animals). The numerical values of variables are called *variates*. Variables that are being considered in an investigation/study are called *study variables*. A variable that is affected by another variable is called a *response* or *dependent* variable, e.g. animal body weight. On the other hand, a variable that is not affected by another variable is known as an *explanatory* or *independent* variable, like food intake. A quantity or number that differs in different circumstances but is constant in the case being considered is called a *parameter*, e.g. prevalence of disease. A parameter may also be a measurable characteristic of a population, e.g. average milk yield of a dairy herd.

9.1 Classification of Data

Data can be classified into two types: qualitative and quantitative.

K. G. Narayan et al., *Veterinary Public Health & Epidemiology*,
https://doi.org/10.1007/978-981-19-7800-5_9

1. **Qualitative data**, also called *categorical data*, describe the property/characteristic of animal, i.e. membership of a group or class, like the breed, sex, and colour of an animal. The aggregates of qualitative data are countable, e.g. the total number of female cows or Red Sindhi cows or black goats. Qualitative data may be of two scales: *nominal* and *ordinal*.
   (a) **Nominal scale**: since categories are nominated names, they are therefore called 'nominal'. A nominal scale is also called classificatory scale, in which the categories cannot be arranged in a logical order. Each category is considered equal to the other. Examples are gender (male/female), blood groups (A/B/O/AB), religion (Hindu/Muslim/Christian/Buddhist/Punjabi), and coat colour (white, brown, black, etc.).
   (b) **Ordinal scale**: here, different categories can be logically arranged in a meaningful order, but the difference between the categories is not 'meaningful'. The following are examples:
   - ***Ranks***, for example 'first/second/third, etc.', can be arranged in either an ascending or a descending order, but the difference between ranks will not be the same. Suppose there is a difference of 10 units between the first and second ranks but may be of 5 units between the second and third ranks. Besides, one cannot say, on the basis of rank, that the first rank is '*X*' times better than the second or third rank. Other examples of ranks are 'good/better/best' and 'no pain/mild pain/moderate pain/severe pain'. In these examples, also a meaningful arrangement (ordering) is possible, but the difference between the categories is subjective and not uniform. 'Best' is not necessarily twice as good as 'better' or four times as good as 'good'.
   - ***Likert scale***: here, the ordering is flexible, for example 'strongly agree/agree/neutral/disagree/strongly disagree', and the order can be easily reversed, viz. 'strongly disagree/disagree/neutral/agree/strongly agree', without affecting the interpretation, but the difference between categories is not uniform.

     In the ordinal scale, any transformation must preserve the order. The physical body score scale can specify 3 as 'good' and 1 as 'poor' or 1 as 'good' and 3 as 'poor', as long as the numbers between 1 and 3 maintain the same order of ranking.
   - ***Visual analogue scale*** (VAS): it uses a straight line of 10 cm, divided into 100 equal divisions, the extreme limits like in the case of the examination of the soundness of a horse (as given below):

     Sound I--I

     Maximum lameness

     Differences between nominal and ordinal scales

     An ordinal scale is 'stronger' than a nominal scale because it includes 'equivalence' as well as 'greater than' and 'less than' properties, but still, an ordinal scale is relatively a 'weak form of measurement'.
2. **Quantitative data**: these relate to amounts, e.g. prevalence, incidence, body weight, milk yield, antibody titre, etc. These data may be *discrete* and *continuous*.

(a) ***Discrete data*** generate counts and have a specified set of values, such as whole numbers (1, 2, 7, 9, etc.), e.g. number of teats on a sow, egg production, etc.

(b) ***Continuous data*** have any value within a defined range (can be infinite), e.g. body weight, the girth of a cow, milk yield, etc. Continuous data, therefore, generate measurements. It may be of two scales—*interval* and *ratio*:

- ***Interval scale***: the values have a meaningful difference and can be ordered, but doubling is not meaningful because of the absence of an 'absolute zero'. For example, in the Celsius scale, the difference between 60 and 50 °C is the same as that between 20 and 10 °C (meaningful difference, i.e. equidistant). Besides, 60 °C is hotter than 50 °C (order). However, 60 °C is not two times as hot as 30 °C and vice versa (doubling is not meaningful).
  In the Celsius scale, the difference between each unit is the same anywhere on the scale—the difference between 62 and 63 °C is the same as the difference between any two consecutive values on the scale (1 unit). Thus, $(5 - 4) = (25 - 24) = (44 - 43) = (100 - 99) = 1$.
- ***Ratio scale***: in this scale, there is an 'absolute zero'; therefore, there is a meaningful difference, and doubling is also meaningful; besides, the values can be ordered in an ascending/descending way. For example, in the Kelvin scale of temperature, 80 K is twice as hot as 40 K; weight: 60 kg is twice as heavy as 30 kg; and height: 90 cm is twice as tall as 45 cm.

9.2 Classification of Data Based on Source

Data may also be classified, depending on their source, into primary and secondary.

1. **Primary data**: they have been collected from first-hand experience and are not yet published and are, therefore, more reliable, authentic, and objective oriented. The validity of primary data is greater than that of secondary data, e.g. information collected through interviews, surveys, the testing of samples, etc.
2. **Secondary data**: they are collected by others and are available in published or unpublished forms, like journals, periodicals, research publications, official records, newspapers, magazines, e-journals, websites, etc. Though this type of data is quick and cheap to collect, it may not fulfil ones' specific research needs and is of poor accuracy.

9.3 Methods of Collection of Primary Data

1. ***Observational study***: a study in which the investigator observes individuals or where certain outcomes are measured without manipulation or intervention
2. ***Experimental study***: a study in which conditions are controlled and manipulated by the experimenter
3. ***Case study***: a comprehensive study of a social unit (a person, family, institution, organisation, or community) to identify and analyse the key issues of the case using relevant theoretical concepts from epidemiology so that a course of action to solve the problem for that particular case can be worked out
4. ***Survey***: an investigation or study in which information is systematically collected from a sample of a population, usually for a short period of time and with a specific aim or conceptual hypothesis
5. ***Questionnaire***: a set of questions meant for collecting information from respondents.
6. ***Interview*:** presentation of questions to respondents either in person, on paper, by phone, or online and noting down their oral/verbal written responses

9.4 Characteristics of Data

- Accuracy
- Refinement
- Precision
- Reliability
- Validity

1. **Accuracy**: it denotes how close or far off a measurement is to its true value. For example, when a cow's weight is 350 kg and a weighing machine records the same, then the measurement is accurate.
2. **Refinement**: it relates to details in a datum. For example, 350 and 350.25 kg may both represent the accurate weight of a cow, but the latter is more refined. Increase in refinement improves the epidemiological value of a descriptive diagnosis, for example mastitis, mastitis caused by bacteria, mastitis caused by *Streptococcus* spp.

   To increase the refinement of a diagnosis, the application of suitable auxiliary tests are required; for example, a complement fixation test (CFT) will detect the types of influenza A virus, but for sub-typing, haemagglutination and neuraminidase tests are essential.
3. **Precision**: it is used in two senses—as a synonym of refinement or, statistically, to indicate the consistency of a series of measurements, i.e. how close or dispersed the measurements are to each other. Therefore, it is a function of the standard deviation (SD) of the data that have been observed. The less the SD is, the more precise the measurement system would be. For example, the prevalence value $10 \pm 2\%$ is more precise than $10 \pm 5\%$.

4. **Reliability**: data are reliable when a test produces similar results when repeated. It is expressed as repeatability and reproducibility:
   (a) ***Repeatability*** denotes the agreement between the results of a test applied on the same animals/samples many times by the same observer
   (b) ***Reproducibility*** is the agreement between the results of a test applied on the same animals/samples by different observers
5. **Validity**: it is the extent to which a test accurately measures what it claims to measure. Sensitivity and specificity are indicators of validity. For example, for the diagnosis of diabetes, physical examination (loss of body weight) is less valid than urine analysis for the presence of sugar, but for the same, blood test is the most valid.

9.5 Bias in Data

Bias is a systematic error, which may be due to the design, conduct, or analysis of a study that makes the results invalid. Important biases are as follows:

1. ***Confounding bias***: an error that causes an incorrect estimation of the association between exposure and outcome. When present, the association between an exposure and outcome is distorted by an extraneous third variable, i.e. confounding variable.
2. ***Interviewer bias***: it is a non-sampling error. Basically, it is human error (consciously or unconsciously) caused by preconceived judgement about an interviewee, which affects the evaluation of the candidate, negatively or positively, thereby making an interview less objective and hence unsuccessful. It can include intentional errors, such as cheating and fraudulent data entry.
3. ***Measurement bias***: it is due to inaccurate measurement (faulty instrument), for example misclassification of animals as diseased and healthy because of low sensitivity and specificity of tests.
4. ***Selection bias***: animals selected from abattoirs are unlikely to have a clinical disease, whereas the general population will have some clinically diseased animals.

9.6 Coding of Data

Data on animals can be divided into two categories:

1. ***Permanent or tombstone data***, which remain unchanged during the animal's life, e.g. species, breed, sex, date of birth/death/calving, etc.
2. ***Descriptors or specifiers***, which vary during life, e.g. lesions, test results, signs, diagnosis, etc.

Table 9.1 Hierarchic numeric code

	Code	Meaning	Category
Treatment	100	General medicine therapy	Broad category
	110	Antibiotic	
	112	Oxytetracycline	Refined category
	120	Parasiticide	
	121	Albendazole	
Species and breed	100	Equine	
	101	Kathiawari	
	200	Canine	
	201	Pomeranian	
	300	Feline	
	400	Bovine	
	401	Tharparkar	

Data are nothing but information that can be represented in both words and numbers. Therefore, it is necessary to make them universal in understanding and acceptance, for which coding is necessary. The coding of data means representing text and numerals in standard abbreviated form, which made data recording consistent, unambiguous, and uniform, as well as economical and easier to handle by a computer.

Coding may be done as follows:

1. Numeric codes (represents text in numbers)
2. Alpha codes (letters)
3. Alphanumeric codes
4. Symbols

- **Numeric codes**: initially, numeric codes were common, e.g. CBPP = 274. Many systems, like the Standard Nomenclature of Veterinary Diseases and Operations (SNVDO), Systemic Nomenclature of Veterinary Medicine (SNOVET), and Systematised Nomenclature of Medicine (SNOMED), etc., were developed using numeric codes. These may be of two types:
  - Consecutive codes: consecutive numbers are drawn up to represent data, e.g. 001 = canine distemper, 002 = hepatitis, 003 = acute cystitis.
  - Hierarchic numeric codes (Tables 9.1 and 9.2).
- **Alpha codes**: these represent plain text through alphabetical abbreviations or acronyms, e.g. F = female, M = male.
  As per Table 9.3, DA PD = displaced abomasum, GL PR = retained placenta, DH B = hepatitis, GU PP = prolapse of uterus.
- **Alphanumeric codes**: these are represented by abbreviations or acronyms that consist of a combination of alphabets and numbers (Tables 9.4 and 9.5).
- **Finger trouble**: four types of error occur during the entry of data onto a computer, which are together called finger trouble:

Table 9.2 Numeric codes for ranges of numbers of helminth eggs per gram (epg) of faeces

Code	Epg	Code	Epg
001	1–500	010	4501–5000
002	501–1000	011	5001–5500
003	1001–1500	012	5501–6000
004	1501–2000	013	6001–6500
005	2001–2500	014	6501–7000
006	2501–3000	015	7001–7500
007	3001–3500	016	7501– 8000
008	3501–4000	017	8001–8500
009	4001–4500	018	8501–9000

Table 9.3 Hierarchic alpha diagnostic code

Axis I (location)		Axis II (abnormality)	
Code	Meaning	Code	Meaning
D	Digestive system	B	Inflammation
DA	Abomasum	E	Exudate
DE	Oesophagus	EBH	Haemorrhage
DH	Liver	P	Position
G	Reproductive system	PD	Displaced
GL	Placenta	PR	Retention
GU	Uterus	PP	Prolapse

Table 9.4 Hierarchic alphanumeric codes for signs. e.g. digestive system

D00		Abnormal appetite
	D01	Decreased appetite
	DO2	Polyphagia (excessive appetite)
	D03	Anorexia (loss of appetite)
	D04	Pica (depraved appetite)
D10		Difficulty in prehension (cannot get food in the mouth)
D20		Chewing difficulty
D30		Signs related to jaw
	D31	Weakness of jaw
	D32	Inability to close jaw
	D33	Inability to open jaw
	D34	Malformation of jaw

- Insertion: extra characters are erroneously added.
- Deletion: characters are omitted.
- Substitution: a wrong character is typed.
- Transposition: correct characters are typed but in the wrong order. For example, the swapping of 4 and 5 to take the list 3456–3546 is a transposition.

To correct finger troubles, there is a check-digit-generated formula. Say, for example, 5029 = anaemia; the first three digits—'502'—relate to anaemia, while

Table 9.5 Standard and universally accepted symbols (FAO-WHO-OIE 1992)

Symbol	Disease occurrence
–	Not reported
?	Suspected
(+)	Exceptional occurrence
+	Low sporadic occurrence
++	Endemic
+++	High occurrence
+?	Serological evidence and/or isolation of causative agent, no clinical disease
+. . .	Disease exists, distribution and occurrence unknown
()	Confined to certain regions
!	Recognised in the country for the first time
<=	Only in imported animals (quarantine)
. . .	No information available

the fourth digit—'9'—is a check digit, which is a function of code numbers. The following formula is used to generate check digit:

$$(\text{First digit} \times 2) + \text{Second digit} - \text{Third digit}/2$$

The computer will not accept the digit 5019 or 5039 as a code for anaemia as neither 501 nor 503 will produce check digit 9. The digits 4229 and 4109 produce check digit 9, but the initial three digits are meant for some other condition and, therefore, not accepted by the computer. It is useful for the validation of check digits and is a mathematical function of the first three digits of the code.

9.7 Important Sources of Veterinary Data

1. Government veterinary organisations
2. Private veterinary practitioners
3. Insurance organisations
4. Abattoirs
5. Poultry packing plants
6. Knacker yards
7. Serum banks
8. Registries: pathology registry
9. Pharmaceutical and agricultural sales: indirect means of assessment of the amount of disease
10. Zoological gardens: International Veterinary Record of Zoo Animals, Geneva (a central registry)
11. Agricultural organisations: BAIF, National Bank for Agriculture and Rural Development (NABARD), dairy co-operatives
12. Commercial livestock enterprises: Venky's, Suguna, Godrej, etc.

9.8 Distribution of Data Set

The distribution of data set means the arrangement of data values, which can be described by its centre, spread (variation), and overall shape. If the left side of a distribution is the mirror image of the right side, then the distribution is *symmetric*, but if not, then it is *asymmetric*.

In symmetric data, the *mean* is used to describe the centre and *absolute deviation* to describe the spread, while in asymmetric data, the *median* is used to describe the centre and *interquartile range* to describe the spread.

The distribution of data may be as follows:

- Normal
- Binomial
- Poisson

1. **Normal distribution**: it is a common probability distribution and is always symmetrical about the mean with a *bell-shaped curve.* The mean and standard deviation determine the shape of normal distribution. If the standard deviation is small, the bell curve will be steeper. If the standard deviation is large, i.e. the data are spread far apart, then the bell curve will be much flatter (Fig. 9.1). The *standard normal distribution* is a special case of normal distribution with a mean of 0 and a standard deviation of 1. The normal random variable of a standard normal distribution is called a *standard score* or *z score*.
   Normal distribution has four characteristics: (a) symmetric, (b) unimodal (i.e. a curve with one peak), (c) asymptotic ('limiting' distribution of a sequence of distributions), and (d) the mean, median, and mode are all equal. A normal distribution is perfectly symmetrical around its centre; i.e., the right side of the centre is a mirror image of the left side. Normal distributions are continuous and have tails that are asymptotic, which means they approach but never touch the *x*-axis.

   In general, in a normal distribution curve, about 68% of the area lies within one standard deviation of the mean; i.e., if $\bar{x}$ is the mean and σ is the standard deviation of the distribution, then 68% of the values fall in the range between $(\bar{x} - \sigma)$ and $(\bar{x} + \sigma)$; about 95% of the values lie within two standard deviations of the mean, i.e. between $(\bar{x} - 2\sigma)$ and $(\bar{x} + 2\sigma)$; and about 99.7% of the values lie within three standard deviations of the mean, i.e. between $(\bar{x} - 3\sigma)$ and $(\bar{x} + 3\sigma)$ (Fig. 9.2).
2. **Binomial distribution**: it relates to discrete data, when there are only two possible outcomes on each occasion, e.g. sex of newborn—male or female, success and failure in examination, or head or tail in coin.
3. **Poisson distribution**: it concerns counts and is applicable when events occur randomly in space and time, e.g. random occurrence of cases of a disease in a unit time or a unit area, distribution of a virus particle infecting cells in tissue culture,

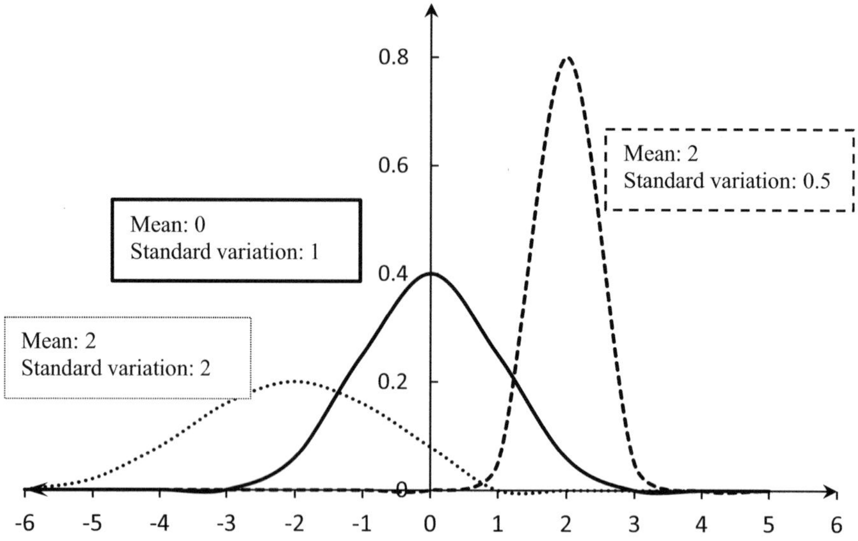

Fig. 9.1 Normal distribution

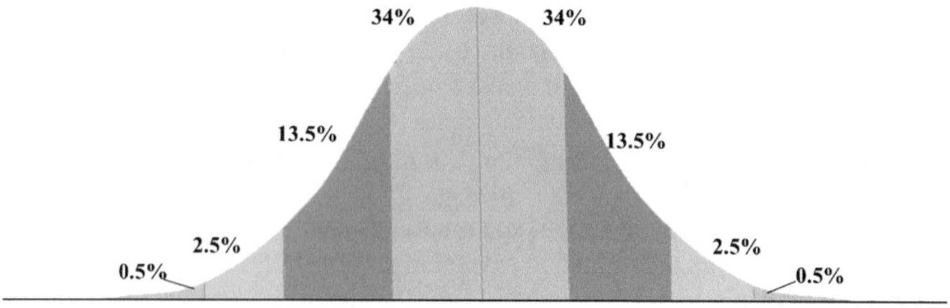

Fig. 9.2 Area under normal distribution curve

etc. Poisson distribution relates to the spatial and temporal distribution of disease; therefore, it has importance in epidemiology.

References

Anonymous (1989) Oxford English dictionary, 2nd ed

FAO-WHO-OIE (1992) Animal Health Yearbook 1991. Food and Agriculture Organization of United Nations, World Health Organization, Office International des Epizooties. Food and Agriculture Organization of United Nations, Rome.

10 Measures of Disease

There may not be a direct measure for health. Indirectly, the absence of disease in a population may be considered a measure of health. The measurement of health is expressed in the form of rates and ratios.

Rate refers to the enumeration of an event in a population during a specified time/ period. It consists of two components: the 'numerator (the event)' and the denominator (the population)'. Both have to be defined precisely.

Rate refers to a proportion representing the probability between 0 and 1 of an animal having a specified disease at a given time. It may be expressed as (10^a) per cent or per 1000 or 100,000, depending on the rarity of the disease.

$$\text{Rate} = \frac{\text{Number of animals affected during a specified time}}{\text{Average population of animals exposed to the risk(population at risk)during the same period}} \times 10^a$$

Ratio refers to relativity. The relative magnitude of two events or observations is measured. There is no need to refer to or relate to the population.

Proportion, often expressed as a percentage (%), is the comparison of a part to the whole. It is a type of ratio in which the numerator is included in the denominator.

When a disease occurs in a population, some are affected, out of which some die. The affected are measured by morbidity, while those who die are measured by mortality. Some of the rates and ratios commonly used in the study of the health and production of animals in a population (herd/flock etc.) are given below.

K. G. Narayan et al., *Veterinary Public Health & Epidemiology*,
https://doi.org/10.1007/978-981-19-7800-5_10

10.1 Morbidity Measures

There are two essential components: the number of cases in a population and the specified period of time. Incidence measures the number of new cases, and prevalence calculates the number of affected. Both are expressed in relation to the population at risk:

$$\text{Incidence rate} = \frac{\text{Number of new cases occurring during a specified period}}{\text{Average population of animals at risk}^{*}} \times 10^{a}$$

*Number at risk at the start of the time period+ number at the end of the time period/2.

$$\text{Cumulative incidence rate} = \frac{\text{Total no.of individuals becoming diseased during a period (new cases)}}{\text{Total no.of healthy individuals (at risk) at the start of observation period}} \times 10^{a}$$

$$\text{Prevalence rate} = \frac{\text{Total no.of cases (new + old) during a specified period}}{\text{Average no.of animals at risk during the same period}} \times 10^{a}$$

$$\text{Point prevalence rate} = \frac{\text{Total number of cases at a given point in time}}{\text{Number of animals at risk at that point in time}} \times 10^{a}$$

Incidence measures new cases, while prevalence measures total (old + new) cases at a given point in time. Annual incidence rate (IR) will include only the new cases reported during the year, while prevalence will report both new and old cases together. Thus, prevalence gives an overall picture of total number of cases.

Prevalence is dependent upon incidence and the duration of the disease and varies with incidence and duration. $P =$ incidence (I) $\times$ duration (D) when I and D remain constant, i.e. when the disease maintains stability and P is small. This formula is useful for the calculation of one component if the other two are unknown. Change in prevalence from one period to another is influenced by (a) incidence, (b) duration, or (c) both. The duration of the disease is measured from the date of detection/diagnosis; it is the same date for recording incidence. The duration of a disease may be affected by the success or failure of therapy. Other reasons for the reduction in prevalence rates may be early deaths (or high case fatality), low incidence, increased cure rate, and migration (in-migration of healthy, out-migration of cases). The opposite will lead to an increase in prevalence rate, which measures the contagiousness of a disease.

The denominator for a dynamic population is measured as 'animal-years' at risk. This is the sum of the periods of observation for each animal at risk (free from disease).

Cumulative incidence rate is an indication of the average risk of developing a disease during a particular period in both the individual and the population, usually calculated for the first occurrence (not multiple) of the disease. It is used in a dynamic population if the period of risk is short and is related to a specific event.

10.1.1 Specific Morbidity Rates

Specific morbidity rates can be calculated based on the same pattern. For example, age-specific incidence rate can be calculated as the number of new cases occurring in a specific age (say 6-month-aged calves)/the average population of calves of 6 months at risk during the same period. Similarly, the prevalence and point prevalence rates can also be calculated. Such specific rates could be specific for sex, a specific physiological group, a specific breed, etc.

10.1.2 Attack Rate

If the population is at risk for a limited period (i.e. the aetiological factor operates for a short time only or the duration of the epidemic is short or the risks are restricted to a certain age group (e.g. imperforate anus, pyloric stenosis)), the incidence rate is represented as an attack rate. The incidence does not change even if the period of observation is increased. Attack rate among the in-contacts of the primary case is called secondary attack rate.

$$\text{Secondary attack rate} = \frac{\text{Total no.of contacts developing disease within the maximum incubation period}}{\text{Total no.of susceptible(if known) exposed to the primary case(i.e. contacts)}} \times 10^{a}$$

For diseases conferring prolonged immunity, the denominator in the secondary attack rate usually excludes individuals who have previously had the disease.

10.2 Mortality Rates

Another parameter for measuring the health of a population of animals is the calculation of mortality rates. These can be the crude death rate (i.e. the total of all deaths, irrespective of cause, age, breed, sex, etc.) or specific death rates (i.e. deaths due to specific causes, say anthrax, specific to sex, specific to an age group, specific to breed, etc.). The numerator consists of the number of deaths and the denominator, the average population during the same period of observation.

$$\text{Crude death rate (CDR)} = \frac{\text{Number of deaths during a specified period}}{\text{Average population of animals during the same period}} \times 10^{a}$$

$$\text{Cause} - \text{specific death rate} = \frac{\text{Number of deaths due to a specific cause(e.g. FMD) during a specified period}}{\text{Average population of animals during the same period}} \times 10^{a}$$

$$\text{Sudden death rate} = \frac{\text{Total number of sudden deaths}}{\text{Total number of deaths}} \times 10^{a}$$

$$\text{Sudden death ratio} = \frac{\text{Total number of sudden deaths}}{\text{Total number of deaths} - \text{Total number of sudden deaths}} \times 10^{a}$$

The crude death rate is a crude measurement. Yet it is valuable in making a comparison of the health status between two populations or in the assessment of a particular package of intervention practices intended to reduce mortality by comparing CDR before and after the introduction of the intervention. However, it is not possible to draw out a conclusion about the natural history of any specific disease in the population under study. For example, a CDR of 12 per 1000 in Farm A is higher than CDR of 9 per 1000 in Farm B, indicating that Farm B maintains better health. Similarly, a CDR of 5 in Farm A in the year 1999 compared to 9 in the year 1997 indicates better attention paid to the control of mortality. Information about the reduction or increase of a specific disease, say anthrax or calf scour among calves (age specific and cause specific), cannot be derived from CDR. Hence, no administrative action can be thought of. The cause-specific, and other specific (e.g., age specific, sex specific, breed specific, etc.) mortality rates would help in deciding specific line of action or directed to a specific group of population as increased death rate is indicative of higher susceptibility of this specific group or some factor operating with this specific population.

$$\text{Breed/Sex/Age-specific death rate} = \frac{\text{No.of deaths in a specific breed/sex/age group due to a specific cause}}{\text{Average of total population of that breed/sex/age group}} \times 10^{a}$$

$$\text{Neonatal}^{*}\ \text{mortality rate} = \frac{\text{Deaths within 4 weeks of birth}}{\text{Number of live births}} \times 10^{a}$$

*Early postnatal = within 48 h of birth.
Delayed postnatal = 2–7 days of age.
Late postnatal = 1–4 weeks of age.

Perinatal = Around birth.

$$\text{Calf/kid/lamb/piglet/pup etc.} = \frac{\text{Number of calves/kids/lambs/piglets/pups etc. dying up to the age of weaning}}{\text{Number of live calves/kids/lambs/piglets/pups etc. born}} \times 10^{a} - \text{mortality rate}$$

The neonatal and young ages (age up to weaning) are defined in the above rates. These are useful and commonly used measures as most mortalities occur in these age groups. The rates used for young age are expressed per thousand.

$$\text{Infant mortality rate} = \frac{\text{Deaths in age group } 0-1 \text{ year in a specified year}}{\text{Total live births in that year}} \times 10^{a}$$

$$\text{Case fatality rate} = \frac{\text{Number of deaths due to a specific cause}}{\text{Total number of cases due to the specific cause}} \times 10^{a}$$

The severity of the disease is measured by case fatality rate. For example, CFR is higher in the case of anthrax than in the case of foot and mouth disease. A veterinary health manager is able to decide priorities with the help of the CFR recorded for different diseases. Also, the virulence of strains of an infectious agent is indicated by CFR. It is expressed in per cent.

10.3 Ratios

The following ratios are useful measures of health and disease:

$$\begin{array}{l}\text{Proportional cause-specific}\\ \text{Incidence/prevalence ratio}\end{array} = \frac{\text{Total number of cases of specific disease}}{\text{Total number of all cases}} \times 10^{a}$$

Note: In the case of incidence, only new cases are counted.

$$\text{Proportional mortality ratio} = \frac{\text{Total number of deaths from a specific cause}}{\text{Total deaths from all causes}} \times 10^{a}$$

These ratios are relative values. However, quite often, population-related figures are not available. One has to depend solely on the record of the hospital, post-mortem laboratory, diagnostic laboratory, or slaughterhouse or on other data. The quality of inferences drawn from these data is not as good as those drawn from the other measures listed earlier.

$$\text{Foetal death ratio} = \frac{\text{Total foetal deaths}}{\text{Total live births}} \times 10^{a}$$

Foetal/neonatal death rate

$$= \frac{\text{Number of foetal/neonatal deaths}}{\text{Total births (live births + foetal/neonatal deaths)}} \times 10^a$$

Zoonosis incidence ratio

$$= \frac{\text{New cases of zoonosis in an animal species at a specific time in an area}}{\text{Average human population at that time in that area}} \times 10^a$$

10.4 Formula for Measuring Production

$$\text{Pregnancy rate} = \frac{\text{Number of females pregnant}}{\text{Number of females checked for pregnancy}} \times 10^a$$

The percentage of conceived that were inseminated is the conception rate.

$$\text{Calving rate} = \frac{\text{Number of females calving (i.e. calves born)}}{\text{Number of females inseminated (exposed to breeding)}} \times 10^a$$

This is also called reproduction rate.

$$\text{Abortion rate} = \frac{\text{Total cows/females that abort}}{\text{Total cows/females that give birth}} \times 10^a$$

Case recovery rate

$$= \frac{\text{Total number of cases treated and discharged as recovered}}{\text{Total number of cases treated}} \times 10^a$$

$$\text{Calf crop} = \frac{\text{Number of calves/kids/lambs/piglets/pups etc. weaned}}{\text{Number of females exposed to breeding}} \times 10^a$$

Kilogram of calf weaned exposed to breeding

$$= \frac{\text{Average weaning weight for herd} \times \text{No of per female calves weaned}}{\text{Number of females exposed to breeding}} \times 10^a$$

This measures productivity in general and reflects quality/level of management. Other measures of economic performance are as follows:

- Age at first calving.
- Per cent females conceiving in the first cycle.
- Per cent females conceiving at first insemination (not missing a cycle).
- Inter-calving interval—short.
- Length of lactation—long, i.e. short dry period.

Table 10.1 Calculation of rate using the 'animal-time' concept in a hypothetical herd of ten cows

Cow No.	Observed healthy for years	Date mastitis recorded	Year remained sick with mastitis	Animal years
01	1	0	0	1 and lost to study
02	2	0	0	2 and lost to study
03	200 (0.57 years)	201st day	0.43	0.57 sold after first year
04	3	0	0	3
05	100 days (0.27 years)	0	0	0.27 lost to study
06	300 days (0.81 years)	301st day	0.19	0.81 sold after first year
07	4	0	0	4
08	4	0	0	4
09	5	0	0	5
10	5	0	0	5
Total			0.62	25.75

In a herd where new animals are included and also some are sold, the population does not remain static. The number of animals keeps changing also due to death. Some of these moving/mobile animals may be lactating cows. The mastitis cases, i.e. the numerator, and the population at risk, i.e. the denominator, are calculated in terms of 'animal-time' or animal-months/years'. 'Animal-time' is the exact exposure time the animals have been available for the study. Each animal on the farm is observed till it shows the disease (mastitis in the present example). The period it shows the disease becomes its 'animal-years'; the sum of such observation periods made for each animal becomes the 'animal-years'. Two animals were observed as healthy (say two lactating cows free from mastitis) for one year. This will make 2 animal-years. One animal remained healthy (say one lactating cow free from mastitis) for 3 years. This will make 3 animal-years (1 × 3). One cow remained free from mastitis for 200 days. This will make 1 × 200/365 or 0.57 animal-years. All these make 2 + 1 + 1 = 4 cows, but animal-years = 2 + 3 + 0.57. This is better explained with the following observations in a herd of ten cows (Table 10.1).

Rate of mastitis in 5 years = 0.62/25.75 × 100 or 2.4% in this herd of 10 cows.

10.5 Explanation and Exercise

A herd of 10 cows observed for 5 years should have made 50 animals under observation, of which two suffered from mastitis. But the calculation is not that straight because animals were either sold and so were lost to studies or brought in different years to the farm, as shown in Table 10.2.

Ratio refers to relativity. The relative magnitude of two events or observations is measured. There is no need to refer or relate to the population.

How is average number at risk calculated? It is measured by the total number at the beginning of the outbreak (say X) + (X—the sum of new cases, recovered cases, and dead due to the same disease during the period)/2. For example, on 1 January 2000, there were 1000 calves on a farm. The calves suffered from calf scour. The first case was noticed on 2 February. The veterinary epidemiologist visited on 10 February. By this date, 102 had died, 32 sick ones were recovering, and 61 had started showing symptoms. There was no sickness before 2 February. The total number of new cases between 1 Jan. and 10 Feb. was, thus, 102 + 32 + 61 = 195. The incidence rate of calf scours for the period 1 Jan. to 10 Feb. (40 days) is calculated; the average population at risk = [(1000–195) + 1000]/2 = 902.5. The incidence rate = 195/905.5 × 40 (time period in days). As the IR is being calculated in the face of an outbreak, the period may be reduced to the date of the first-case reporting and the date of observation, i.e. 2 Feb. and 10 Feb. (8 days). As the total number of calves (1000) remained the same also on 2 February, the calculation would, therefore, be 195/905.5 × 8 days. This incidence rate is the measure of the speed at which the disease is spreading. The denominator is indicative of the total time that each animal in the population was at risk of getting the disease. In contrast, the conventional formula is called the cumulative incidence rate (CIR).

$$\text{CIR} = \frac{\text{Total number of new cases}}{\text{Total number at risk at the beginning of the observation period}} \times 10^{a}$$

$$\text{Prevalence rate} = \frac{\text{Total number of cases (new + old) during a specified period}}{\text{Average number of animals at risk during the same period}} \times 10^{a}$$

$$\text{Point Prevalence rate} = \frac{\text{Total number of cases at a given point in time}}{\text{Number of animals at risk at that point in time}} \times 10^{a}$$

Table 10.2 Animals available to studies during the 5 years of observation

Cow No.	First year	2nd year	3rd year	4th year	5th year
01					+
02				+	+
03	+	Sold after	Recovery		
04	+	+	+		
05	+sold after 100 days				
06	+	Sold after	Recovery		
07		+	+	+	+
08	+	+	+	+	
09	+	+	+	+	+
10	+	+	+	+	+

Table 10.3 Cases of mastitis according to the date of reporting and recovery during 1999 in a farm

Cases	Date of reporting	Date of recovery	Duration
01	Continuing since 1998	28 January	56 days
02	Continuing since 1998	16 January	42 days
03	10 June	15 August	65 days
04	15 June	10 August	56 days
05	20 June	26 July	35 days
06	30 June	20 August	50 days
07	2 August	28 August	26 days
08	2 October	15 November	44 days
09	15 November	Continuing	Continuing
10	18 December	Continuing	Continuing
Total cases = 10			Average = 46.75 days or 0.1271 years

Table 10.4 Number of lactating cows (population at risk) month-wise during 1999

Months	Number
January	990
February	998
March	1000
April	997
May	999
June	1000
July	999
August	998
September	999
October	997
November	998
December	1000
Average for the year	11,975/12 = 996

Incidence measures new cases, while prevalence measures the total (old + new) cases. Annual incidence rate will include only the new cases reported during the year, while prevalence will report both new and old cases together. The latter is a cross-section of what prevails. Prevalence for a particular time, say total cases on January 2020, will be calculated as a point prevalence rate for January 2020 (Tables 10.3 and 10.4).

Prevalence rate for 1999 = 10 (8 new +2 old cases)/996 × 10^2 = 1.004%.

Point prevalence for the month of August = 4 (one new + 3 old)/ 998 × 10^2 = 0.4%.

Incidence rate = 8 (all new cases)/996 × 10^2 = 0.8%.

Average duration of sickness = 0.1271 years.

Prevalence is approximately the product of incidence rate × duration. Duration is measured in the same unit of time as incidence is.

In this case, the prevalence rate (*P*) is 1.004. It should be = (*IR*) or 0.8 × (*D*) or 0.1271 years = 1.016

Exercise: For learning methods of assessing the health, production, and disease of livestock maintained in a farm (closed population)

- Defining the numerator and denominator for specific purposes.
- Collecting information from the records and tabulating.
- Calculating different rates and ratios.
- Deriving inferences/hypotheses.
- Maintaining farm records for useful purposes.
- Preparing a status report.
- Presentation of report.

A dairy farm is maintaining Sahiwal and Tharparkar cows and calves. The total strength of the animals during the year 2000–2001 (1.4.2000 to 31.3.2001) was 2500. There were 300 cases of sickness and 105 deaths. The animals were maintained separately as follows: neonates, 1–3 months age group, 4–12 months age group, and the remaining animals. The farm veterinary doctor maintains the detail records.

(a) Hence, any information may be collected from the record. Ask for it. See Appendix for data.
(b) You are asked to calculate the following rates and ratios
(c) Draw inferences, and comment on the status of the health, production, and disease of the animals on the farm:
    (i) Morbidity rates: prevalence rates—point prevalence on 30 June 2000, period prevalence for the third quarter (October–December 2000), and annual prevalence rate for Johne's disease.
    (ii) Incidence rates for the diseases recorded; neonatal incidence rates, broken up in each of the four weeks; and incidence rates in the calves (1–3 months, 4–12 months, and other age groups)
    (iii) Incubation period, secondary attack rate, and the duration of ephemeral fever.
    (iv) Mortality rates: crude and specific death rates (specific diseases and specific age groups), abortion rates, and case fatality rates.
    (v) Ratios: proportional cause-specific-incidence/prevalence ratio and proportional mortality ratios.

Calculate the above rates also with 'animal years of risk' as the denominator.

Calculation of Rates and Ratios.

(a) **Morbidity measures.**
(b) **Mortality measures.**
(c) **Calculation of rates using 'animal years of risk'.**

A dairy farm is maintaining Holstein-Friesian and cross-bred cows and calves. The total strength of the animals during the year 2000–2001 (1.2.2000 to 31.1.2001) was 2200. There were 292 cases of sickness and 84 deaths. The animals were maintained separately as follows: neonates, 1–3 months age group, 4–12 months age group, and the remaining animals. The farm veterinary doctor maintains the detail records.

(a) Hence, any information may be collected from the record. Ask for it. *See Appendix for data.*
(b) You are asked to calculate the following rates and ratios.
(c) Draw inferences, and comment on the status of the health, production, and disease of the animals on the farm:
    (i) *Morbidity rates*: prevalence rates—point prevalence on 30 June 2000, period prevalence for the last quarter (October–December 2000), and annual prevalence rate for Johne's disease.
    (ii) *Incidence rates* for the diseases recorded; neonatal incidence rates, broken up in each of the four weeks; and incidence rates in the calves (1–3 months, 4–12 months, and other age groups).
    (iii) Incubation period, secondary attack rate, and the duration of ephemeral fever.
    (iv) *Mortality rates*: crude and specific death rates (specific diseases and specific age groups), abortion rates, and case fatality rates.
    (v) *Ratios*: proportional cause-specific-incidence/prevalence ratio and proportional mortality ratios.

Calculate the above rates also with 'animal years of risk' as the denominator.

Strategies of Epidemiology

11

There are four strategies of epidemiological investigations, often termed types of epidemiology.

1. Descriptive.
2. Analytical.
3. Experimental.
4. Theoretical or mathematical.

11.1 Descriptive Epidemiology

Descriptive epidemiology is used to classify diseases based on person, place, and time. The information related to person includes who is affected with respect to variables like age, sex, physiological status, race, and breed and, in the case of humans, socio-economic status, etc. The characteristics related to place include geographical location, which may be municipality, city, state, country, etc. for humans, while in the case of husbandry practices (intensive vs extensive rearing), housing, etc. for animals. Finally, time-related information is recorded, such as days, weeks, season, day vs night, etc.

Thus, it deals with the description of epidemic, whereas a detailed description of the cases and healthy individuals during an outbreak/epidemic is made. Answers to the cardinal questions—who, what, when, where, why, and how—are sought. Precise, authentic, correct, and unbiased information help in the development of valid hypotheses and inferences. The methods of collecting information could be through direct interviews, questionnaires, or available records in the form of.

K. G. Narayan et al., *Veterinary Public Health & Epidemiology*,
https://doi.org/10.1007/978-981-19-7800-5_11

11.1.1 Surveys

I. Surveillance records.
II. Others: farm records, general insurance claims, records on the use of vaccines and drugs; environmental and ecological data; certain events peculiar to the epidemic, such as the use of certain consignments of feed, import of animals, methods of transport of animals or import of contaminated products of animal origin, etc.

These pieces of information are then grouped with respect to person, place, and time.

Surveys are made on an identified population or in an identified area for a defined purpose, for example a survey made on cattle (identified animals) located in a village (identified area, also called local survey) and for recording repeat breeders (defined purpose). This may be called 'active survey'. The same information, along with additional information, may be collected and recorded by a village dairy cooperative. The data on repeat breeders collected from the records of the village cooperative may be useful in epidemiological studies on 'repeat breeders'; this is passive survey. In the case of an investigation of an epidemic, the data collected by active and passive surveys are useful. A survey made once only (single point in time) is called cross-sectional. This gives information on what 'exists' at that particular time. On the other hand, if a survey is made more than once, i.e. a population is being followed for a specified purpose (e.g. repeat breeders), it is called longitudinal. Compared to this, the survey may be made periodically or continuously (periodic and continuous survey).

11.1.2 Surveillance

Surveillance is an ongoing systematic collection, collation, analysis, and interpretation of data on health and disease, formulation of recommendations, timely dissemination of these to those who need to know, and their implementation and evaluation. The final link in the surveillance chain is the application of these data for prevention and control (CDC 1986). Surveillance is active search for disease—clinical signs of disease or antibody, i.e. infection. If the disease is found, actions follow. This means that surveillance is conducted to confirm that the disease is absent. The objective of surveillance is, thus, to demonstrate a state of freedom from disease or infection or to confirm that it has been reintroduced. This is in contrast to 'disease monitoring' and 'disease reporting'.

11.1.3 Monitoring

Monitoring is an ongoing systematic collection, analysis, and interpretation of data essential to planning, implementation, and evaluation. It is the continuous follow-up of activities to ensure that they are proceeding according to plan. It is applicable to health and production or any programme. It is often confused with ‘surveillance’. In the case of ‘disease monitoring’, it is presumed that the disease is existing and the objective is to search actively to determine its incidence or prevalence.

11.1.4 Reporting

Disease reporting is a passive process. There is no active search for disease or infection. There is no presumption about the existing status of a disease. It is the responsibility of the health care provider and not the patient to report a disease when it is diagnosed by a doctor or laboratory. Every country has a list of notifiable diseases. The reporting of a notifiable disease is mandatory.

Disease reporting and disease surveillance are complimentary. The international recognition of ‘freedom’ from disease status requires effective ‘disease reporting’ and ‘disease surveillance’.

Surveillance calls for immediate action and proper intervention to intercept the cycle of transmission of infectious diseases. This is equally applicable to non-infectious diseases. Although it was coined for public health, it is equally important and useful for diseases in animals, including zoonoses. Surveillance has been a successful tool in the eradication of animal diseases, like rinderpest (RP), foot and mouth disease, and also rabies, in many countries. The control of smallpox, yellow fever, and plague are similarly good examples of success made in public health. Two important developments in modern science have made ‘surveillance’ a very efficient tool. These are (a) rapid methods of specific diagnostic tools, like deoxyribonucleic acid (DNA) probes, polymerase chain reaction (PCR) tests, monoclonal-antibody-based diagnostics, like enzyme-linked immunosorbent assay, and (b) fast modes of communication, such as ‘bioinformatics’. Thus, rapid disease diagnosis and reporting have become possible. The Ministry of Agriculture of the Government of India collects and compiles data on animal diseases through its Livestock Health Surveillance Units and brings out a monthly bulletin called Animal Disease Surveillance Bulletin.

11.1.5 Formulation of Hypotheses

Epidemiology looks for patterns after attributes related to person, place, and time are analysed and studied with respect to differences, similarities, and correlations among two or more attributes. Hypotheses explaining the observed association of attributes with disease are made. For example, a hypothetical hypothesis is ‘among unvaccinated Holstein Friesian cows and without previous exposure, the inhalation of ten particles of FMDV will result in an attack rate of 60% within a period of 15 days’. Logical methods for the formulation of hypotheses are as follows:

1. Method of agreement.
2. Method of difference.

3. Method of analogy.
4. Method of concomitant variation.

Method of agreement: a factor or an attribute common to patients drawn from a population that is heterogeneous is sought out. For example, increased incidence of cases of *Salmonella* poisoning mainly due to sausage eating with isolations of *S. weltevreden* from stool of patients and increased isolation of *S. weltevreden* from sausages in routine laboratory examination of foods indicate that the three observations *agreed* that 'sausage contaminated with *S. weltevreden* might be on the increase and caused increased human salmonellosis'. This happened in England, leading to an investigation, which confirmed that there was increased incidence of sausage contamination with *S. weltevreden*, revealing the source of contamination and its spread.

Method of difference: this method requires comparing factors present in affected (patients) and not affected (control) subjects. The two groups may *differ* in some or a few of the factors. This method is useful particularly in situations where the population is homogenous. Snows' investigation into cholera in the Broad Street lamp episode is a good example to remember. The affected population differed from the unaffected one only in the source of water supply to their houses (Southwark vs. Lambeth Water Supply Company). The difference in source of water help in identification of the contaminated water supply (as the cause) leading to the outbreak of cholera. It is remarkable that an effective intervention method was found to prevent waterborne infectious diseases even before the discovery of *Vibrio cholerae*, and this proves the importance and relevance of epidemiology. Effective prevention can be achieved even before the 'sufficient and necessary cause' is identified.

Method of analogy: an analogy is drawn between the disease under investigation and a disease that has been well studied in order to formulate a hypothesis. The search for an animal reservoir of *Leishmania donovani* in India is based on the method of analogy. A similar approach led to the discovery of desert gerbils as reservoirs of *L. tropica* in India.

Method of concomitant variation: a quantitative variation in attribute leads to a corresponding quantitative change in the disease. This dose-response-like phenomenon yields the most acceptable hypothesis. An example could be toxicities.

A good hypothesis should elucidate the cause-effect relationship. It should be biologically and statistically valid. It should be universal, i.e. reproducible.

11.2 Analytical Epidemiology

Analytical epidemiology is used to study the etiology of disease and identify whether any causal association exists between the etiology (exposure) and the disease through a critical evaluation of hypotheses. Here, an attempt is made to answer 'why'. Analytical epidemiology is, thus, used to test a hypothesis by either accepting or rejecting one that is formulated. The trends of the pattern of the disease in nature are *observed*, and so this is also called 'observational study'.

11.3 Experimental Epidemiology

Here, an experiment(s) is/are conducted to prove or disprove the hypotheses. This is more stringent than 'analytical epidemiology', where the hypotheses proven or rejected by the analytical studies are further confirmed.

Study is optional, and it may not be possible in all cases to conduct an experiment. Most epidemiological studies end at the analytical level. Many experimental studies cannot be conducted on the population. Simulated experimental studies can be conducted in the laboratory—on laboratory animals. The trial of a vaccine/drug in a population is often carried out under experimental epidemiology. The experiment has a strength that no other observational/analytical study can match.

Observational vs. experimental studies: in an experiment, the direct association between an attribute and the disease can be established with almost absolute certainty. Experimental studies are prospective, consisting of a test and a control group. The attribute(s) under test is/are manipulated. The principle of 'double blind' techniques is applied to avoid any bias.

In an observational study, nature provides the experiment. But the difference between the test and control groups is not sharp. It may be controlled or uncontrolled. The test group (those possessing the attribute) and the control (those not possessing the attribute) are first selected after some of the attributes, like age, sex, race/breed/strain, etc., between the two groups are matched. They are observed till the outcome, the frequency of which is recorded. In uncontrolled studies, there are no explicit controls. Judgement is made as to whether the attributes of the cases (diseased) differed from those of the non-cases (not diseased/healthy), and both groups are drawn from the same population. Then the data are analysed. As the population and also the attribute are not under the control of the experimenter and also various factors might affect the study, the inferences drawn are not as dependable as in the case of an experimental study.

11.4 Theoretical or Mathematical Epidemiology or Modelling

Theoretical or mathematical epidemiology helps explain how an infectious disease progresses in a population, the role of different factors, and the likely outcome of an epidemic. It will help in formulating the preventive/control intervention(s) as well as future predictions and behaviour.

Lowell Reed and Wade Hampton Frost, medical research scientists at Johns Hopkins University, developed a mathematical model in the 1920s to describe accurately how diseases spread through populations. This is known as the 'Reed-Frost Measles Epidemic Model'. Their purpose was to sensitise medical students to the variability of the epidemic process. This model is accurate. The relationship between the suspected causal factors (attribute) and the disease is quantified. Measles spreads rapidly in school settings when a child with measles (i.e. ill/case) attends a class and infects susceptible children (exposed group) in the class (closed population). This model explains the biological continuum, herd/population immunity, and the basis of mass vaccination. The model is based on certain assumptions. These are the following:

1. An ill individual is infectious and transfers infection through adequate contact (and in no other way) with the susceptible.
2. The susceptible are infected.
3. In turn, they become infectious to others and also become immune.
4. Each individual has a defined probability of coming in contact with an infectious individual within a one-time interval. The time interval is equal to the average period during which a new case was infectious.
5. The individual(s) of this exposed group is/are segregated from the others outside (closed population).
6. These conditions remain constant during the epidemic.

Certain parameters are set initially, and these are as follows:

- Size of the population (100 in this example).
- Number of individuals already immune (0 or all of 100 are susceptible).
- Number of cases set initially (usually set at 1).
- Probability of adequate contact—corresponds roughly to $R_{o,}$ It is the basic reproduction number an infective is expected to produce. $R_o = \text{In}(1/1 - p)$ new cases.

Each infectious (or infective) independently infects the susceptible with certain probability '*p*' of adequate contact for transmission in generation time '*t*', resulting in a new case (*It*). '*St*' is the number of susceptible individuals at time *t*, and '*q*' is the probability of specified individuals who avoid adequate contact with the infective (infected/new case(s)).

The average number of cases produced at time '*t* + 1' is the product of *St* and the probability of adequate contact with an infectious case and is arrived at using the formula

$$It + 1 = St\ \left\{1 - (1 - p)^{It}\right\} \text{ or } St\left\{1 - q^{It}\right\}$$

and

$$St + 1 = St\ (1 - p)^{It}$$

Assume that the introduction of one case of measles in a population of 100 susceptibles initiates an infection cycle. Each case is able to infect two susceptibles ($p = 0.02$ and $q = 0.98$), who, in turn, become immune. The average number of cases produced and the number of susceptible at time interval '*t* + 1' can be calculated.

The calculation of the infected (*It*), susceptible (*St*), and immune with $R_o = 2$ and the formula $It + 1 = St\{1 - (1 - p)^{It}\}$ for *It* + 1, *It* + 2, and *It* + 11 are presented

Table 11.1 Calculation of the infected (*It*), susceptible (*St*), and immune

Infection at time *t* (cycle)	Calculation	New cases (*It*)	Susceptible (*St*–*It*)	Summation of *It* or infected (hence immune)
It + 1	$100\{1 - (1{-}0.02)^1\} = 100\{1{-}(0.98)^1\} = 100\{0.02\} = 2$	02	98	02
It + 2	$98\{1 - (1{-}0.98)^2\} = 98\{1{-}0.9604)\} = 98\ (0.0396) = 3.88$ or 4	04	94	06
It + 11	$22\{1 - (1{-}0.98)^1\} = 22\{1{-}0.98\} = 22\ (0.02) = 0.44 < 1$ or 0	0		79

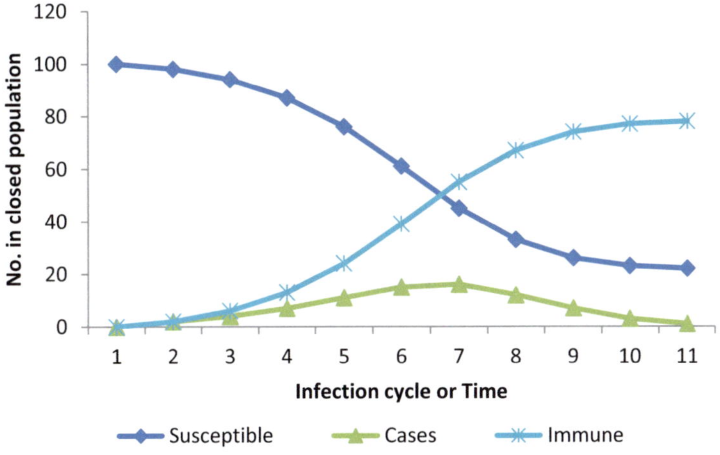

Fig. 11.11 An epidemic curve of a disease ($R_o = 2$) showing number of susceptible population (Initially 100), cases and immune animals simulated by Reed- Frost Model

(Table 11.1) for learning. Complete the calculation for the remaining. Learn to interpret the results from the figure below (Fig. 11.11). Practice varying the values for R_o, *St*, and *p*.

After a peak in the number of infected/cases (16) is reached, the number of infected starts declining.

At the end of the 11th cycle, 21 susceptible (St) and 79 immune (It) individuals remain. Each infective finds themselves surrounded by more of the immune and less of the susceptible.

The infection cycle cannot proceed further for want of susceptibles. The mass vaccination programme aims at attaining a situation (>75% immune population) where the introduction of infective individuals/carriers fails to set up a chain of infectious cycle. The immune population would not allow infection to proceed.

Mathematical models are useful for the public, public representatives, public health administrators, and policymakers. Measles, like several others, is a vaccine-preventable disease. Anti-vaccine lobby, lack of access to vaccines, and avoidance/hesitancy lead to reversing the measles-free status of several countries in 2018. Mass vaccination and surveillance succeeded in eradicating RP and smallpox. The rapid mass vaccination of pets against rabies led to the control of urban rabies and the pushing of the virus to its wildlife habitat in several countries.

The mathematical models may be (a) deterministic and (b) stochastic (probabilistic). The deterministic model is used as a first approximation model, assuming that for a given number of susceptibles and infectives and for a given attack rate a definite number of new infections will occur at any specified time. This predetermined or known causal values of determinant(s) of disease, i.e. 'inputs' influence the 'outcome', i.e. the nature and quantity of disease (morbidity) and mortality in the case of the deterministic model. The Reed-Frost model is deterministic in nature. A model of bovine mastitis-Markov chain is another example.

In stochastic models, the probability distribution of the number of susceptibles or infectives occurring at any instant replaces the point values of the deterministic treatments. The stochastic model functions on the basis of randomness or probability in regard to various determinants (factors), i.e. 'input'. It is possible to prepare a simulation model and also predict an epidemic.

11.5 Types of Epidemiological Studies

'Observational studies or analytical epidemiology' is carried out by any of the following methods based on whether comparisons between two groups are being made or not:

1. No comparison: cross-sectional.
2. Comparison: longitudinal.
   (a) Cohort.
   (b) Case control.

11.5.1 Cross-Sectional

A study/survey made once only (single point in time) is called cross-sectional. This gives information on what 'exists' at that particular time. Usually, the event/prevalence of the disease is observed with respect to certain fixed characters, for example the prevalence of thalassemia versus blood group. In a 2×2 contingency table, the total population is only known in this study.

11.5.2 Longitudinal

A survey is made more than once on the same population; i.e., the population is being followed for the specified (e.g. repeat breeders) purpose for which measurement is taken repeatedly; this is called longitudinal.

Longitudinal studies, thus, require repeated observations made on the same population at more than a single point in time. This enables one to observe the changes over a period of time, i.e. in between the two observations.

11.5.2.1 Cohort Studies

In this type of study, a group of individuals, i.e. a cohort, is observed for changes in health status over a period of time. When the observation is made from present time to future, the study is known as a prospective cohort study. But when the study period is from past time to present time, it is called a retrospective cohort study. While in a prospective study cohorts with similar features exposed to one attribute are followed till the outcome (disease) is seen, in a retrospective study, the exposure and outcome are already there and the investigator needs to look backwards. Let us consider this hypothesis to be tested through an observational study: 'Pups born of *Toxocara canis* infected pregnant bitches get infected with *T. canis*'. The attribute to be tested is 'infection during pregnancy' and the outcome, i.e. the event or disease is 'toxocariasis' in newly born pups (intrauterine infection). The observer (not the experimenter) selects bitches (sampling frame) and performs a laboratory examination of the stool of each to determine which of these are infected with *T. canis.* Thus, two groups of bitches, one infected and the other non-infected, are identified. Next, he examines all these for pregnancy. He then selects 50 each of pregnant and infected (study cohort) and pregnant non-infected (comparison cohort). As both groups have been drawn from the same sampling frame, they match in most of the attributes. These two cohorts are followed till the pups are born. The study has proceeded 'forward', and the observer is 'looking forward' to the outcome. This study is, therefore, called forward looking and 'prospective'. When the pups are born, all are examined for *T. canis* infection (contracted from the mother). The data are tabulated, as in Table 6. The incidence of *T. canis* infection in pups born of infected bitches and also non-infected bitches are calculated as $a/a + b$ and $c/c + d$, respectively. The two rates are compared. The relative risk is calculated. The relationship between the attribute under study and the outcome is established. Further, a statistical test, chi-square (X^2), is applied, and a statistically significant association, too, is confirmed. *The essence of this study is that cohorts possessing and not possessing the attribute under study are selected and followed till the outcome.*

The prospective cohort study is time-consuming, expensive, and beset with certain limitations. Diseases with low incidence would require a selection of a large number of cases. Chronic, rare, and slow-developing diseases would require a long period of follow-up and are associated with dropouts and the aging of cases from the cohort. Nonetheless, this method provides a direct measure of relative risks, is more accurate, and is less prone to bias.

In case records of a past epidemic (historical) are available and information about the 'exposure, *i.e.*, the attribute/factor' and the disease happen to be recorded, a cohort study can be carried out. There is no need to follow up prospectively. It saves time, which otherwise would have been required for selecting a sampling frame as well as study and comparison cohorts and for waiting till the outcome. It maintains the *essence of the prospective study*, although it is historically retrospective as the event has already occurred in the past. Since a 'past epidemic' is being investigated, it is also called 'retrospective prospective study' (note it sounds contradictory). It takes less time and is less expensive but can be used for rare diseases as records are already available for analysis.

11.5.2.2 Case-Control Study

This type of study uses the subjects selected on the basis of their having (cases) or not having (control) the outcome or disease. These groups are then compared in order to find out the differences in exposure affecting the outcome or disease. Case-control studies are inherently retrospective and, thus, inexpensive and fast. They are useful in the study of rare diseases since the cases and controls are already there. The hypothesis that 'Pups born of *T. canis* infected pregnant bitches get infected' can be tested by a 'case-control' study also. The observer has to select newly born *T. canis* infected pups. These are called 'cases' ($a + c$). Suitable matching 'controls' are selected. These should be pups of the same (matching) age and not infected with *T. canis* ($b + d$). Now, the mothers of the cases and controls are studied; that is, records of their being infected with *T. canis* during their pregnancy are studied. The infected and non-infected are distributed ($a + b$ is distributed into 'a' and 'b'; $b + d$ are distributed into 'b' and 'd') so as to prepare a 2 × 2 table. The rates of attribute in the 'cases' ($a/a + c$) and 'controls' ($b/b + d$) groups are calculated and compared. Thus, RR = 30/35 divided by 20/65 = 39/14 = 2.78. The relationship between the attribute and the disease is established.

It is obvious that the approach is indirect. A case (the outcome or the effect of the attribute is already manifested) is followed up backwards to trace the factor/attribute. Therefore, the study is also called 'retrospective'. The case-control study is most common as it is easy (the manifestation of the factor is visible, unlike the invisible factor in the cohort study), economic, less time taking, and less cumbersome. The value of the RR obtained is usually low. The measurement is indirect only, and the study is prone to suffer from 'bias'. It is, therefore, suggested that the case-control study is taken up first, followed by the cohort study.

The merits and demerits of the two methods have been compared in Table 11.2.

11.6 Exercise: Study the Attributes of a Herd Disease

Objective: To study the distribution of the disease in time and space and formulate a hypothesis.

Table 11.2 Comparison of the cohort and case-control methods of study

Cohort study	Case control study
Cumbersome	Simple
Difficult	Easy
Less convenient	More convenient
Large number of subjects required	Less number of subjects required
Less prone to bias	Prone to bias
Direct estimates of risk available, both *RR* and *AR* can be calculated	Indirect estimates only, *RR* can be calculated
More accurate	Less accurate
Longer time taking	Less time taking
Useful for acute diseases, difficult with chronic and slowly developing diseases, and not practical for infrequent diseases	Useful for acute, chronic, and slowly developing diseases; also practical for infrequent diseases
Compares a group or cohort exposed to/possessing a suspected cause with a cohort that is not exposed to/possessing that cause	Compares individuals with disease (cases) with those without the disease (healthy/not down with the same disease, i.e. control)
Tests if the frequency of disease is more in the group possessing the suspected cause than in the group not possessing the suspected exposure	Tests if the frequency of the suspected cause among the cases is more than among the controls
Prospective study	*Retrospective study*
Cohort is drawn from a population sampling frame. Hence, results can be generalised. The subjects of study are followed, and the outcome (disease) is recorded; i.e., incidence rates are recorded	A reference population/population at risk is not available; hence, neither incidence nor prevalence rates can be calculated. Results are difficult to generalise

Table 11.3 Observed and expected cases

	Number of cases observed on days of the week					
Class	1	2	3	4	5	6
Observed cases	0	0	10	8	0	0
Expected cases	0	0	0	0	0	0

From the following data on the distribution of disease X in time and space, plot the epidemic curve and distribution in spaces and match them with the geographical map/road of the area.

Logically explain the disease distribution. Comment on the possible cause, origin, and spread of disease × through the information given in Tables 11.3 and 11.4 and Fig. 11.2.

A. Epidemic of X disease.

Table 11.4 Outbreaks of X disease observed in different farms and the source of feed supply

Feed supplier	A	B	C	D	E	F	G	H	I
1	+	+	+		+		+		
2				–		–		–	–

Disease X was reported from farms A, B, C, E, and G. Feed was supplied to these farms by supplier 1. Farms D, F, H, and I received feed from supplier 2

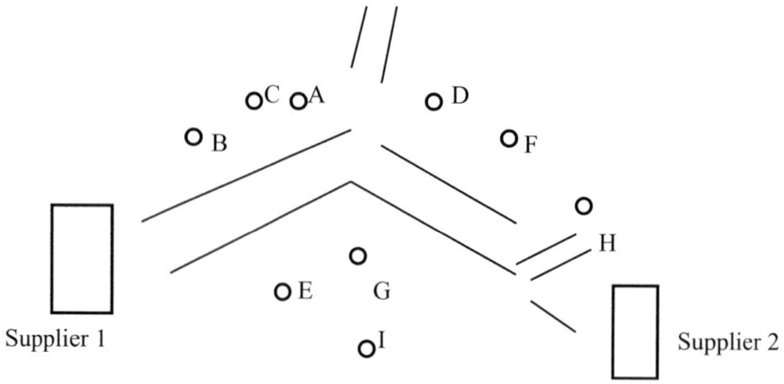

Fig. 11.2 Road map and distribution of farms

Reference

Centers for Disease Control (1986) Comprehensive plan for epidemiologic surveillance. Centers for Disease Control, Atlanta, Ga, USA

12 Sampling Techniques

Sampling is a statistical method to select a subset or sample from a population for the purpose of making certain observations to draw inferences regarding the population under study. It is difficult to study an entire population for an attribute, say a disease condition. Reducing the number of individuals in any study reduces the cost, time, and workload, besides providing high-quality information that can be extrapolated for the entire population. At times, it becomes difficult to locate and/or reach the entire population. Therefore, a representative group of individuals, i.e. a sample, is selected from the population to make any observation and analysis. It is of utmost importance that the sample is a true representation of the population so that the inferences arrived at after analysis can be applied to the population from which it has been drawn. Any bias leading to improper/non-representative drawing of the sample will give a result that cannot be applied to the population under study. Using sampling techniques eliminates any bias in choosing the subset.

Sample: it is a subgroup of individuals drawn from a population to estimate the characteristics of the entire population (Fig. 12.1).

Target Population: it is the population at risk about which information is to be generated and applied.

Study population: it refers to the population from which a sample is drawn.

Sampling frame: it is a list of all the members/sampling units of a study population (e.g. student roster, list of phone numbers, stock register of a farm).

Sampling unit: it pertains to each member of the sampling frame (e.g. household, dairy farm).

Observational unit: it is the element to be measured (e.g. individual people in the household, individual cow in the dairy farm).

Stratum: it refers to a group of elementary units having a common characteristic, like age, breed, or body weight.

Sampling fraction: it is the ratio of the sample size to the population size; e.g., out of 900 cows, 30 are drawn as samples, in this case the sampling fraction will be $30/900 = 0.033$.

K. G. Narayan et al., *Veterinary Public Health & Epidemiology*,
https://doi.org/10.1007/978-981-19-7800-5_12

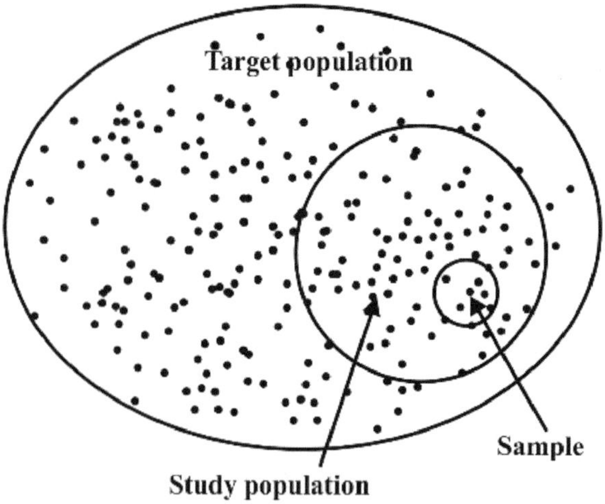

Fig. 12.1 Target and study population and sample

Table 12.1 Difference between probability and non-probability sampling

Factors	Probability sampling	Non-probability sampling
Sample frame	Necessary	Not necessary
Sampling unit information	Each unit identified	Details on the habits, activities, traits, etc. required
Sampling skill	Required	Little skill required
Time required	More time	Less time
Cost per unit sampled	Medium to high	Low
Estimates of population parameters	Unbiased	Biased
Representativeness	Good and assured	Suspect and undeterminable
Accuracy and reliability	High	Unknown
Sampling error measurement	Statistical measures available	No true measures available

Sampling technique: depending upon the use of random selection, the sampling technique is of two types:

(i) **Probability sampling**: this is a sampling method that uses random selection; therefore, all units in the population have an equal chance/probability of being chosen.
(ii) **Non-probability sampling**: in this method, the selection of the sample unit is dependent on the choice of the investigator (Table 12.1).

12.1 Classification

A. **Probability sampling technique**: it may be of four types:
   1. Simple random
   2. Systemic
   3. Stratified random
      (a) Proportionate
      (b) Disproportionate
   4. Clustering
      (a) One stage
      (b) Two stage
      (c) Multi-stage

B. **Non-probability sampling**: it may be of six types:
   1. Convenience
   2. Quota
   3. Purposive
   4. Snowball
   5. Volunteer
   6. Sequential

12.2 Probability Sampling

Simple random sampling: when a population is small, homogeneous, and readily available, then simple random sampling is feasible. First of all, a sampling frame enlisting each unit/element of the population should be prepared. The sample selection is made with the help of either a 'table of random numbers' or a 'lottery system'. This technique is easy to use and does not need prior information about the population. However, this method is impracticable when the sampling frame is large.

Whether the selected unit is replaced or not, the simple random sampling technique is of two types:

i. **Simple random sampling with replacement**: the unit selected at any particular draw is replaced in the population before the next draw.
ii. **Simple random sampling without replacement**: here, the unit selected at any particular draw is not returned to the population before the next draw.

For example, in a calf unit of a dairy farm, we draw a calf, measure the body weight, and immediately return it to the calf unit before drawing the next calf; this is with a replacement design. Here, one might end up catching and measuring the same calf more than once. However, if we do not return the calf, then it is without a replacement design.

Systemic sampling: first of all, the unit/element of the study population is arranged following some ordering scheme and then the unit/element is selected at regular intervals based on that ordered list. Systematic sampling involves a random start and then proceeds with the selection of every n^{th} (n = sampling interval) element from then onwards. It is more common in production units for quality control. Suppose we have 200 cows and the sampling interval decided is 8. Now, arrange cows serially, then by lotterymethod first cow selected is number 7, then the next cow at number 15 has to be selected, followed by 23 and so on.

The advantages of this method are as follows: the sampling frame can be made easily, the sample unit is evenly spread over the entire reference population, and the sample is easily selected, which is cost-effective too. The disadvantages are the following: if hidden periodicity in a population coincides with that of selection of sample, it results in biasness; here each element does not have equal chance to get selected, and there is ignorance of all elements which fall between sampling interval.

Stratified random sampling: in a stratified random sample, the study population is divided into exclusive groups/strata based on common characteristics, e.g. breed, herd, body weight, milk yield, gender, socio-economic status, nationality or geographical regions, etc., and then the sampling unit is randomly selected from all individual strata. The advantages of this method are as follows: control of sample size in strata, the provision of data to represent and analyse subgroups, the use of different methods in strata, and increased statistical efficiency. The disadvantages are increased error if the subgroups are selected at different rates and that if the strata of the population have to be created, it would be expensive.

Based on the proportionate share of each stratum to the total population, stratified random sampling can be as follows:

a. **Proportionate stratified sampling**: here, the sample from each stratum is drawn in proportion to its share in the total population.
b. **Disproportionate stratified sampling**: when representation is not given to strata according to their share in the total population that results either over-representation to some strata or under-representation to other, while sampling.

Clustering sampling: based on geography/place/location contiguity, population is divided into many clusters; from which using random technique clusters are selected. All observations in the selected clusters are included in the sample. This method requires a sampling frame on a cluster level. Here, the variability within clusters is maximum but is minimum between clusters. Basically, cluster sampling is an example of *two-stage sampling*. In the first stage, a sample of areas is chosen, and in the second stage, a sample of respondents within those areas is selected. Here, the sampling units are groups rather than individuals.

Advantages: if properly carried out, cluster sampling provides an unbiased estimate of population parameters. It is more economic, easier, and more efficient than simple random sampling.

Disadvantages: Since clusters/subgroups being homogenous rather than heterogenous which results in lower statistical efficiency, higher standard errors and provide less information per observation than simple random sampling.

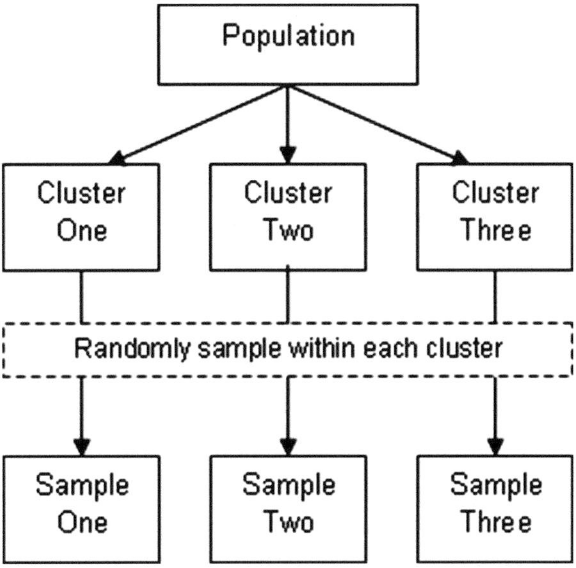

Fig. 12.2 Multi-stage clustering sampling

In *multi-stage clustering sampling*, the sample is selected in various stages, but only the last sample of subjects is studied.

In *multi-phase sampling*, the process is the same as in multi-stage clustering sampling, but here, each sample is adequately studied before another sample is drawn and all samples are researched (Fig. 12.2).

12.3 Non-probability Sampling

Convenience sampling: Non-probability sampling is also known as convenience/grab/opportunity/accidental/haphazard sampling because the selection is based on ease of accessibility and proximity to the researcher; therefore, the samples are biased and least reliable, though it is the cheapest and easiest method. Examples of this include informal pools of relatives, friends, and neighbours; people responding to an advertised invitation; and 'on the street' interviews.

Quota sampling: it is based on 'quota' fixed by the researcher or as per their proportion in the target population regarding demographics, attitudes, behaviours, etc. The samples drawn contain specific subgroups in the desired proportions, which reduces biasness. It is an easy and quick method. Since sample selection depends on subjective decisions, which may be biased, it is therefore not possible to generalise.

Purposive sampling: this is also known as *judgmental selection* because the average of the selected sample's quantitative characteristics (e.g. weight) or the distribution of qualitative characteristics (e.g. sex and breed) is similar to those of the target population. Although sample selection is based on an experienced individual's belief, biasness cannot be ruled out.

Volunteer sampling: here, the respondent/individual himself volunteers to be the unit of sample to provide information, e.g. vaccine or pharmaceutical trials.

Snowball sampling: when it is difficult to gain access to the population, this technique is applied. The contact with an initial group is used to communicate with others and so on; thus, this method is also called *chain referral sampling*. It is useful in qualitative research. However, the sample selected will not be representative of the population, which leads to biasness.

Sequential sampling: here, the researcher picks a single or group of subjects in a given time interval, conducts his study, analyses the results, then picks another group of subjects if needed, and so on.

12.4 Steps in Random Sampling

1. Define the target population.
2. Specify the sampling unit.
3. Prepare the sampling frame.
4. Select the sampling method.
5. Determine the sample size.
6. Select the sample.

Statistical and non-statistical deliberations have an impact on the sample size. Statistical considerations include the desired precision of the estimate of prevalence and the expected frequency of the disease, while non-statistical deliberations include the availability of manpower and sampling frames.

12.5 General Rules on Sampling

1. A smaller percentage is required for a larger population.
2. Studies using a population of less than 100 should use the entire population.
3. A population of approximately 300 requires a sample size of 50%.
4. A population of over 100,000 would require only 384 individuals in the sample.
5. The higher is the level of confidence, the larger is the sample size.
6. More the absolute precision desired, larger the sample size.

12.6 Sample Size for Different Types of Studies

(a) Experimental studies: at least 30 individuals in each group.
(b) Correlational study: minimum of 30 number of individuals in each sample.
(c) Descriptive study: based on a 95% level of confidence with 5% desired absolute precision; the sample size will be given in Table 12.2.

Table 12.2 Sample size of different populations

Population	Sample size	Population	Sample size	Population	Sample size	Population	Sample size
10	10	60	52	150	108	2000	322
20	19	70	59	200	132	5000	357
30	28	80	66	300	169	10,000	370
40	36	90	73	500	217	50,000	381
50	44	100	80	1000	278	100,000	384

12.7 Exercise

12.7.1 Selection of Population for Study and Methods of Sampling

Objective: Selection of suitable population, sampling frame, strata, and subjects for epidemiological studies.

12.7.2 Surveillance and Monitoring

Techniques for collecting quality information at minimal cost within the limitations of developing countries have been developed. These are taken from ADMAS-technical Bulletin-2 (2000). Information will provide the following, and these in turn will enable the formulation of selective/strategic/smart and efficient disease control programmes:

- Identify the diseases existing in the country.
- Determine the level and location of diseases.
- Set priorities for disease control.
- Plan, implement, and monitor disease control programmes.
- Respond to disease outbreaks.
- Meet the reporting requirements of the Office International des Epizooties (OIE).
- Demonstrate disease status to trading partners.

12.7.3 Definitions (as per OIE)

Surveillance refers to (continuous) investigation programmes executed in a given population *to detect the occurrence of disease for control purposes*, which may involve the testing of a part of the population.

Monitoring pertains to ongoing programmes aimed at the *detection of changes in the prevalence* of disease in a given population and in its environment.

Surveillance may be 'active' and 'passive'.

An active surveillance system is a structured disease survey to collect high-quality information quickly and inexpensively. Its advantages include as follows: (a) problems of under-reporting are avoided, (b) it represents the true disease situation in a population, and (c) information is collected from known population size, and hence the calculation of disease rates and proportions is possible and can be related to the population.

A passive surveillance system is such in which no active effort is made; e.g., a Subdivisional Animal Husbandry Officer waits for the disease report to reach his office. The report is then passed on to the District A.H. Officer, who then transmits the same to the directorate. The report is compiled and sent to the central authority. A national-level report is thus prepared. The quality of the report is such that it has limited utility, for example (a) it meets the basic requirements of the OIE, (b) it responds to the outbreak of a disease, and (c) it identifies the presence and location of a disease. Passive surveillance reports are not useful for meeting all the requirements of the 'Disease monitoring and surveillance' listed above.

12.7.4 Disease Survey

12.7.4.1 Explanation of Certain Terms of Interest

Survey: it gathers reliable information quickly and inexpensively. Trained persons examine a small proportion of the population, called a sample. The survey involves the examination of a small group (a sample) of elements (unit of interest) drawn from all the elements of interest (the population).

Inference: it is the process of estimating the true value of the disease status of the population based on the results observed in the sample. Inference runs a risk of error. This can be minimised by taking/examining a 'representative sample'. A 'representative sample' has to be chosen (selected) and must be similar to the population. The selection of a sample systematically different from the population introduces a 'selection bias'.

Bias: this is the difference between the average estimate from the survey and the real value in the population. It is caused by a systematic error, which means the same type of error in each observation, e.g. measuring with a defective scale.

Random sampling: it means that every element (unit of interest) in the population has the same probability of being selected in the sample. It is the only way of selecting a representative sample.

Estimates; sample characteristics are attributed as population characteristics and are reported as 'population estimates'.

Sample size: it is the number of animals selected in the sample. The larger is the sample, the more precise are the results.

Confidence interval: it measures the precision of the estimates. A confidence interval indicates how close the estimates are to the real population. It also states how confident the experimenter is that his estimates are correct. A 95% confidence interval indicates that one is 95% sure that the true population value lies within a 95% confidence interval.

The results of survey II are more dependable (Table 12.3). Repeated survey yield results that differ slightly each time. This difference is called 'random error' and if the differences are small, the random error is low and results are considered precise. A large sample size yields low random errors and precise results.

Table 12.3 Illustrative example: results of surveys I and II with two different sample sizes

Survey no.	Sample size	Prevalence (estimated)	Per cent confidence interval
Survey I	20	75%	51–91%
Survey II	200	75%	73–77%

In case the results of repeated surveys are always different from the true value by about the same amount and in the same direction, the error is called 'systematic error', and the results are biased.

12.7.4.2 Random Sampling Techniques

- Physical randomisation uses dice and black cards.
- Random numbers use a random number table or are computer aided. Random numbers have been so generated that for each digit, the chance of it being any number between 0 and 9 is the same.
- Systematic sampling is used when individuals can be organised in some order and making a list of individuals and numbering them is difficult. It involves selecting individuals in some defined order, e.g. every tenth individual. The animals are confined in a yard and allowed one by one. Every tenth is selected. Ten is called the sampling interval. The number of animals selected in this way, say 25, becomes the sample size (stop the selection once the sample size is achieved).
- Probability proportional to size sampling (this will be explained later).

12.7.4.3 Sampling Frame

Every unit of interest in the population has the same chance of getting selected in the case of random sampling. Prepare a list of units of interest in a population, and using a random table, make a random selection. A random list of units of interest is thus obtained. This is called a sampling frame. It should contain every unit of interest in the population. Properties of a good sampling frame are the following: (a) no unit of interest is omitted, (b) no unit of interest is duplicated, and (c) every unit of interest is uniquely identified. Things making up a population, cattle, buffaloes, human beings, etc. are units of interest. Additional information available with sampling frames is also useful, e.g. 'village' as a sampling frame, with information about villages in that area, the population of animals, etc.

In the absence of a 'sampling frame', one can

- Build a sampling frame.
- Perform two-stage sampling.
- Do random geographic coordinate sampling.

Building a sampling frame (of animals in a village): list and identify every animal in the village. One may conduct a census by visiting each house, which will take too much time, and a chance of missing some animals is there. Alternatively, one may conduct an interview with the villagers/livestock owners, asking them the number of animals they have. Use this information to make a 'sampling frame'. An interview enables one to collect other related information, for example about the outbreak. It is possible to explain the purpose of the interview and seek cooperation and participation. For example, (a) ask them the number and species of animals they possess, (b) ask if any livestock owner is not attending the meeting, and (c) inquire from those present and make a group estimate of the animals kept by the absentees. Continue till it is ascertained that none is missed.

Table 12.4 Data recording sheet

Sl. no.	Name of the owner	Cattle	Buffalo	Total	Cumulative total	Random no.	Selected
1	A	5	–	5	5	3	3
2	B	2	3	5	10		
3	C	–	4	4	14	12	2
4	D	8	2	10	24	17, 20	3, 6
...	...	...	...	...	...	...	...
24	ZX	5	3	8	118		

Table 12.5 Animal identification number (ID no.)

Serial 1, A					Serial 2, B					Serial 3, C			
1	2	3	4	5	6	7	8	9	10	11	12	13	14

Serial 4, D									
15	16	17	18	19	20	21	22	23	24

The list thus prepared is the 'sampling frame'.

In selecting the 'number' of animals, a random number table or computer may be used.

When using a random number table, use the following as guides.

The cumulative total in the data-recording sheet (Table 12.4) represents the identification number of each animal in a village. The animal number in Table 12.4 at Sl. no. 1,A, has animals with ID Nos. 1–5, the owner 2, B, has animals with ID No. 6–10 and like this (Table 12.5).

With a random number table, pick 20 random numbers, which must be between 1 and 118, i.e. the total number of animals in the village/sampling frame. For purposes of demonstration, let us pick number 12. Search ID No. 12 from the Animal ID No. and locate its owner. In the above example, the owner is at Sl. No. 3, C. Record this in the data-recording sheet.

How is animal No. 12 identified? Owner No. 3 has four animals: 11, 12, 13, and 14. Animal 12 is the second animal of owner C. Record this (2) in the last column—'selected'—of the data-recording sheet.

Repeat the above steps till the required number of animals (20) is selected. If the same animal is selected twice, discard and select another random number.

The animal owner is asked to count loud all the animals he has. The owner has thus assigned the temporary number himself. Check which number is required, and then proceed for examination (clinical)/collecting specimen (e.g. serum).

Two-Stage Sampling

Stage 1. A group of animals (e.g. a number of cattle farms/villages) is selected. The 'unit of interest' is the farm/village, and the 'population' is all the farms/villages in the country.

Stage 2. Individuals are selected from the selected group. The 'unit of interest' is cattle and the 'population' of the cattle in each selected farm/village.

At each stage, the sample is selected by random method. Stratification can be used, especially at the first stage, e.g. stratifying farms/villages by size or districts. In the second stage, create a sampling frame of cattle in each selected village through interviews, as above.

This method is simple, easier, and more practical. However, results may not be as precise as those obtained by simple random sampling, and analysis is complicated.

Random Geographic Coordinate Sampling

This is a method used when it is not possible to create a sampling frame. For example, the goat population is mobile, and so records of 'unit of interest' are not available. Infrastructure may also not be available.

Stratification

It is useful and becomes a necessity in some situations. Stratification by states provides estimates for the whole population and also for the states. It is convenient. The workload gets distributed. It may provide more precise results (a) if the animals selected within each stratum are as similar as possible with respect to the characteristic in question, (b) if animals in different strata are as different as possible with respect to the characteristic in question, and (c) the distribution of characteristics in the population is unknown. Stratification of the factor linked to the characteristic will help increase precision.

Probability Proportional to Size Sampling (PPS)

The chance of a unit of interest being selected is proportional to some measure of the unit of interest's size. For example, a survey of districts in a large state uses PPS to select districts based on their village population. The population in this case is from all the districts in the state. The unit of interest is district. Records of the total number of villages in each district are collected and used as a sampling frame. Districts with a large number of villages have more chances of being selected than districts with a small number of villages. The procedure is as follows.

Pick up a random number representing a village and select the district that contains the village.

The total number of villages in the four districts of the state is 594 (Table 12.6), assuming that the above represents the entire population of districts in the state. A number between 1 and 594 is selected, say 256. Searching down the list, the second district contains the number 256. This district will be included in the sample. Continue until the required number of units of interest has been selected.

Table 12.6 Probability proportional to size sampling

Name of district	Size of unit of interest (number of villages)	Cumulative total of villages
X	232	232
Y	89	321
Z	144	465
Q	129	594

Reference

ADMAS Technical Bulletin No. 2. Compiled by Rajashekhar M, Sudhindra, Yathinder PV, Gangadhar NL, Isloor S, Suresh KB, Renukaradhya GJ, Veere Gowda BM, Gowda L, Nagaraju NR, T. R. Nagaraja, Mohan P. PD-ADMAS, Bengaluru. 2000

13 Measurement of Causal Association

There is a causal association between an agent (a factor/attribute) and a disease (effect). In biological science, this association has to be biologically feasible. It is not sufficient that the association is statistically significant. It has to be logical. Chance, bias, and confounding associations have to be excluded. The common criteria are as follows:

Time sequence: cause precedes effect.

1. Dose-response: when increasing the dose, severity increases, and the reverse is also true.
2. The presence of cause and effect is there: remove the cause, and the effect vanishes.
3. The association fits into the logical and prevalent theories/concepts.
4. The strength of the association between cause and effect—(relative risk).
5. Similarity/consistency with results in other similar studies: an example is variant Creutzfeldt-Jakob disease (vCJD). Pathological brain lesions in mad cow disease/ bovine spongiform encephalitis (BSE) in bovines and humans with vCJD are similar. But the oral route of transmission in humans could only be 'a probability', unlike the 1987 BSE epidemic, which was thought to be associated with the use of a dietary protein supplement and meat and bone meal (MBM) of infected carcasses of other cattle (Wilesmith et al. 1991). This 'plausible association' was later found to be true, and BSE was finally controlled by banning the use of ruminant proteins as cattle feed. It was concluded that the human epidemic was related to the bovine epidemic and was caused by the same infective agent—prion. Policies were amended with respect to blood donation and the use of disposable surgical instruments.

The example given in Table 13.1 also illustrates an *experiment*. Two groups of pregnant bitches are selected. One group is infected with *T. canis*. The other is not, and this serves as the control group. Both are observed till pups are born. The pups

K. G. Narayan et al., *Veterinary Public Health & Epidemiology*,
https://doi.org/10.1007/978-981-19-7800-5_13

Table 13.1 Relationship between *Toxocara canis* infection in pregnant bitches and its infection in neonates

		Prenatal infection of pups		
Group	*T. canis* infection in pregnant bitches	Present	Absent	Total
A	Present (stool +)	a (30)	b (20)	$a + b$ (50)
B	Absent (stool −)	c (05)	d (45)	$c + d$ (50)
Total		$a + c$ (35)	$b + d$ (65)	$a + b + c + d$ (100)

are examined for *T. canis* infection. The infected and non-infected ones are counted, and the incidence rates in both groups are calculated. The status of infection of the 100 bitches is known only to the experimenter. The administration of infection to bitches is done in a way that the administrator is unable to make out which bitch received infection and which received *placebo*. In the case of human volunteer experiments, the volunteers do not know this. This is called a double-blind technique. The observer of the pups also does not know which of the pups are born of the experimental group and which are born of the control group. The experiment is, thus, more stringent and free from bias.

13.1 Risk and Its Measurement

The measurement of risk can be made in terms of strength, effect, and total effect. The measures of strength are relative risk (RR), population relative risk (RR_{pop}), odds ratio (OR), and population odds ratio (OR_{pop}). The measures of the effect of the factor are attributable rate (AR), attributable fraction (AF), and estimated AF. The total effect of the factor can be measured by population attributable rate (PAR), population attributable fraction (PAF), and estimated population attributable fraction.

13.2 Measures of Strength

13.2.1 Relative Risk

It is the ratio of incidence in exposed and unexposed groups, i.e. $\{a/(a + b)\}/\{c/(c + d)\}$. It is expressed in times. If RR is >1.0, then the attribute in question does have a causal association. With the values of RR 1 or less, the causal association is not inferred. RR is not applicable to case-control studies.

As per Table 13.6, the incidence of prenatal toxocariasis in pups born of infected bitches is $a/a + b = 30/50$.

The incidence of prenatal toxocariasis in pups born of non-infected bitches is $c/c + d = 5/50$.

Then $RR = (30/50)/(5/50) = 0.6/0.1 = 6$.

Inference: The chances of prenatal toxocariasis in pups born of infected bitches are six times more than the pups born of non-infected bitches.

13.2.2 Odds Ratio (OR)

This is the ratio between the odds of a disease. The odds that cases were exposed can be calculated by the 'probability that cases were exposed' divided by the 'probability that cases were not exposed', i.e. $[(a/a + c)]/[(c/a + c)] = a/c$.

The odds that controls were exposed can be calculated by the 'probability that controls were exposed' divided by the 'probability that controls were not exposed', i.e. $[(b/b + d)]/[(d/b + d)] = b/d$.

Therefore, the odds ratio $= (a/c)/(b/d)$ or ad/bc.

As per Table 13.1, (30 × 45)/(20 × 5) or 13.5.

Inference: The prenatal toxocariasis may occur 13.5 times more in pups born of infected bitches (exposed) than pups born of non-infected bitches (non-exposed).

The *RR* and *OR* values should be nearly equal. Imagine in the above table if 'a' = 2, the total $a + b = (2 + 48)$ tends to be equal to 'b' = 48. Similarly, if 'c' is =1, then the total $c + d = (1 + 49)$ tends to be equal to 'd' or 49. Then $RR = 2$ and OR = 2.04. The odds ratio is applicable in all study types.

13.2.3 Population Relative Risk (RRpop)

It is only used in cross-sectional studies and calculated using the formula $\{(a + c)/n\}/\{c/(c + d)\}$.

As per Table 13.1, (35/50)/(5/50) = 0.7/0.2 = 3.5.

Inference: The rate of toxocariasis in neonatal pups is increased 3.5 times because of *T. canis* infection in bitches.

13.2.4 Population Odds Ratio (ORpop)

It is only used in cross-sectional studies, or if controls are representative of a non-diseased population, then in case-control studies also. It can be calculated using the formula $\{d \times (a + c)\}/\{c \times (b + d)\}$.

Putting the value from Table 13.1, 45 × 35/5 × 65 = 1575/325 = 4.85.

Inference: The rate of toxocariasis in neonatal pups is increased by 4.85 times because of *T. canis* infection in bitches.

13.3 Measures of Effect

13.3.1 Attributable Risk

It is also known as attributable difference or absolute difference and attributable proportion (describing the difference in relative terms). It is not applicable to case-control studies. It is the absolute difference between the incidence of disease in the 'exposed' and the incidence of disease in the 'unexposed'. It is useful in cross-sectional studies when the morbidity in a population is known; data on prevalence rates are available.

$$AR = a/(a+b) - c/(c+d)$$

As per Table 13.1, (30/50) – (5/50) or 0.6 – 0.1 = 0.5 or 50 per 100.

Inference: The rate of toxocariasis in neonatal pups that may be attributed to *T. canis* infection in bitches is 50 per 100.

A positive risk difference value indicates that exposure is associated with disease, while a negative risk difference value indicates that exposure is not associated with disease.

13.3.2 Attributable Fraction (AF)

It is the proportion of incidence in exposed animals attributable to exposure to risk. It can be calculated by either of the two formulae given below:

(i) $RR - 1/RR$, i.e. 6 – 1/6 or 5/6 or 0.83 or 83%.
(ii) $AR/\{a/(a+b)\}$ = 0.5/(30/50) or 0.5/0.6 or 0.83 or 83%.

Inference: 83% of toxocariasis in neonatal pups is attributable to *T. canis* infection in bitches.

13.3.3 Estimated AF

It is calculated by the formula $(OR - 1)/OR$. After putting the value from Table 13.1, (13.5 – 1)/13.5 = 0.92 or 92%.

Inference: 92% of toxocariasis in neonatal pups is attributable to *T. canis* infection in bitches.

13.4 Measures of Total Effect

13.4.1 Population AR (PAR)

It is the excess risk of disease in the total population attributable to exposure. It helps in determining exposures relevant to public health in the community. It can be calculated by either of these two formulae:

(i) $\{a + c/n\} - \{c/c + d)\}$
(ii) $\{a + b/n\} \times AR$.

The first formula is the difference between the incidence of disease in the total population and the incidence of disease in the unexposed group.

So, (35/100) − (5/50) or 0.35 − 0.1 = 0.25 or 25 per 100

As per the second formula, $(a + b/n) \times AR$, i.e. (50/100) × 0.5, or 0.5 × 0.5 = 0.25 or 25 per 100.

Inference: The rate of toxocariasis in neonatal pups that may be attributed to *T. canis* infection in bitches is 25 per 100; i.e., we would expect the rate of toxocariasis in neonatal pups to decrease by 25 per 100 if bitches were not infected with *T. canis*.

13.4.2 Population Attributable Fraction (PAF)

It can be calculated by either of the below two formulae:

i. $PAR/\{(a + c)/n\}$ or 0.25/(35/100) = 0.25/0.35 = 0.71.
ii. $(RR_{pop} - 1)/RR_{pop}$, i.e. (3.5 − 1)/3.5 = 2.5/3.5 = 0.71.

Inference: 71% of toxocariasis in neonatal pups is attributable to *T. canis* infection in bitches.

13.4.3 Estimated PAF

It can be calculated using the formula $(OR_{pop} - 1)/OR_{pop}$, i.e. (4.85 − 1)/4.85 = 3.85/4.85 = 0.79.

Inference: 79% of toxocariasis in neonatal pups is attributable to *T. canis* infection in bitches.

13.5 Relationship Between AR and RR

AR can be expressed as *n* terms of *RR*. $AR = (RR - 1) \times \{(c/c + d)\}$ or (6 − 1) × {5/50} or 5 × 0.1 = 0.5.

RR can be measured from any of the main types of study. It is fairly consistent in a wide range of populations. It is independent of *AR*. *RR* is more valuable than *AR*. However, attributable risk provides a better indication than the relative risk of the effect of a preventive campaign, which removes the factor.

13.6 Statistical Association

The observed association between the attribute under study and the disease is subjected to statistical test(s) to determine if the observed association is significantly independent of or dependent upon each other. The commonly used statistical tests are chi-square, correlation analysis, regression analysis, and multivariate analysis. The general formulae are as follows

13.6.1 Chi-Square

The *chi-square* is used to test the independence of attributes. It is calculated using the formula.

$$X^2 = \frac{O - E}{E}$$

where $O =$ observed frequency of the event (disease) and $E =$ expected frequency of the event (disease). The proportion of pups that were infected = total infected/ universe (N) or $(a + c)/(a + b + c + d)$ or 35/100. This applied to the population (n), or the group possessing the attribute $(a + b)$ will give the expected value for 'a'. Once 'a' is determined, the rest in the 2 × 2 table can be determined as follows: 'b' $= (a + b) - a$; 'c' $= (a + c) - a$; and 'd' $= (b + d) - b$. Otherwise, the expected values are calculated as per the formulae given below:

$$E \text{ for } a = \frac{(a+b)(a+c)}{N} \text{ or } \frac{(30+20)(30+05)}{100} \text{ or } 17.5$$

$$E \text{ for } b = \frac{(a+b)(b+d)}{N} \text{ or } \frac{(30+20)(20+45)}{100} \text{ or } 32.5$$

$$E \text{ for } c = \frac{(c+d)(a+c)}{N} \text{ or } \frac{(05+45)(30+05)}{100} \text{ or } 17.5$$

$$E \text{ for } d = \frac{(c+d)(b+d)}{N} \text{ or } \frac{(05+45)(20+45)}{100} \text{ or } 32.5$$

The total population is normally indicated by N. The following table (Table 13.2), similar to the one above, is remade.

Apply the formula

Table 13.2 The observed and expected frequencies of disease (toxocariasis in pups) according to the study attribute

T. canis infection in mother bitches	Toxocariasis in pups		Total	Groups
	Present O (E)	Absent O (E)		
Present	30 (17.5)	20 (32.5)	50	A
Absent	05 (17.5)	45 (32.5)	50	B
Total	35	65	100	

$$X^2 = \frac{O-E}{E} \quad \text{or} \quad 8.98 + 4.80 + 8.98 + 4.8 = 27.456$$

The value is compared with the probability/test of significance table at one degree (the 2 × 2 table has a degree of freedom equal to 1) of freedom.

The *chi square* distribution

P	0.1	0.5[a]	0.01	0.005[b]	0.001	0.0001	0.00001	0.000001
X^2	2.71	3.84	6.64	7.88	10.83	15.19	19.51	23.92

[a]Any value >3.84 is considered significant; i.e., chance occurs five times in 100

[b]Any value >7.88 is considered highly significant; i.e., chance occurs five times in 1000

In the present case, the pups born of *T. canis* infected pregnant bitches get infected *by chance* will have a probability of even <1 in 106 as the calculated value 27.456 is >23.92 the tabulated value.

The association is highly significant and hence cannot be independent but dependent.

Yates correction for significance is applied for the estimation of *chi-square* only in case the value of N is up to 40 and the expected frequency is less than 5. However, many authors agree that Yates correction may be applied even if no theoretical cell frequency is less than 5 (Gupta and Kapoor 2000).

$$X^2 = \frac{N\{(ad - bc) - N/2\}^2}{(a+b)(c+d)(a+c)(b+d)}$$

Instead of the expected values, the observed values are used in the above formula. Therefore,

$$X^2 = \frac{100\{(30 \times 45 - 20 \times 05) - 100/2\}^2}{50 \times 50 \times 35 \times 65} \text{ or } \frac{100\{(1350 - 100) - 50\}^2}{5{,}687{,}500} \text{ or }$$

$$\frac{144{,}000{,}000}{5{,}687{,}500} \text{ or}$$

25.31

The observed value of 25.31 is >23.92. The inference is the same as above.

13.6.2 Correlation Analysis

The relationship between the attribute under study and the disease is established by this analysis. It also helps in determining that a change in the attribute also influences the change in the pattern of occurrence of disease. The co-efficient of correlation 'r' is determined. The value of 'r' varies between +1 and − 1. If the attribute has a definite influence on the disease, a value of 'r' up to +1 is obtained. Higher values indicate a stronger correlation. A negative value (−1 or up to −1) would indicate that an increase in attribute would decrease disease occurrence.

$$r = \frac{ad - bc}{(a+b)(c+d)(a+c)(b+d)} = \frac{X^2}{n}$$

13.6.3 Regression Analysis

The relationship between the attribute under study (x) and the disease (y) can also be obtained through regression analysis. The values of attribute x are predetermined and so are called independent variables, and the values of y (i.e. disease) is dependent and so are called dependent variables. The regression of 'y' on 'x' is determined. The regression values are indicated by estimating the 'coefficient of regression' (b). Precaution against 'bias' is taken. Knowledge of regression to the mean is essential.

13.6.4 Multivariate Analysis

The relationship between several variables, r factors, may be established by using this method. Path analysis, factor analysis, and discriminant analysis also determine the relationship among various factors associated with disease occurrence. For example, studies on hydatidosis used path analysis.

13.7 Synergy in Multifactorial Causation of Diseases

If two or more risk factors acted together (synergistically), independently in exposed persons/population. The answer may be found following the method presented by Cole and MacMahon (1971). It is possible to compute the attributable risk percentage for persons or populations exposed to a suspect aetiological/risk factor using data from case-control studies. Accordingly, when estimates of absolute disease frequency are available, the attributable risk percentage among the exposed is determined as follows:

Table 13.3 Several measures of bladder cancer risk according to single and multiple exposure categories, men aged 20–89

High-risk occupation[a]	Cigarette smoking[b]	No. of cases	No. of controls	Relative risk (*RR*)	Estimated annual rate/10^5	Attributable annual rate/ 10^5	*RR* – 1
No	No	43	94	1.0	20.3	0	0
No	Yes	173	189	2.0	40.6	20.3	1.0
Yes	No	26	20	2.84	57.7	37.4	1.84
Yes	Yes	111	72	3.37	68.4	48.1	2.37
Total		353	375	–	41.8	–	–

[a]*Yes = has ever worked in an industry shown in this study to be associated with increased risk*
[b]*Yes = has smoked at least 100 cigarettes in his life*

$$\text{Ae\%} = (\text{Re} - \text{Ro})/\text{Re} \times 100\% \text{ and } \text{Ae\%} = R - 1/R \times 100\%$$

where Ae % is the attributable risk percentage among the exposed, Re = absolute risk among the exposed, Ro = absolute risk among the unexposed, and R = relative risk.

They used the following data (Table 13.3) to validate the utility of the method.

The attributable risks are excess relative risks and are additive, unlike relative risks. The excess of disease among persons exposed to multiple factors may be caused by each of the factors operating independently. The tabulated data show this in the last column (*RR* – 1), and attributable risk is shown in the last but one column. The excess relative risks 2.37 (observed) is compared to the 2.84 (1*plus 1.84) expected, and the observed attributable risk 48.1 is compared to the 57.7 expected.

The two exposures (smoking and occupation) do not act synergistically.

Simple additivity of excess risks implies that the different factors belong to the same constellation* of the causes of disease; i.e., they are indicative of the type of multiple causalities in which different constellations of causes are producing manifestations, which if not identical are not distinguishable on the basis of current knowledge.

*Constellation = a set of/group of. For example, *Mycobacterium tuberculosis* (the agent and its attributes are constellation 1) affects lung tissues of humans (host's attributes—constellation 2) working in silica mines (environmental factors—constellation 3). Thus, each factor, i.e. agent, host, and environment, has its own constellation which functions as disease determinant. *M. tuberculosis*, say the MDR strain, caused tuberculosis in those working in silica mines as miners (and not as clerks). Alteration in this 'interacting basic constellation' may change the effect/outcome, e.g. 'miners working with mask or other protective device' may not get the MDR-TB

Synergism may suggest that different factors are part of the same constellation of causes that are responsible for a common single final mechanism for the induction of the manifestations. This stems from (a) the logarithmic form of many dose-response curves and (b) the supposition that the two independent factors may be acting as a single factor or that one of the factors increases the availability of the other. In each case of promoting we find, the logarithmic increase in response to an arithmetic increase in dose e.g., age at risk and occupation (butcher/vet) are independent factors, but one is promoting the other (a child cannot be working as a butcher or a vet).

13.8 Exercise

13.8.1 Estimation of Risk: Calculation of *RR, AR,* and *OR*

Objective: Establishing a causal association between attribute and disease.

While going through the reports on foot and mouth disease (FMD) epidemics during 1999 in villages and farms in and around Patna, you came across certain interesting recorded events. A summary of the same is tabulated below (Table 13.4).

You have read that FMDV has been recovered from the nasal mucosa of human beings attending clinical cases of FMD for 28 h after contact

1. Formulate your hypothesis
2. What is the method of the formulation of hypothesis you used?
3. Calculate *RR* and *AR*.
4. Calculate X^2 to determine statistical association.
5. Which type of observational study is this and why?
6. Suggest how to control FMD and how to prevent it in future.

13.8.2 Determination of Additivity/Independence of Factors Causing Disease

Objective: When it is observed that two factors are operative, it is desired to determine whether they have additive effects.

Table 13.4 Observation of two farms—A and B—under the same establishment

Class	Farm A	Farm B
Number of cattle in all age groups	600	750
Number of FMD vaccinated	300	650
Number of unprotected	(600 − 300) = 300	(750 − 650) = 100
Animal attendants	20	25
Incidence of FMD	60% (180 cases)	10% (ten cases)
In the attendants' village, there was an FMD epidemic; four attendants owned FMD-infected animals during the same period	They attended to the animals	No such attendant attended to the animals

Table 13.5 Observation in two farms—A and B—under the same establishment

Class	Farm A	Farm B
Number of cattle in all age groups	400	500
Number of FMD vaccinated	200 with one case of FMD	400 with one case of FMD
Number of unprotected	(400 – 200) = 200	(500 – 400) = 100
Animal attendants	20	25
Incidence of FMD	60% (120 cases/ 200 unvaccinated)	10% (10 cases/100 unvaccinated)
In the attendants' village, there was an FMD epidemic; four attendants owned FMD-infected animals during the same period	They attended to the animals	No such attendant attended to the animals

Using the recorded observation in Table 13.4, with modifications tabulated (Table 13.5), determine the additive effect of the 'absence of vaccination' and 'exposure to vector attendant'.

The factors affecting FMD incidence are (a) the status of the animals with respect to vaccination against FMD and (b) exposure to farm attendants who owned and attended to FMD cases in their respective homes. Study the data in the table above. Following combination of risk factors, cases and healthy (i.e. not ill animals) can be made out:

- Farm B has 400 animals for which risk no. 1, viz. vaccinated, is absent, so risk is absent, and so also risk no. 2, viz. exposure to vector attendant, is absent (risks 1 and 2 absent).
- Farm A has 200 animals for which risk no. 1 is absent, viz. vaccinated, and so risk is absent BUT risk no. 2 is present; viz., exposure to animal attendants is acting as vectors (risk 1 absent, risk 2 present).
- Farm B has 100 animals for which risk no. 1 is present, viz. unvaccinated, BUT risk no. 2, viz. exposure to vector attendant, is absent (risk 1 is present and risk 2 absent).
- Farm A has 200 animals for which risk no. 1 is present, viz. unvaccinated, and also risk no. 2 is present; viz., exposure to animal attendants are acting as vectors (both risks 1 and 2 are present).

Relative risk for animal attendant acting as a vector of FMD in the unvaccinated group of animals = 120/200 divided by 10/100 = 6.

Relative risk for animal attendant acting as a vector of FMD in the vaccinated group of animals = 1/400 divided by 1/200 = 2.

If risks 1 and 2 were operating independently, the risk of having both exposures (87.56) should have been the sum of the risk for 1 and risk for 2, viz. 0.037 + 14.56 (Table 13.6). The two factors do not seem to be operating synergistically/additively. This indicates that these belong to different constellations

Table 13.6 FMD in farms A and B (same establishment) according to the risk of being unvaccinated and exposed to vector attendants

Risk 1 (un-vaccinated)	Risk 2 (vector attendant)	Cases	Comparison	Total	Incidence	Relative risk	Estimated rate in %	Attributable rate in %	*RR* − 1
Absent	Absent	1	399	400	0.0025	1	0.0365	0	0
Absent	Present	1	199	200	0.005	2	0.073	0.037	2–1 = 1
Present	Absent	10	90	100	0.1	40	14.6	14.56	40–1 = 39
Present	Present	120	80	200	0.6	240	87.6	87.56	240–1 = 239

13.8.3 Evaluation of an Intervention Measure

Objective: Application of the epidemiologic method in the evaluation of intervention measures

1. The evaluation of a new vaccine or chemoprophylactic/chemotherapeutic agent requires that the trial be double blind. Selection of a population and the precise parameters of measurements are required.
2. Design an experiment for the trial of a recent drug (X) against theileriasis.
3. Design a field trial of a molluscicidal agent, 'Y', in the control of liver fluke.
4. Design a field trial of a recent vaccine, 'Ab', against brucellosis.
5. This practical also explains 'experimental epidemiology'.

Steps in the study are taken from MacMahon and Pugh (1970).

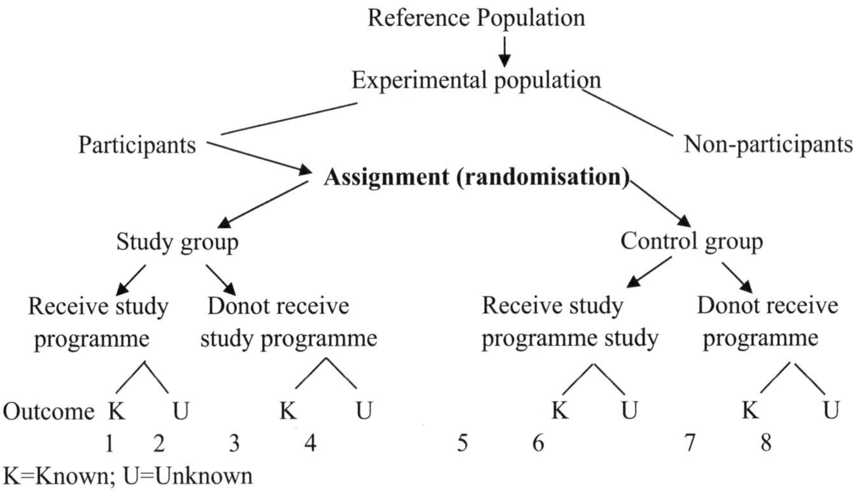

The study group is administered the 'study programme/intervention measure'; the control group is administered a 'placebo'.

The 'reference population' may be universal (benefits of the study applicable to all—mankind), restricted to certain regions/cultural groups, or limited to certain ages/sex, etc., to which the results are going to be applied.

The experimental population is the actual population on which the experiment/study is to be conducted. It should have demographic attributes similar to the reference population. It should be accessible and convenient for the study, providing certain medical resources, etc. The disease in question must be prevalent. The higher the incidence, the smaller size of the experimental population may be adequate for the study. Take the help of statisticians to decide the sample size for the study. It is dependent upon the estimated incidence of the disease, the estimated difference the 'intervention measure' is likely to bring about, and the degree of confidence (say 95%) desired. It is advisable to enlist much more than the statistically defined size of the population for the study for various reasons, such as to account for many dropouts during the course of the study.

The participants in the study need to be explained about the study, its purpose, the procedure, and its possible advantages and dangers, if any. These participants should be representing the reference population in respect of demographic attributes. The participants are randomised and assigned into study (experimental) and control groups. Systematic (sampling) selection is not recommended. An alternative method is to 'randomise' the 'intervention programme'. The assignment has to be 'double blind'. The study staff and recipient of the 'intervention programme' must not know 'what is administered' till the outcome is recorded. The 'vaccine vial' and the 'placebo vial' are indistinguishable apparently. The epidemiologist alone can de-codify and identify. If the disease in question varies appreciably between sexes, ages, etc., select the strata (particular age group/sex) for obtaining study and control groups that are equally distributed with respect to such variables. Randomisation within the strata should be done prior to the assignment of individuals. This is also called 'blocking'. This increases efficiency in calculation.

The study requires a 'follow-up', which may be of short or long duration, depending upon the expected outcome. The observer does not know which group to which the participant belonged—experimental or control. In order to overcome the difficulty arising out of dropouts and also the possibility of 'stopping' the study prematurely, a 'sequential design' may be planned. In this case, the entry of participants in the study, the administration of the programme, and the recording of observation are concurrently done.

Analysis requires the comparison of the outcome of the study between the experimental and control groups. An ideal comparison is 1 + 3 versus 5 + 7 in the above outline.

References

Cole P, MacMahon B (1971) Attributable risk percent in case-control studies. Br J Prev Soc Med 25(4):242–244. https://doi.org/10.1136/jech.25.4.242

Gupta SC, Kapoor VK (2000) Fundamentals of Mathematical Statistics. 10th Revised Edition. Sultan Chand & Sons, New Delhi

MacMahon B, Pugh TF (1970) Epidemiology—Principles and Methods. Churcill/Livingstone, London

Wilesmith JW, Ryan JB, Atkinson MJ (1991) Bovine spongiform encephalopathy: epidemiological studies on the origin. Vet Rec 128:199–203

14 Investigation of an Outbreak

The definitions of outbreak and epidemic are more or less the same. An outbreak of a disease is limited or localised to a smaller geographic area, like a village, town, or closed institution (e.g. hostel, farm, prison). However, when the magnitude of the disease involves wider geographic areas, even beyond one district, then it is called an epidemic. The investigation of an animal disease outbreak/epidemic requires teamwork, where the veterinarian's role is to report the occurrence, mobilise and educate the community, and assist and advise the municipal/district/animal husbandry authorities in carrying out appropriate control and preventive measures. The procedure depends upon the objective of the investigation, the availability of the resources, and the facilities and tools for investigation. The most common objectives of any disease outbreak investigation are to identify

i. The causal factor(s) of the disease.
ii. The origin of these factor(s) and.
iii. The mode of disease transmission/spread.

The information obtained after the investigation will help develop appropriate managemental measures to prevent and control the occurrence of the disease in future.

Theoretically, the investigation of an outbreak starts with descriptive epidemiology, which helps in the formulation of a causal hypothesis, followed by analytical epidemiology, to evaluate the proposed hypothesis, and if it is found sound, then it can be proved by experimental epidemiology, report writing, and submission. The step-wise description of the entire exercise can be as below

K. G. Narayan et al., *Veterinary Public Health & Epidemiology*,
https://doi.org/10.1007/978-981-19-7800-5_14

14.1 Descriptive Epidemiology

1. First of all, the disease should be defined, which means the characteristic signs and symptoms are seen in the diseased animals, the case histories of the affected animals are obtained on an individual basis, the cases and controls (not affected) among the affected population are identified, and the source (factors) of exposure is determined. A good case definition will help in the identification of the animals inflicted with the primary disease under investigation as well as in excluding those that are healthy or may be sick but from an unrelated disease. Clinical and morbid samples are collected from the diseased as well as healthy animals for laboratory tests to further confirm the diagnosis.
2. It is essential to confirm whether it is an epidemic. That means the number of animals affected must be more than what is expected normally. For this, the frequency of disease (prevalence) in the affected population should be compared with a similar group of animals under similar conditions or with the previous year's prevalence. First, a count of the affected animals and the total number of animals at risk is obtained to calculate the attack rate (AR) for the population under investigation, which is compared to the attack rate in other similar populations in the previous year to confirm the outbreak/epidemic. If it is an outbreak/epidemic, then it should be determined whether it is point or propagative. The pattern of the disease is described on the basis of collected and collated information.
3. The distribution of the disease in relation to time (temporal distribution), i.e. days, months, seasons, lactation number, stage of lactation, and relationship with calving or weaning time or the time of change of pasture, feed, shed, vaccination, and therapy, needs to be established.
4. Likewise, the distribution of the disease to space (spatial distribution) should be established, i.e. related to a particular herd, flock, pen, shelter, village, district, etc. The role of farm management practices in the causation of the disease should be critically examined.
5. The demographic distribution, i.e. whether the disease affects animals of a particular age, sex, species, and breed, needs to be determined. The addition of new animals or the temporary/permanent withdrawal of an animal from a herd, vaccination, dipping, and particular therapy have significant roles in the causation of the disease.
6. The role of collateral factors like water, feed (grass, roughage, concentrates, etc.), vectors, air (ventilation), biological factors, and drugs should be examined. Sample of feed, water, as well as vector specimens should be taken to confirm their role in the disease causation.

14.1.1 Formulation of Hypothesis

On the basis of the information collected, under descriptive epidemiology, a causal hypothesis should be formulated, which should be appropriately one or two, not more, which will help in easily identifying the cause. The steps and the points for consideration are as follows:

1. Necessary preliminary evaluation of data for (a) reliability, accuracy, and freedom from bias, as well as (b) statistical validity.
2. Analogy and its dangers.
3. Statistical association: (a) common factor(s) of agreement—(i) qualitative agreement and (ii) quantitative agreement, also called concomitant variation; (b) factors of disagreement; and (c) statistical association vs. causal relationship.
4. Exploitation of unusual opportunities: (a) incubation period, (b) period of communicability, and (c) exception to the general rule.
5. The problem of mixtures: (a) simultaneous occurrence of multiple diseases, (b) multiple cases of the same disease, and (c) multiple manifestations of the same disease.

14.1.2 Evaluation of Hypothesis

1. The value of the hypothesis is inversely related to the number of acceptable alternatives. Inconsistencies between what is actually found and the expectation of what will be found based on a hypothesis may be due to (a) multiple causes, (b) crudity of the disease classification used, and (c) errors of observations.
2. New hypotheses to be formed may be evaluated in the light of clinical, pathological, and laboratory observations.
3. The stronger a statistical association is, the more useful it is as a basis for a hypothesis.
4. A change in the frequency of a specific disease over a period of time may be one of the variables that most support a hypothesis.
5. An isolated or unusual case may offer a clue to the hypothesis.
6. Depending upon the result, the hypothesis may be accepted or rejected. If rejected, another hypothesis is explored by re-examining the collected data.

14.2 Analytical Epidemiology

Observational studies are designed for testing the hypothesis to draw out the relationship between the occurrence of the disease and the factors related with the host, environment, etc.

1. Disease distribution in time.
2. Disease distribution with respect to the distribution of susceptible hosts.
3. Distribution of cases with respect to the distribution of possible vectors/sources, etc.
4. Calculation of rates among those exposed and those not exposed to determine causal relationship: for example, if the attack rate of diarrhoea is high in the groundnut-cake-fed group (exposed) and low in those not-fed-GN-cake group (non-exposed), groundnut cake (factor) is more likely to be the cause of the

diarrhoeal outbreak. It is particularly helpful to calculate the difference between the attack rates for exposed and non-exposed groups.

14.3 Experimental Epidemiology

This is optional. It may not be possible in all cases to conduct an experiment. Most epidemiological studies end at the analytical level because it may not be possible to conduct an experiment on the population. Simulated experimental studies can be conducted in the laboratory on laboratory animals. The trial of vaccines/drugs in a population is often carried out under experimental epidemiology. The experiment has a strength that no observational/analytical studies can match.

14.4 Report Writing and Submission

A detail report should be prepared step by step, incorporating data analyses, photographs, laboratory test results, maps, charts, and experimental findings, and based on the findings, appropriate measures should be recommended to prevent future outbreaks. The report should be submitted to concerned authorities for implementation and communicated through media to make the public at large aware. The report will be a part of the veterinary record and a useful educational tool for livestock owners, veterinary students, and practitioners.

An investigation of an outbreak of *Salmonella choleraesuis* in a pig farm (Choudhury et al. 1982) covers most of the steps/procedures stated above. A case is defined at the beginning of an investigation for syndromic surveillance. The following is an example from the article 'Outbreak of Rift Valley Fever—Saudi Arabia, August–October, 2000' (https://www.cdc.gov/mmwr/preview/mmwrhtml/mm4940a1.htm).

14.5 Exercise

14.5.1 Investigation of Food Poisoning Outbreak

Objective: Learn how to investigate an outbreak.

Students are expected to learn the following:

- Cause (attribute) and effect (disease) relationship.
- Calculation of the incubation period.
- Calculation of the duration of the disease.
- Frequency of symptoms.
- Application of the strategies of epidemiology.

On 22 May 2001, the Infectious Disease Hospital in the city reported that a large number of cases of suspected food poisoning have been admitted. The hospital has sought help in investigating this outbreak.

1. *Descriptive epidemiology*: collect all relevant information/data on the food poisoning.
2. Verify and establish the existence of an outbreak.
3. *Formulate a hypothesis* regarding the possible association of food with the outbreak.
4. Collect information and tabulate it to calculate the incubation period and frequency distribution of the salient symptoms and signs of the disease.
5. *Analyse.* Tabulate the distribution of cases in time and plot. Analyse the incubation period, signs, and symptoms and draw an analogy with known food poisoning to draw a hypothesis and continue further investigations, such as interviews with cases and others sharing the exposure, tabulating and calculating food-specific attack rates and their combination, and collecting specimens for laboratory diagnosis and dispatch. Attempt to trace the source of contamination.

14.5.1.1 Observation, Analysis, and Inferences

The number of admissions with symptoms of nausea and vomition on the night of 22–23 May 2001 was 91.

This far exceeded the number of cases with similar symptoms admitted during the previous four weeks. This verifies and established the existence of an outbreak.

All 91 cases were *similar/related* and admitted during less than 24 h (22nd, night, to 23rd, morning). This plotted on a graph presents a 'holomiantic epidemic curve' and fits into the definition of an outbreak. The pattern of the epidemic is explosive and suggestive of exposure to a single common factor/source, i.e. food.

An outbreak is defined as an episode in which two or more cases of the same disease have some relationship to each other. The relationship may be between 'the time of onset, the place where food is eaten, persons' age, sex, occupation, ethnic group, food preference, food ingestion history. A food borne outbreak is such an episode in which there was an exposure to a common food containing pathogen/toxin/poisonous substance.

A sporadic case is a case of specific disease that is unrelated, as far as is known, to any other case of that disease.

Attack rate is a kind of incidence rate in which the period of risk is limited. The etiologic factor operates for only short time or the risk is restricted to certain group (say certain age group, e.g., *imperforate anus, cleft palate) so that even extended period of observation does change the number of cases.*

Menu for the four parties was different. There were common items.

The victims and those attending them were approached. One of the four parties, party B, cooperated. The data so collected were tabulated (Tables 14.1, 14.2, 14.3, 14.4, and 14.5) as follows.

Table 14.1 Food-specific attack rate

	Those who ate				Those who did not eat				
Food item	Ill	Not ill	Total	%	Ill	Not ill	Total	%	Difference
Soup	20	15	35	57.1	15	10	25	60	−2.9
Pulao	5	30	35	14.2	3	2	5	60	−45.8
Chicken curry	31	19	50	62.0	5	5	10	50	+12.0
Paneer butter masala	20	30	40	50	11	9	20	55	−5.0
Ice cream	*39*	*11*	*66*	*59*	*0*	*10*	*10*	*0*	*+59.0*

Table 14.2 Modified figures of Table 14.1 for two items

	Those who ate				Those who did not eat				
Food item	Ill	Not ill	Total	%	Ill	Not ill	Total	%	Difference
Chicken curry	31	22	53	56.6	10	13	23	43.5	+13.1
Ice cream	39	27	66	59	2	8	10	20	+39.0

Table 14.3 Food combination attack rate

		Chicken curry Who ate Who did not (B) eat (A–B)			Total (A)
Ice cream	Who ate	Ill	31	8	39
		Not ill	22	5	27
		Total	53	13	66
		Percent	56.6	61.5	59
	Who did not eat	Ill	0	2	2
		Not ill	0	8	8
		Total	0	10	10
		Percent	0	20	20
	Total	Ill	31	10	
		Not ill	22	13	
		Total	53	23	
		Percent	56.6	43.5	

Table 14.4 Incubation period

Party	Time of admission of cases	Time dinner was served	Difference = incubation period
A	11:30 pm–2:00 am	8:30 pm	3–5.5 h
B	11:30 pm–3:30 am	9:30 pm	2–6 h
C	1:30 am–5:00 am	11:00 pm	2.5–6 h
D	2:30 am–5:30 am	12:30 am	2.0–5.30 h

The food-specific attack rate for those who ate ice cream was 59.0% compared to 0 for those who did not eat it. Therefore, the responsible food item seems to be ice cream.

In order to learn how to overcome the confounding situation, let us assume the following figures for chicken curry and ice cream.

Table 14.5 Frequency of the signs and symptoms observed in 50 cases

Signs and symptoms	Number (50)	Percent
Nausea and vomition	48	96
Headache and giddiness	20	40
Diarrhoea	8	16
Abdominal pain	6	12
Fever	1	2

Table 14.6 Duration of illness

Duration in hours	Number (91)	Cumulative number
0–6	1	0
7–12	30	31
13–18	50	81
19–24	8	89
>24	2	91

Note that those who ate ice cream alone and fell sick (A–B) had an attack rate of 61.5%.

The time dinner was served was 8:30 p.m. for party A, 9:30 p.m. for party B, 11:00 p.m. for party C, and 12.30 a.m. for party D. The time of admission of each case is taken from the admission register. The difference indicated the incubation period (Table 14.4).

Now use the method of analogy to formulate your hypothesis about the cause of 'food poisoning'.

The short incubation period, symptoms, and duration suggest a similarity with food poisoning due to staphylococcal enterotoxin.

Accordingly, specimens of the suspected food item and vomitus need to be sent to the laboratory for laboratory diagnosis, indicating therein that the specimen be examined for *Staphylococcus aureus* and its enterotoxin, besides other pathogens.

14.5.2 Searching Causal Factor

Objective: Learning steps in investigating an outbreak.

A hypothetical situation in a pig farm introduced an infection. A large number of young piglets fell sick. The outbreak continued, causing heavy mortality until the investigation identified the cause and implemented measures of control.

Symptoms observed were diarrhoea, high rise of temperature, and subcutaneous haemorrhages located specially on the hind legs and mostly the inner side. Initially, death occurred in three to four days. The recovery was slow, except for those given high doses of antibiotic chloromycetin. Pigs older than 240 days were not affected.

Post-mortem pathology: carcasses showed mainly septicaemia, petechiae on mesenteric lymph glands, 'turkey egg' kidneys, lesions in the intestines, and ulcers.

Calculate the attack and death rates, feed (item)-specific attack and death rates, and age-specific attack and death rates from the following tabulated (Tables 14.7 and 14.8) data.

Table 14.7 Observed illness and death in different age groups

	40–80 days			81–120 days			121–160 days			161–200 days			201–240 days		
Feed item	ate	ill	dead	ate	ill	dead	ate	ill	dead	ate	ill	dead	ate	ill	dead
Wheat bran ++	50	15	08	50	16	10	50	10	08	50	06	03	50	05	02

++A combination of wheat bran, ground nut cake, and fish meal was fed

Table 14.8 Results of experimental feeding

Feed item	40–80 days			81–120 days			121–160 days			161–200 days			201–240 days		
	ate	ill	dead	ate	ill	dead	ate	ill	dead	ate	ill	dead	ate	ill	dead
Ground-nut cake	50	02	0	50	02	0	50	02	0	50	01	0	50	0	0
Fish meal	50	15	10	50	20	15	50	10	06	50	08	04	50	06	01

The group fed with wheat bran and the control group fed with decontaminated feed (autoclaved feed) did not show any sickness and/or deaths.

What is your tentative diagnosis? Identify the determinant of the disease. Calculate the strength of the association of the determinant with the disease.

Reference

Choudhury SP, Singh SN, Narayan KG (1982) Outbreak of *salmonella cholerae suis* infection in a pig farm. Indian J Anim Sci 52(10):910–915

15 Diagnostic Test and Its Evaluation

A disease has multidimensional impacts on animal husbandry; therefore, an early, quick, and accurate diagnosis of the disease is essential. A diagnostic test helps in making a decision to start or withhold treatment or cull the animal. At the herd level, a diagnostic test helps in measuring the frequency and distribution of the disease, which in turn enables formulating prevention and control strategies. It is necessary to understand the difference between screening and diagnostic tests. A screening test is used to detect the diseased in an apparently healthy population and should be easy to conduct. A screening test begins with presumably healthy individuals while a diagnostic test with diseased individuals. A diagnostic test is used to distinguish between animals that have the disease in question and those that have other diseases on a differential list (White 1986). The diagnostic test is usually applied after an animal is found positive through a screening test. Depending upon the nature of the population used to standardise the test and disease prevalence, a test may be used as screening or diagnostic. Test results may be interpreted and expressed as positive or negative (nominal scale), strong or weak positive (ordinal scale), or titre (interval scale).

The term 'gold standard test' is used for a diagnostic test which gives the true disease or health status, e.g. the isolation and identification of causative organisms like *Brucella* spp. in brucellosis, post-mortem examination, biopsy, etc. It functions as a quality control device. It provides the basis for determining the value of other diagnostic tests, treatment strategies, and prognoses. Gold standard test means the best available test under reasonable conditions. For example, for a brain tumour diagnosis, magnetic resonance imaging (MRI) is considered the gold standard test, though biopsy is superior to MRI. Since the sensitivity and specificity of MRI are not 100%, therefore, it is called an 'imperfect gold standard' or 'alloyed gold standard' (Spiegelman et al. 1997).

Except for the gold standard test, none of the tests is perfect; therefore, evaluation of tests is essential. The merit of a diagnostic test depends on its reliability and validity. The following properties of a diagnostic test are used for evaluation.

K. G. Narayan et al., *Veterinary Public Health & Epidemiology*,
https://doi.org/10.1007/978-981-19-7800-5_15

Table 15.1 2 × 2 Contingency table

Test result	Disease/infection Present	Absent	Total
Positive	a	b	$a + b$
Negative	c	d	$c + d$
Total	$a + c$	$b + d$	$a + b + c + d$ (n)

Table 15.2 Analytical sensitivity of a few serological tests

Test	Protein (μg/mL)
Gel diffusion	30
Ring precipitation	18
Bacterial agglutination	0.05
Complement fixation	0.05
Passive haemagglutination	0.01
Haemagglutination inhibition	0.005
Immunofluorescence	0.005
ELISA	0.0005
Bacterial neutralisation	0.00005

15.1 Properties of Diagnostic Test

15.1.1 Reliability

When a test produces similar results when repeated, it is reliable. It is measured in terms of the following:

(a) **Repeatability**: it is the degree of agreement between the sets of observations made on the same animal/sample by the same observer.
(b) **Reproducibility**: it is the degree of agreement between the sets of observations made on the same animal/sample by different observers; i.e., the test must produce identical results on repeated trials by different workers. Its precision value must be high.

15.1.2 Validity

If a test measures what it seems to measure, it is valid. The indicators of validity are sensitivity and specificity, which are the absolute properties of a test. For example, in the case of diabetes, validity increases as one goes for physical examination > urine analysis > blood analysis. With the help of a 2 × 2 contingency table, the sensitivity and specificity of a test can be measured (Table 15.1).

(a) **Sensitivity**
   i. **Analytical sensitivity**: it is the ability of a test to detect very small amounts of antibodies or antigens. The analytical sensitivity of a few serological tests used for antibody detection is given in Table 15.2.

ii. **Diagnostic/clinical sensitivity**: it is the ability of a test to give a positive result if the patient has the disease (no false negative result). It is expressed in per cent (%).

$$\text{Diagnostic sensitivity} = \frac{\text{True positive}}{\text{Total positive}} \times 100$$
$$= \frac{a}{a+c} \times 100$$

(b) **Specificity**

i. **Analytical specificity**: it is the ability of a test to detect a substance (e.g. antibody) without interference from cross-reacting substances.

ii. **Diagnostic/clinical specificity**: it is the ability of a test to give a negative result if a patient does not have a disease (no false positive result).

$$\text{Diagnostic specificity} = \frac{\text{True negative}}{\text{Total negative}} \times 100$$
$$= \frac{d}{b+d} \times 100$$

(c) **Predictive value**: it is the probability that a test result reflects the true disease status. Predictive value is the relative property of a test because it depends upon sensitivity, specificity, and the prevalence of disease in a herd/population. The sensitivity and specificity of a test are innate characteristic that is why fixed means does not change at defined cut-off point but prevalence of a disease in a population being tested will affect the predictive value of test. Even high sensitivity and specificity are not expected to make a dramatic improvement in predictive value.

i. **Positive predictive value**: it is the probability of disease in an animal with a positive test result. A highly specific test improves the positive predictive value; i.e., it gives fewer false positive results. A lower prevalence of disease results in a lower positive predictive value.

$$= \frac{\text{True positive}}{\text{Test positive}} \times 100$$
$$= \frac{a}{a+b} \times 100$$

ii. **Negative predictive value**: it is the probability that an animal does not have the disease when the test result is negative. A highly sensitive test improves the negative predictive value of the test; i.e., it gives fewer false negative results. A lower prevalence of disease results in a higher negative predictive value.

$$= \frac{\text{True negative}}{\text{Test negative}} \times 100$$
$$= \frac{d}{c+d} \times 100$$

15.1.3 Accuracy

It is an indication of the extent to which a test conforms to the truth, i.e. able to detect the true morbidity levels in herds. Accuracy expresses the overall performance of a diagnostic test. Factors influencing accuracy are cross-reactivity, inhibitory substances, and agglutinins, which yield false positives or negatives.

$$\begin{aligned}\text{Accuracy} &= \frac{\text{True positive} + \text{True negative}}{\text{Total sample tested}} \times 100 \\ &= \frac{a+d}{n} \times 100\end{aligned}$$

15.1.4 Likelihood Ratio

This is the measure that can summarise a test performance if a given result is observed.

(a) **Likelihood ratio for a positive test result**: it is the ratio of the likelihood of a positive result in patients with the disease to the likelihood of a positive result in patients without the disease, which can be calculated by the formula:

$$\text{Sensitivity}/(1 - \text{Specificity})$$

(b) **Likelihood ratio for a negative test result**: it is the ratio of the likelihood of a negative result in patients without the disease to the likelihood of a negative result in patients with the disease, which can be calculated by the formula:

$$(1 - \text{Sensitivity})/\text{Specificity}$$

An ideal test would have a likelihood ratio of 'infinity' (100%/0%) for a positive test and a likelihood of '0' (0%/00%) for a negative test.

15.1.5 Multiple Testing

Since none of the serological tests has 100% sensitivity or specificity, therefore to arrive at a clinical diagnosis and herd testing, more than one test is used. Multiple tests are done either in parallel or serially.

(a) **Parallel testing**: this is when two or more tests are conducted on a sample/animal simultaneously and the sample/animal is considered to be diseased if found positive to any of the tests. Therefore, parallel testing increases the sensitivity and predictive value of a negative test result. Here, the chances of missing the disease are minimised, but the chances of a false positive diagnosis are increased.

(b) **Serial testing**: here, tests are conducted sequentially based on previous test results; i.e., only those samples/animals that are positive in the first test results are tested by a second test and so on. Only those samples/animals positive to all tests are declared diseased. Therefore, serial testing increases the specificity and predictive value of a positive test result. The first test used in serial testing must have the highest specificity to minimise the number of samples/animals tested further.

15.1.6 Concordance

It is the proportion of all test results on which two or more different tests agree. However, with an increase in the number of different tests applied to the same sample, there is a decrease in the likelihood of an agreement between all tests.

$$\text{Concordance } (\%) = \frac{\text{Sample positive in both tests} + \text{Sample negative in both tests}}{\text{Total number of samples tested}} \times 100$$

15.1.7 Selection of Cut-Off Point

Selection can be made in several ways and must take into consideration the distribution of results in two different populations, i.e. normal and diseased; the prevalence of the disease in the population to be tested; and, most importantly, the cost of false negative and false positive test results. The most common approach is to take two or three standard deviations greater than the mean of the test values of known negative samples or unaffected animals, depending on the prevalence of the disease in the population under consideration. The optimum cut-off point also depends on the frequency distribution of the test variables in healthy and diseased populations. However, when a cut-off point is determined, there is usually an inverse relationship between the sensitivity and specificity of a particular test. An increase in the cut-off point leads to an increase in specificity and a decrease in sensitivity and vice versa.

15.1.8 Receiver-Operator Characteristic (ROC) Curve

A ROC curve is one of the ways to compare diagnostic tests, which is nothing but a plot of the true positive rate (sensitivity) on the vertical or *Y* axis against the false positive rate (1 − specificity) on the horizontal or *X* axis. A ROC curve indicates

- The relationship between sensitivity and specificity. For example, an increase in sensitivity results in a decrease in specificity and vice versa.

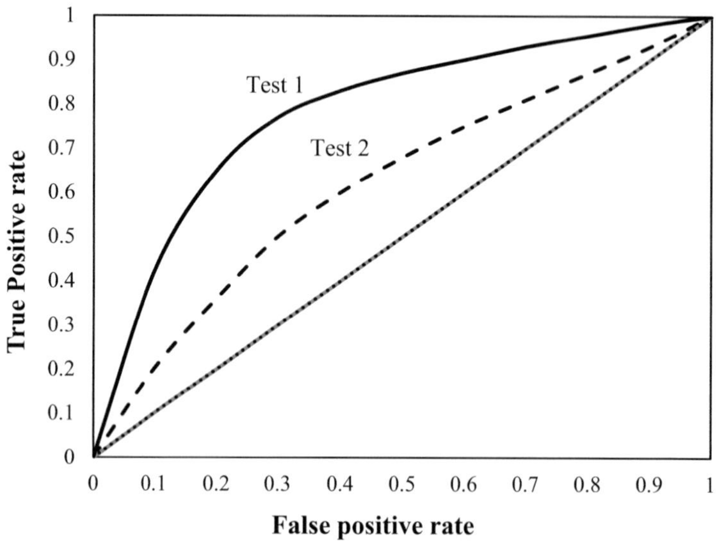

Fig. 15.1 ROC curve

- Test accuracy: if the graph is closer to the top and left-hand borders, the test is more accurate, and if the graph is closer to the diagonal, the test is less accurate. Therefore, for a perfect test, the graph would go straight from 0 up the left corner and then straight across the horizontal axis. Test accuracy is also represented as the area under the curve. A more accurate test has a greater area under the curve. A perfect test has an area under the ROC curve of 1.

The ROC curve helps in the determination of the optimum cut-off value. The ROC curve is a series of likelihood ratios corresponding to each cut-off value. As likelihood ratios are independent of disease prevalence, the ROC curve is a standard way to evaluate test performance (Greiner et al. 2000; Hajian-Tilaki 2013). A graph showing the ROC curves of two tests is illustrated in Fig. 15.1. Test 2 is closer to the diagonal; therefore, it is less accurate than Test 1.

15.2 Exercise

15.2.1 Validity of Screening Test

Objective: To evaluate a sero-diagnostic test for its suitability for use in an epidemiological study.

Pullorum testing has been used in screening poultry for the prevalence of pullorum disease. A drop of a pullorum antigen is mixed with a drop of blood taken from the wing vein of a bird on a glass slide. The immediate appearance of agglutination is diagnostic of pullorum disease. In this experiment, a 'pullorum test' was carried out on 200 birds. All the birds were sacrificed. A thorough post-mortem pathology, followed by a bacteriological examination, was done. There were 110 birds from which *Salmonella pullorum* was isolated. These were, therefore, considered to be 'true positive'. The remaining 90 birds did not show any lesion of pullorum disease, and no *Salmonella* was isolated. These were considered to be 'true negative'. The 'pullorum test' was able to detect 100 of the 110 'true positives' and 85 of the 90 'true negatives'.

Calculate the sensitivity, specificity, and positive and negative predictability of the pullorum test. Which of the two—higher 'sensitivity' or higher 'specificity'—would you prefer and why? What are the other parameters of the screening test?

References

Greiner M, Pfeiffer D, Smith RD (2000) Principles and practical application of the receiver-operating characteristic analysis for diagnostic tests. Prev Vet Med 45:23–41

Hajian-Tilaki K (2013) Receiver operating characteristic (ROC) curve analysis for medical diagnostic test evaluation. Caspian J Intern Med 4(2):627–635

Spiegelman D, Schneeweiss S, McDermott A (1997) Measurement error correction for logistic regression models with an "alloyed gold standard". American J Epidemiol 145(2):184–196

White ME (1986) Evaluating diagnostic test results (letter). JAVMA 188:1141

Surveillance 16

'Surveillance' is a French word—'sur' means over and 'veiller' to watch (Brachman 2009)—that means 'close and continuous observation of one or more persons for the purpose of direction, supervision, or control' (Merriam-Webster 1976). The 21st World Health Assembly adopted the concept of population surveillance and defined it as 'the systematic collection and use of epidemiologic information for the planning, implementation, and assessment of disease control' (WHO 1968). More appropriately, surveillance can be defined as continuous scrutiny or watchfulness over the distribution and spread of infection/disease, predicting the development of potentially dangerous situations and collecting data of sufficient accuracy and completeness that are pertinent to effective disease control.

The aim of surveillance is to follow up on specific diseases in terms of morbidity and mortality in time and place and to follow the spread of infection/disease in the susceptible population. For meaningful surveillance, four steps must be followed: (i) keeping a close eye over the distribution and spread of the disease, (ii) creating a suitable method for collecting epidemiological data with reliability and precision, (iii) giving early warning and forecasting for future trends of the disease, and (iv) recommending suitable control measures.

As a health strategy, epidemiological surveillance may be divided into (a) *monitoring*, which is a routine observation of health, productivity, and environmental factors and the recording and transmission of these observations for the specified purpose of protecting and improving the health of the population, and (b) *health surveillance*, which is the collation and interpretation of the data collected from monitoring with a view to detecting any changes in the health status of the population.

Therefore, monitoring is a specific and essential part of surveillance, which requires careful planning of data collection through a recognised procedure over a long period of time, while surveillance requires professional analysis and the interpretation of data, which will lead to the recommendation of fruitful control measures.

K. G. Narayan et al., *Veterinary Public Health & Epidemiology*,
https://doi.org/10.1007/978-981-19-7800-5_16

In a national disease surveillance programme, priority should be given to a disease.

(a) That has a high incidence rate.
(b) That has the highest case fatality rate.
(c) That has a high economic impact.
(d) For which effective control measures exist and.
(e) That has geographical distribution and potential to spread in the country, region, and the world.

16.1 Set-up for National Disease Surveillance

The basic requirements to set up national disease surveillance of important animal diseases are as follows:

1. Well-organised health and epidemiological services.
2. An adequately equipped and suitably staffed laboratory diagnostic service.
3. A central agency to collect, analyse, and disseminate the consolidated information and.
4. A budget for the implementation of surveillance activities.

Surveillance involves a systematic collection and careful evaluation of data from reporting centres and the prompt dissemination of consolidated information to all those who contributed to its collection and also to those who have responsibilities for the control of diseases at local, national, and international levels (Fig. 16.1).

Surveillance is meant to know the health status of animals in the country and the diseases identified in order to take appropriate action. Since the 1990s, animal disease surveillance approaches have changed significantly. It is because of the development of comprehensive population databases, better data management due to better analytical tools, and statistical techniques, besides improvement in the understanding of concepts of risk in surveillance.

16.2 Why Surveillance Is Required

After the implementation of the World Trade Organization (WTO) on 1 January 1995, the surveillance of animal diseases has become more important. The purpose of surveillance varies according to the country's needs and situation. There are two situations in a country, i.e. whether a particular disease is present or absent.

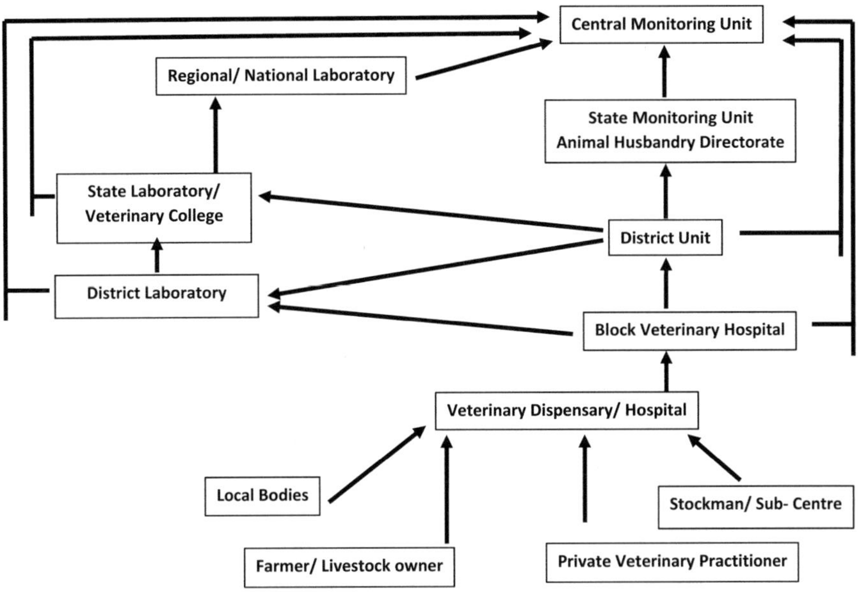

Fig. 16.1 National animal disease reporting system

16.2.1 Diseases Not Present

(a) Exotic disease (a known disease that exists in other countries).
(b) Emerging disease (a disease that is changing in its importance due to increased host range, pathogenicity, or spread).
(c) New disease (a disease that has not been previously reported).

The purpose of surveillance is to maintain freedom from the above disease(s) and to detect these early on.
1. *Demonstrating freedom from disease*

It is difficult to declare freedom from disease. A single infected animal is enough to prove that a disease is present in a country. However, after screening hundreds or thousands of animals and finding all are uninfected not enough to prove that the disease is absent, because chance of a small number of infected animals that have not yet been examined and identified is there.

A country (or a zone or compartment within a country) with an absence of disease carries with it a number of benefits, viz. permission to export animals, stoppage of disease control measures (such as a vaccination programme), public health safety, and political gain. The veterinary authorities must be sure of the 'freedom from disease status'.

2. *Early detection of disease*

It helps in early response, which prevents the further spread of the disease, thereby decreasing the cost of control or eradication and increasing their effectiveness.

16.2.2 Diseases Present

These include endemic diseases. Surveillance measures their level or detects cases.
1. *Measuring the level of disease*

The measures of disease are prevalence, incidence, and mortality rates. The strategy may be single (a cross-sectional study) or multiple (a longitudinal study).

A single measure helps in the prioritisation of disease and in risk analysis, while multiple measures assess the spatial and temporal distribution of disease. Spatial distribution helps in understanding spatial risk factors and in establishing a disease-free zone. Temporal distribution helps in monitoring control programmes and the early detection of changes in the endemic disease due to changes in the agent, host, or environment.

2. *To find cases of the disease*

Surveillance as part of a disease control programme, like for contagious bovine pleuropneumonia or tuberculosis, aims to find either infected herds or infected animals within herds and their segregation.

16.3 Characteristics of Surveillance

Some important characteristics of surveillance include the following:

(a) **Timeliness**: this refers to the *rapidity* (i.e. how rapidly the surveillance system is able to produce information) and *periodicity* of surveillance, e.g. ongoing (data are being gathered all the time), *regular* (e.g. at monthly intervals), and ad hoc (occasionally or as per needed).
(b) **Population coverage**: this is the proportion of the population covered by the surveillance system. Some surveillance (e.g. surveys) covers only a sample, i.e. relatively small proportion of the population, while other systems, like a census, covers the entire population.
(c) **Representativeness**: this means that the animals under surveillance are representative of the population.

16.4 Classification

The classification of surveillance is based on various criteria, all of which have their own advantages and disadvantages, as described below.

16.4.1 Based on Who Makes the Primary Observation

1. **Active surveillance:** Veterinarians or personnel of veterinary services makes the primary observation. It is a structured disease survey to collect high-quality information quickly and inexpensively. The advantages are as follows: (a) problems of under-reporting are avoided, (b) the true disease situation in the population is represented, and (c) information is collected from a known size of the population, and hence the calculation of disease rates and proportions is possible and can be related to the population.
2. **Passive surveillance:** This happens when farmers/livestock owners report the primary observation. No active effort is made. The system generates data; e.g., a Subdivisional Animal Husbandry Officer waits for the disease report to reach his office. The report is then passed on to the District A.H. Officer, who then transmits the same to the directorate. The report is compiled and sent to the central authority. A national-level report is thus prepared. It has limited utility—(a) meets the basic requirement of the Office International des Epizooties (OIE), (b) responds to the outbreak of a disease, and (c) identifies the presence and location of the disease. Passive surveillance reports are not useful for meeting all the requirements of 'disease monitoring and surveillance'; therefore, a **survey** is required to compensate for this, which is able to collect reliable information quickly and inexpensively for certain terms of interest. Trained persons examine a small proportion of the population, called a sample. A survey involves the examination of a small group (a sample) of elements (unit of interest) drawn from all the elements of interest (the population).

16.4.2 Based on the Frequency of Observations

1. **Continuous surveillance:** Animal owners see their animals frequently, at least once every day. It helps to.
   - Detect the appearance of exotic, new, or emerging diseases and
   - Identify the major diseases present in the country.
2. **Periodic or ad hoc surveillance:** Veterinarians or the personnel of veterinary services come into contact with animals intermittently and cannot be in full-time contact. It helps to.
   - Measure the level of disease.
   - Detect changes in the level of disease over time.
   - Detect the differences in the level of disease in different geographical areas.
   - Identify other factors influencing the disease.

- Demonstrate freedom from the disease and.
- Find cases as part of a control programme.

16.4.3 Other Approaches

1. **Participatory disease surveillance (PDS):** Under PDS, veterinary services visit farmers/livestock owners to ask about their observations rather than wait for farmers to report the problem themselves.
2. **Syndromic surveillance:** Here, the observations of non-veterinary reports (e.g. farmers') are recorded and analysed to detect abnormal patterns, which leads to the initiation of an investigation. The primary observer is still the farmer, but this approach optimises the use of resources by launching a detailed investigation only when there is evidence that something unusual is happening. Historically, during the Texas cattle fever, farmers' observation led to experimental studies to describe the role of tick-borne bovine babesiosis and insects (vectors) in the disease causation/spread.
3. **Laboratory surveillance:** The confirmation of diagnosis by laboratory tests will improve the quality of information from the field. However, the initial report on the disease still comes from the farmer, and samples are collected for testing during the follow-up investigation.
4. **Zero reporting:** This is based on farmers' observations that the disease is not present in their animals.
5. **Sentinel veterinary practices:** Small sentinel herds or flocks are being identified, placed in a fixed strategic location, and monitored over time. The herds are tested regularly by clinical examination or serologically for specific antibodies or examined for a specific disease agent. Sentinel herds act as indicators for the rest of the population to warn them that disease is present and established in areas considered as high risk of infection.
6. **Telephone hotline or SMS reporting:** The development of a communication system helps overcome the slow transmission of disease reports through a hierarchical reporting system and allows urgent reports to be passed directly to the central level. The Dutch Cattle Watch telephone hotline is an example.
7. **Indirect surveillance:** It uses related data, which may be an indirect indicator of disease; e.g., data on sales of antibiotic feed additives may increase when farmers perceive a disease problem.

   The integration of the Geographic Information System (GIS) will help in quick and reliable disease monitoring and surveillance, which provides information on the location of the disease and the population at risk. GIS, cell phones, and other related technology have been integrated to make customised apps, such as Arogya Setu in India, to track and trace infected individuals, the population at risk, and hot spots. Mobile GIS applications and Global Positioning System (GPS) records of cars may be used to track the contacts of the first case. Aerial photography using drones and satellites may also be used for surveillance.

References

Brachman PS (2009) Chapter 2. Public health surveillance. In: Brachman PS, Abrutyn E (eds) Bacterial infections of humans: epidemiology and control. Springer, New York, NY, USA

Merriam-Webster. (1976) Merriam-Webster's dictionary of English usage. Merriam-Webster, Springfield, Mass, USA

World Health Organization. Report of the Technical Discussions at the 21st World Health Assembly on National and Global Surveillance of Communicable Disease. Geneva, Switzerland; 1968

Prevention, Control, and Eradication of Disease

17

Conceptually, the three strategies for the management of herd disease are applicable to three different situations. Situation number one is characterised by the absence of disease X in a population. All measures taken to prevent its entry into this population are classified under '**prevention**'. Situation number two is characterised by the presence of disease X in a population, and this disease is causing a serious loss in terms of morbidity, mortality, and loss of production. The measures required to contain, i.e. to control disease X, so that the loss is reduced to a minimum are called '**control measures**'. In other words, it is the management of cases, latent carriers, and patent foci of infection and the promotion of healthy environmental conditions. In the third situation, measures are taken to push out a disease prevailing or recently making its appearance in a population. These measures are grouped under the term '**eradication**', which means the reduction of the prevalence of infectious disease in a specified area to a level at which transmission does not occur and intervention measures are no longer needed. It requires proactive measures and active surveillance to successfully detect a disease very recently entering into a population and 'stamp it out'. The eradication of a disease may be at the local/state/country/global level. The eradication of foot and mouth disease (FMD) from the USA and many European countries and the global eradication of smallpox (WHO 1980) and rinderpest (RP) (FAO and OIE 2018) are examples of eradication.

The problem of control/prevention of infectious diseases gets accentuated because of the free, fast, and global movement of animals and produce of animal origin in the international open trade, as well as ecological changes and the migration of wildlife and birds. The transmission of infection is facilitated.

K. G. Narayan et al., *Veterinary Public Health & Epidemiology*,
https://doi.org/10.1007/978-981-19-7800-5_17

17.1 Prevention

The goals of veterinary public health are to promote and preserve health, for which prevention is the most important step. Prevention has three levels—primary, secondary, and tertiary.

Primary prevention involves interventions that are applied before there is any evidence of disease or injury. Examples include immunisation, preserving good nutritional status, physical fitness, improving housing, or chemoprophylaxis. The strategy is to remove causative risk factors (risk reduction), which protects health and so overlaps with health promotion.

Secondary prevention is concerned with detecting a disease in its earliest stages, before symptoms appear, and intervening to slow or stop its progression. Earlier intervention will be more effective and cheaper. It includes the use of screening tests (tuberculin testing, pullorum testing, etc.) or other suitable methods to detect a disease as early as possible so that its progress can be arrested and the disease, if possible, can be eradicated. To be detectable by screening, a disease must have a long latent period during which the disease can be identified before symptoms appear.

Tertiary prevention means to 'minimise the consequences of disease'; therefore, such interventions are applied that arrest the progress of an established disease and to control its negative consequences, i.e. to reduce disability and handicap, to minimise suffering caused by existing departures from good health, and to promote patients' adjustment to irremediable conditions. This extends the concept of prevention into the field of clinical medicine and rehabilitation.

17.2 Methods of Disease Prevention

(a) Quarantine.
(b) Mass vaccination.
(c) Environmental measures.
(d) Chemoprophylaxis.
(e) Early detection and.
(f) Education.

17.2.1 Quarantine

It is a restraint on the movement of animals, man, plants, and even goods suspected of being carriers or vehicles of infections or having been exposed to infection. Quarantine may be imposed at the local, national, and international levels. In order to prevent the spread of the plague, passengers of a ship were forcibly restrained at the port of Marseilles for 40 days. The word 'quarantine' has its origin from this '40 days' restraint. In order to prevent the spread of diseases, the International Sanitary Commission (1851) identified six diseases—smallpox, yellow fever, louse-borne typhus, louse-borne relapsing fever, cholera, and plague—and formed regulations, such as compulsory vaccination against these before travelling abroad. In 1890, the first International Livestock quarantine introduced in the USA held imported cattle for 90 days and sheep for 15 days, which kept surra and *Brucella melitensis* out of the United States for many years. Australia has kept its cattle free from FMD since 1872, while England has kept rabies out since 1919 due to strict quarantine. The Office des International Epizooties (OIE), Paris, is the international regulatory authority overseeing disease control. The inherent principle of quarantine is that if imported animals were infected, they may manifest the disease clinically after the completion of incubation period. This method is coercive in nature and requires the assistance of a regulatory authority.

In India, 'The Livestock Import Quarantine Rules called the Model rules of 1961' consist of a number of schedules. Under Schedule I, the certificate issued by appropriate authorities in various countries exporting animals to India is accepted. The diseases of horses, asses, mules, bulls, bullocks, cows, buffaloes, sheep, goats, pigs, poultry, dogs, and cats are listed in Schedule II. Freedom of animals from diseases for 30 days before embarkation is necessary. In Schedule III, specific diseases are listed, e.g. brucellosis, tuberculosis, Johne's disease, glanders, fowl typhoid, pullorum, and psittacosis. These must be absent on testing 30 days prior to the actual date of embarkation.

17.2.2 Mass Vaccination

An immunised individual is protected against the disease for which he is vaccinated. He carries this protection wherever he moves, including the place where the disease is endemic. A vaccine is administered once a year or every six months, depending upon the period of immunity it confers. Mass vaccination aims to cover most of the individuals of a population as it may not be possible to vaccinate all. Normally, 80% of the population vaccinated keeps the infection out. Objections to mass vaccination may be acceptability of the vaccine, imperfect protection, sensitisation, difficulty to administer, the risk of spread of infection if the batch of the vaccine is contaminated, improper storage, and inadequate cold chain facility, affecting the potency of the vaccine. A number of developments in vaccinology have alleviated most of such fears and made mass vaccination easy. These are pure antigen, sub-unit vaccine (VP1 peptide of FMDV capsid), anti-idiotypic antibody vaccine (e.g. hepatitis virus B, poliovirus type II, *Listeria monocytogenes*, *Schistosoma mansoni*), syringe with a Gispen valve, disposable syringes, aerosol vaccine (Newcastle disease, distemper), oral vaccine (e.g. polio, rabies), vaccine incorporated into water, and even syngenic plants containing protective antigens or multiple antigens (which combine vaccines for more than one disease, like rabies-canine distemper-hepatitis and two serotypes of *Leptospira*).

17.2.3 Environmental Measures

This method is based on the principle of altering/modifying the environment in a way that it becomes unsuitable for the infectious agent and healthy for the population, and those exposed to such environment or living in such environment do not fall ill. This method has the greatest acceptability as it is not coercive, and the individuals sharing the environment do not know of the alteration made, for example the chlorination of water to prevent waterborne diseases, the disposal of sewage and excreta, pest control, fogging and using insecticide spray to control insect vectors, food inspection, improved housing, swimming pool sanitation, etc.

Portable calf pens, the McLean County system, and deep litter systems are examples of environmental measures to prevent infection/disease.

17.2.3.1 Portable Calf Pen

Here, the gastrointestinal parasitic infections spread through the contaminated grazing field or infected soil of the pen. The eggs of parasites are laid in the pen or on a grazing field by infected adult animals. These undergo development to become infective stage larvae. If these do not find susceptible hosts (calves) to infect, they perish. The 'rotational grazing system' or 'portable calf pens' rotate the calves at such intervals as to allow them to escape infection.

17.2.3.2 McLean County System

This system of pig rearing prevents infection and mortality in piglets. The care starts with the pregnant sows, which are held in well-sanitised farrowing pens during the last week of expected farrowing. The farrowing takes place in a well-sanitised state, and all care is taken to prevent deaths, e.g. due to trampling or inadequate feeding. Subsequent care is taken till the piglets are weaned.

17.2.4 Chemoprophylaxis

It is the use of chemicals to prevent infections, such as coccidiostat/coccidiocidal agents in drinking water to keep coccidia out in poultry, iodine in salt to prevent goitre, fluorine in water, etc. Anti-nematode/anti-fluke blocks of urea-molasses and suitable anthelmintics are being tried at the National Dairy Development Board (NDDB) biotechnology laboratory.

17.2.5 Early Detection

The identification of infection/disease in its early stage enables one to take immediate action to prevent further spread. Mass screening and multi-phasic screening are the methods for early detection. Examples are tuberculin testing, pullorum testing, multi-phasic screening of the serum of one individual against as many antigens as possible and especially for important diseases.

17.2.6 Mass Education/Awareness

Public support is essential in the implementation of any health programme. Educating the public before initiating a health programme assures acceptability and cooperation. Educated farmers can take care of their animals and also demand their desired preventive health programme.

17.3 Disease Control

Methods to control diseases aim at reducing the opportunity for disease transmission. These are (a) reservoir control, (b) vector control, (c) test and slaughter, (d) mass treatment, and (e) miscellaneous.

17.3.1 Reservoir Control

An infectious agent perpetuates in nature in a reservoir host. The death of the host is suicidal for the infectious agent. Development of immunity in the host is also determental for infectious agent. The infectious agent must, therefore, infect another susceptible in order to perpetuate in nature. The continuity of this process of transmission to susceptible hosts is in the interest of the infectious agent. This continuity of transmission is dependent on the high density of the susceptible reservoir host. The disease spreads from the reservoir host to domestic animals, pets, or human beings. Therefore, the control of the reservoir population is a method for the control of disease. The control of street dog populations is a method for the control of rabies.

17.3.2 Vector Control

In the case of vector-borne diseases, increased vector density increases the opportunity for transmission. Mosquito density influences the spread of malaria, dengue, and Japanese encephalitis. Similarly, tick density governs the incidence and prevalence of blood protozoan disease in animals and Kyasanur Forest disease (KFD) in human beings. Vector density increases seasonally and so also the incidence of these diseases. Spraying and fogging of insecticides keep vector density low and consequently the prevalence of diseases.

17.3.3 Test and Slaughter

A diseased individual sheds the infectious agent, which spreads, increasing disease prevalence. Those in contact with the diseased may be infected but not manifest symptoms. Such animals, too, are infectious or are likely to become infectious. The identification of such animals requires testing, for example, the collection of the oesopharyngeal fluid of cattle for the examination of FMDV, the testing of the cough/milk/urine of cows for acid-fast bacilli, and the examination of uterine discharges for *Brucella abortus* and the serum of in-contacts for *Brucella* agglutinin. The method of eradication of tuberculosis and brucellosis uses detection of infected and slaughter. Scandinavian countries succeeded in controlling these two diseases this way. Where slaughter is not possible, testing and segregation may be the alternative.

17.3.4 Mass Treatment

Chemotherapeutic agents are used to treat a case and also to clean the host's body system of an infectious agent. Thus, the treated individual ceases to be infectious to others, and the transmission cycle is broken. The use of tetracycline in the treatment of pet birds to control chlamydiasis (psittacosis-ornithosis) is an example.

17.3.5 Miscellaneous

A variety of methods may be used to control disease. For example, freezing beef and pork controls taeniasis and trichinosis and pasteurising milk controls milk-borne diseases, including tuberculosis and Q fever. Certain breeds have become resistant to certain endemic infections and diseases through selection. Zebu cattle are resistant to blood protozoan diseases. Evidence of genetic resistance to diseases, like infectious bronchitis, Marek's disease, infectious bursal disease, and infectious bronchitis, is available. Thus, it seems that breeding disease-resistant transgenic animals is possible.

17.4 Disease Eradication

The eradication of disease is achievable. The study of the natural history of diseases provides examples from which one may learn lessons. French West African soldiers brought bancroftian filariasis (*Wuchereria bancrofti*) along with vector mosquitoes in Lebanon during World War II. After the army (West African soldiers) left, the disease also vanished. The local mosquitoes failed to sustain the infectious agent. Visceral leishmaniasis (*Leishmania donovani*), i.e. kala-azar in India, is not a zoonosis, although it is so elsewhere. Experimental infection in dogs is set up (i.e. dogs are susceptible), but the infection fails to get established in the canine population because the vector (*Phlebotomus argentipes*) refuses to feed on dogs. It is, thus, evident that efforts on two important fronts, the reservoir hosts and the vectors, can succeed in eradicating a disease. The weapons therefore may be (a) the testing and slaughter of hosts and (b) vector eradication.

17.4.1 Test and Slaughter

It is a method that requires strong public and administrative support. Mass education and adequate compensation to animal owners may help in implementing this drastic and coercive measure. Bovine contagious pleuropneumonia (BCPP), dourine, fowl plague, and bovine tuberculosis from the Netherlands, Denmark, and Finland were eradicated following testing and slaughter. A newly imported infectious agent is stamped out through prompt action.

17.4.2 Vector Eradication

This is possible. Insecticides may be used as spray of the animal premises, dipping of animals or dusting of animals. Mechanical picking of vector (Tick, Lice etc.) from individual animal also helps at the individual animal level. Chemicals may also be used for sterilising males, which on release would fail to impregnate females. Therefore, future crops of insects may not be born. Ultraviolet rays (caesium-137 and cobalt-60) have also been used for the sterilisation of male insects. This method (sterile male technique) was used jointly by the World Health Organization (WHO) and the Indian Council of Medical Research (ICMR) from 1964 to 1974 to control the mosquito population. Biological methods of controlling vectors are eco-friendly. They hit only the target species without affecting the ecological balance. Having knowledge of parasites and the predators of vector insects is useful in this regard. Entomophagous microbes grow, develop, and feed upon insect vectors. Such microbes are called entomogenous. *Hunterella hookeri* is a wasp used to control ticks in Africa. The tick *Dermacentor variabilis* is parasitised and controlled. *Bairamlia fuscipes* (wasp) parasitises the flea *Xenopsylla cheopis*, as seen in Russia and England. *Coelomyces* (fungus) affects the larvae of *Anopheles gambiae* in Zambia. *Australorbis glabratus* is a snail intermediate host of *Schistosoma mansoni*. An omnivorous snail, *Marisa cornuarietis*, destroys the eggs of *A. glabratus*. *Gambusia affinis* and tilapia fish feed upon the larvae of *Anopheles*. This has been used in India in malaria control programmes. Similarly, *Wolbachia* spp. is a common bacterium of mosquitoes that stops the virus from replicating inside *Aedes aegypti*, a major carrier of dengue. Mosquitoes infected with *Wolbachia* spp. are not infected with the dengue virus and hence do not transmit the virus. Australian researchers bred mosquitoes that are infected with the *Wolbachia* bacteria, which were released in places where they could naturally breed in over 66 km^2 in Townsvilla, Queensland, which has a human population of 187,000. In four years since then, no new cases of dengue have occurred. The community welcomed the project. It is self-sustaining and is ongoing in 11 countries. The World Mosquito Program in India is part of a global, not-for-profit initiative that is working to protect local communities from mosquito-borne diseases. The Indian Council of Medical Research (ICMR) is a partner.

Sequential Steps in a 'Disease Elimination/Eradication Programme'.

1. Planning.
2. Organising the campaign creation of infrastructure facilities and listing supporting institutions.
3. Implementing specific measures of control and eradication.
4. Continuing the action taken in no. 3.
5. Monitoring of achievements and reduction in the prevalence of disease or infection.
6. Surveillance and selective action.

The last step is continued till zero prevalence for three consecutive years is observed, meeting the OIE requirement for the declaration of 'elimination of diseases/infection'. Eradication has been further explained at the conference on 'Global Disease Elimination and Eradication as Public Health Strategies', held in February 1998 in Atlanta, Georgia. There are four stages: (a) the elimination of disease, (b) the elimination of infection, (c) eradication, and (d) extinction. These are defined as follows.

- Elimination of disease is the reduction to zero of the incidence of a specific disease in a geographic area as a result of deliberate efforts; continued intervention measures are required to maintain this status, e.g. neonatal tetanus.
- Elimination of infection is the reduction to zero of the incidence of infection caused by a specific agent in a defined geographical area as a result of deliberate efforts; continued measures are required to prevent the re-establishment of transmission, e.g. measles and polio.
- Eradication is the permanent reduction to zero of the worldwide incidence of infection caused by a specific agent as a result of deliberate efforts; intervention measures are no more required, e.g. smallpox and rinderpest.
- Extinction is a state when a specific agent no longer exists in nature or laboratories. Note that smallpox and rinderpest viruses are preserved in laboratories today.

17.5 Integrating the Concept of Disease Process and Principles of Disease Management

The disease process, starting from 'natural nidus' to a population of human beings or their domestic and pet animals, has been discussed earlier. The sequence of events may be described under three main heads: pre-pathogenesis period, period of infection, and period of pathogenesis (Fig. 17.1). The pre-pathogenesis period covers conditions that favour 'exposure', e.g. earthquakes/floods, creating conditions for susceptible hosts and reservoirs/carriers of infection to come in close contact. Flood favoured infectious hepatitis in the outbreak in Najafgarh, Delhi. The 'period of infection and pathogenesis' cover the host's response to the infectious agent.

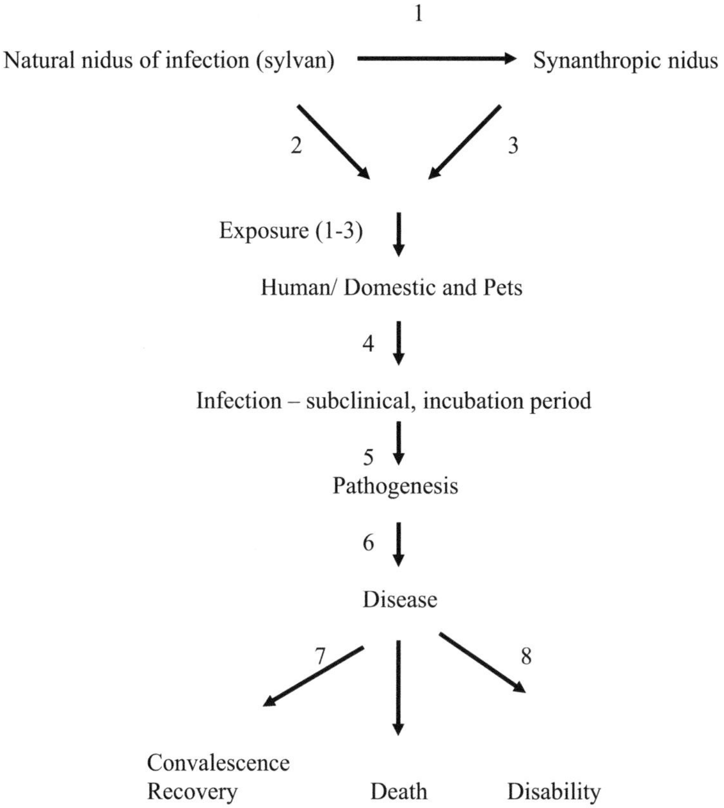

Fig. 17.1 Stages of the disease process and sites of intervention (Arabic numbers). Identification of (1–3) and the application of appropriate methods of prevention would be the approach. Exposure may or may not result in infection. (4) Methods of prevention, like mass vaccination and chemoprophylaxis, may not allow 'exposure', which leads to infection. Sub-clinical cases (e.g. mastitis) and incubatory carriers (e.g. RP, FMD) may spread the disease. (5) Methods like 'early detection' and 'chemotherapy' (as in mastitis) and 'quarantine' (for incubatory carriers) should be helpful. A diseased animal is infectious to others. (6) Methods like 'isolation/segregation' to stop transmission as well as 'chemotherapy' to reduce the period of infectivity may be useful. (7) Care and the treatment of clinical cases: specific therapy and intensive management tactics, such as life support systems for critical patients, help in recovery. Surgical management may help remove 'disability', such as prosthetic limbs in humans. This follows rehabilitation. (8) Death is inevitable. Proper disposal of dead bodies and terminal disinfection are important in controlling the spread of disease.

A natural nidus of infection is a 'support system for the infectious agent' (refer to 'rodent-flea-*Yersinia pestis*', landscape epidemiology). The Surat plague in 1994 was preceded by an earthquake in Latur. The residents of earthquake-damaged houses shifted to new ones. Some of them used old, damaged houses where bags of grain were left for storage, which facilitated the uncontrolled breding of rodents and mixed with field rats infected with plague bacilli infected flea. A nidus of plague was created, infecting the residents who went to collect grains. A few of them worked in Surat. They carried *Y. pestis*, which infected local rats. Outbreak of plague occured, initially in bubonic form followed by pneumonic form, resulted in epidemic.

Chain of transmission from the infectious agent to the susceptible through contact or by air is another method. 'Social distance between infectious and susceptibles' and portals of exit and entry of infectious agents are determinants. Airborne or contact-borne infections, like measles, spread in a crowd, such as in a school setting. Ebola spreads in 'cremation-aggregation'. The maintenance of other infectious agents and the sustenance of infection depends upon the density of the susceptible population, e.g. rabies and echinococcosis. A threshold population is necessary. Infectious agents spill over to humans.

The above are just guidelines for disease management. Rehabilitation, as applied to human beings, includes hospital and community facilities like shelters, the education of both the victims and the employer/non-governmental organizations (NGOs), work, physiotherapy, etc. In animals, test and slaughter or selective slaughter, sending animals to gosadans to save and protect the remaining uninfected stock, the creation of replenishment stock, terminal disinfection of the premises, checking for complete freedom from infectious agents before reusing the premises, etc. are the methods.

References

FAO & OIE. 2018. Global Rinderpest Action Plan: Post-Eradication. Published by the Food and Agriculture Organization of the United Nations and the World Organisation for Animal Health.2018. https://www.woah.org/app/uploads/2021/03/global-rinderpest-action-plan-2018.pdf

WHO. 1980. https://www.who.int/health-topics/smallpox#tab=tab_1

18 Economics of Disease

Disease or disability causes loss due to a reduction in the total output of ill or disabled animals. The summation of such a loss in the case of outbreaks and epidemics is huge as animal resources are affected. Epidemiological studies remain incomplete without the assessment of the cost of outbreaks or epizootics. Economic evaluation is essential for influencing policymakers.

The sum of output losses due to disease and control expenditures to contain the disease can be a measure of the economic cost of a disease. Depending upon the situation, there are different approaches to estimating economics in animal farms.

18.1 Partial Farm Budget

The purpose of a partial farm budget is to evaluate whether a change in farm practice is profitable and can increase the net farm income, for example contracting out the rearing of replacement heifers in a dairy unit, which will significantly reduce the costs associated with labour, feed, and provision of housing and bedding, but it must account for the extra cost of paying the contract rearer.

In the case of capital investment, the partial budget should include the projected extra revenue, which can be used to calculate payback time and the expected return on investment. The profit is measured by taking into account all cash and non-cash items incurred for the changes. There are four components of a partial farm budget:

(a) Additional revenue realised (r_1)
(b) Reduced costs (c_1)
(c) Increased costs (r_2)
(d) Cost of implementing the change (c_2)

Profitability in a partial budget is usually measured by estimating the average change in the annual profit. A positive value, i.e. $r_1 + c_1 > r_2 + c_2$, means the net farm

K. G. Narayan et al., *Veterinary Public Health & Epidemiology*,
https://doi.org/10.1007/978-981-19-7800-5_18

income is increased and, thus, change is profitable, while a negative value, i.e. $r_1 + c_1 < r_2 + c_2$, indicates that the net farm income is decreased and, therefore, the change is not economically viable.

The partial budget takes one change at a time. Hence, to measure the most profitable change, many partial budgets related to the changes have to be done and then compared. Thus, a partial farm budget is a simple description of the financial consequences of a particular change in farm management practice.

18.2 Measures for Selecting a Control Campaign

There are four important measures used for the selection of a disease control campaign:

1. Net present value (NPV).
2. Benefit-cost ratio (B/C).
3. Internal rate of return (IRR), and.
4. Payback period.

18.2.1 Net Present Value (NPV)

It is the difference between the present value of benefits (*Bt*) and the present value of the costs (*Ct*) incurred. The formula to calculate NPV is:

$$\text{NPV} = \sum_{t=0}^{n} \frac{Bt - Ct}{(1 + r)^t}$$

where.

Bt = value of benefits gained in time t.
Ct = value of costs incurred in time t.
r = discount rate.
n = life of the project.

A positive NPV indicates that the project is viable. NPV is affected by the scale of the project, and it does not indicate how much benefits may outweigh the cost in percentage terms.

18.2.2 Benefit-Cost Ratio (B/C)

It is the ratio of the present value of benefits to the present value of costs. B/C ratio > 1 indicates that the project is beneficial.

$$B/C = \sum_{t=0}^{n} \frac{Bt}{Ct}$$

where.

Bt = value of benefits gained in time t.
Ct = value of costs incurred in time t.

18.2.2.1 Illustrations (Schwabe 1969)

Cost of a Single Case of Dog Bite in California in 1981

The cost was $105,790. The breakdown is as follows:

Hospital billing for anti-rabies treatment	$92,650
Veterinary services	$2849
Animal rabies vaccination clinic supplies	$1341
Animal control	$6015
Sutter-Yuba county Health Department overtime	$2935

These are the amount spent on control. Not included in this are costs for lost workdays, livestock losses, transportation expenses, compensation for the mental anguish of persons bitten and their families and friends, and laboratory services.

Cost of Brucellosis in India (1970)

The average annual prevalence was 4%. Expected abortion was one third. The breedable female cattle and buffaloes were 75 million. Three million would thus be infected, and one million of these would abort, resulting in the loss of one million calves, or Rs. 50 million (conservative estimate). About 20% of infected animals, i.e. 600,000, would be rendered sterile, and at Rs. 150 per animal, the annual loss would be Rs. 90 million. Brucellosis causes a reduction in milk yield—an expected loss of 25% of the normal production and, at the then prevailing price, Rs. 100 million per year. The total comes to Rs. 240 million/year.

Zoonotic consequences: 75% of 500 million Indian populations live in villages and are thus exposed to infected animals. An estimated 20% of the villagers suffer from pyrexia of unknown origin per year. Of this, 1–2% may be assumed to be due to brucellosis, which is a protracted illness, may be running for a month, average 30-man days would be lost annually, i.e. 30 million-man days. Invisible losses include sub-clinical cases and infection in other species of animals, like sheep, goats, and pigs, which in turn would be spreading the infection further to human beings and animals. Monetary value can be assigned to these also.

Unlike in Table 18.1, the cost of control is not estimated. The economic cost of disease and also the selection of a cost-effective strategy for control in a given situation can be estimated.

Table 18.1 Benefits and costs of the control of zoonoses (Grace 2014)

Disease	Perspective	Country	Cost considered	Benefit-cost ratio	References
Brucellosis	Ex ante	Nigeria	Livestock only	3.2	McDermott et al. 2013
	Ex ante	Mongolia	Human health and livestock	3.2	
	Ex post	Czech Republic	Livestock only	7.1	
	Ex ante	Cyprus	Not specified	6.5–21.7	

18.2.3 Internal Rate of Return (IRR)

It is the rate of return (r) that equates the present value of the costs with the present value of the benefits and is calculated based on the equation for NPV. If IRR is greater than the actual interest rate, the project is economically viable.

18.2.4 Payback Period

It refers to the time period which gives the total flow of the return from the investment that is equal to the total cost incurred. There is a direct relationship between IRR and payback period; i.e., the higher the IRR is, the smaller is the payback period.

18.3 Definitions

A. Tangibles and intangibles benefits: benefits that can be quantified in terms of monetary units are called tangible, whereas benefits that are subjective and cannot translate into monetary terms are called intangible (e.g. decrease of noise level).

B. Discounting: when costs and benefits spread over several years and have to be compared, they must be adjusted to calculate their present value. The process of adjustment is called discounting, which is the opposite of compounding. Here, the rate of interest used in the calculation is adjusted to exclude the effect of price inflation. It can be calculated by the formula:

$$\text{Rate} = (1 + r)^t$$

where r = rate in per cent and t = time (year/month).

In discounting, the amount (cost and benefit) should be divided by the rate, while for compounding, the amount (cost and benefit) should be multiplied by the rate. Usually, discounting is done when a project is completed and the benefit-cost ratio is calculated now, i.e. past to present, while compounding is done when a project will be completed in future and the benefit-cost is calculated now, i.e. present to future.

References

Grace D (2014) The business case for one health. Onderstepoort J Vet Res 81(2):725, 6 pages. https://doi.org/10.4102/ojvr.v81i2.725

Mcdermott J, Grace D, Zinsstag J (2013) Economics of brucellosis impact and control in low-income countries. Rev Sci Tech Off Int Epiz 32(1):249–261

Schwabe CW (1969) Veterinary medicine and human health. Williams Wilkins Co., Baltimore

19 World Organization for Animal Health (WOAH)/Office International Des Epizooties (OIE)

The Office International des Epizooties (OIE) was established on 25 January 1924 following an epizootic of rinderpest in Belgium in 1920 with the following objectives: (a) to promote and coordinate research on the surveillance and control of animal diseases throughout the world, (b) to inform government veterinary services of the occurrence and course of epizootics which would endanger animal and human health, and (c) to issue warning to the member countries to act rapidly should the need arise.

It is an intergovernmental organisation of the United Nations from 1945 with headquarter at Paris. It is recognised as a reference organisation by the World Trade Organization (WTO). In 2003, it was renamed the World Organisation for Animal Health (WOAH). Since 28 May 2022, the OIE has had a new name, WOAH, and has unveiled a new identity and logo (WOAH 2022). With the passage of time, the organisation's objectives and functioning have undergone changes. The revised objectives include—(a) transparency in the global animal diseases situation—essentially retains the original three objectives and manages through sharing of information via e-mail, Disease Information and the World Animal Health Information System Interface (WAHIS Interface), (b) scientific information, (c) international solidarity, (d) sanitary safety, (e) promotion of veterinary services, and (f) food safety and animal welfare.

19.1 Organization Set-up

The World Organisation for Animal Health is under the authority and control of the World Assembly of Delegates, which is composed of delegates from the government of each member country. These delegates elect a director general for a term of five years. WOAH has one council, five regional commissions (Africa; the USA; Asia, the Far East, and Oceania; Europe; and the Middle East), and four specialist

K. G. Narayan et al., *Veterinary Public Health & Epidemiology*,
https://doi.org/10.1007/978-981-19-7800-5_19

technical commissions (Terrestrial Code Commission, Scientific Commission, Laboratories Commission, and Aquatic Animals Commission).

The warning system functions as follows: the affected country reports to the WOAH Central Bureau within 24 h on the incidence of a listed disease or any other disease that has a great impact on public health and/or the economy. The WOAH Central Bureau then transmits this information immediately by fax/telex/telegram/e-mail to countries directly at risk and by mail to all other countries, as well as publishes it on the online weekly publication 'Disease Information'.

A network of 246 WOAH Collaborating Centres and Reference Laboratories prepared Guidelines on the methods used to control and eradicate diseases, which are disseminated through various works and periodicals published by the WOAH, notably the Scientific and Technical Review (three issues/year). Other important and useful publications are the bimonthly OIE Bulletin and an annual publication entitled 'World Animal Health'.

WOAH publishes health standards for international trade in animals and animal products, which safeguard world trade. These standards are adopted by the World Assembly of Delegates and are recognised by the World Trade Organization as reference international sanitary rules.

The WOAH develops normative documents containing rules by using which the member countries can protect themselves from the introduction of diseases and pathogens without setting up unjustified sanitary barriers. The main normative documents produced by the WOAH are (1) the Terrestrial Animal Health Code, (2) the Manual of Diagnostic Tests and Vaccines for Terrestrial Animals, (3) the Aquatic Animal Health Code, and (4) the Manual of Diagnostic Tests for Aquatic Animals.

19.2 How WOAH Functions

There are 'Specialists Commissions' and 'Working Groups', supported by 'Collaborating Centres' and 'Reference Laboratories', to accomplish the tasks of promoting research and coordinating disease surveillance and control. This is supported by meeting of experts and scientific publication.

As per need, the 'International Committee' decides creation of a 'Specialist Commission' and also for the time to solve a specific problem.

The 'Specialist Commission' studies problems of epidemiology and concerns about the control of animal diseases, as well as issues related to the harmonisation of international regulations. The Foot and Mouth Disease and Other Epizootics Commission assists in identifying the most appropriate strategies and measures for disease prevention and control. The commission also convenes 'expert groups', particularly during 'emergencies', such as foot and mouth disease (FMD), African horse sickness, and bovine spongiform encephalopathy. The 'Standards Commission', 'Fish Disease Commission', 'International Animal Health Code Commission', and others hold regular scientific meetings in their respective areas. There are 'Working Groups', e.g., on (a) Biotechnology, (b) Informatics and Epidemiology,

(c) Veterinary Drug Registration, and (d) Wildlife Diseases. The 'Working Groups' meet to review the progress made in their respective fields and ensure that the member countries benefit rapidly from this progress. Worldwide surveys are undertaken, and results are published. Scientific meetings, training courses, and seminars are organised to disseminate knowledge/information.

'Reference Laboratories' and 'Collaborating Centres' extend scientific and technical assistance and expert advice pertaining to disease surveillance and control through the sending of experts, supply of diagnostic kits, and reference reagents, besides organising meetings, seminars, and workshops.

The principal concern of WOAH is to prevent the transfer of pathogens to animals and human beings via the international trade of animals and animal products while avoiding unjustified sanitary barriers to trade. Earlier animal diseases were listed under A and B. the animal industry in an exporting country suffers from the imposition of bans on export once a disease under List A is detected in any locality; e.g., bird flu/FMD detected in one locality of India resulted in the total ban of export from India.

In 2005, WOAH organised an Ad Hoc group, which examined the diseases under Lists A and B, as per the adopted criteria for listing diseases. The Ad Hoc group proposed a new list of diseases meeting the criteria, which came into force in 2006. The list of diseases is reviewed on a regular basis, and in an annual general session, these modifications are adopted by the World Assembly of Delegates. The new list comes into force on 1 January of the following year. For the year 2019, the list includes 117 animal diseases, infections, and infestations.

The WOAH codes are available in its publications. The WOAH Terrestrial Animal Health Code, for example, provides standards for the improvement of animal health and welfare and veterinary public health worldwide through standards for safe international trade in terrestrial animals (mammals, reptiles, birds, and bees) and their products. The health measures in the Terrestrial Code should be used by the veterinary authorities of importing and exporting countries to ensure early detection, reporting, and control of agents that are pathogenic to animals or humans and to prevent their transfer via international trade in animals and animal products while avoiding unjustified sanitary barriers to trade. This supports the member countries by providing the information needed to take appropriate action to prevent the transboundary spread of important animal diseases, including zoonoses. This is achieved through transparent, timely, and consistent disease notification.

Disease notification is based on a diagnosis by a laboratory recognised by an authority and through an approved method. Reporting can be done by anyone.

The spillover of pathogens from laboratories may lead to an outbreak. Tissues like semen or embryos or tissues for transplant can be a source of or a mode of transfer of pathogens. There are guidelines that must be followed.

The safeguards implemented at the research laboratories should guarantee containment (premises of categories P1 to P4) and biological containment (classification of the risk of an escape from I to IV for live organisms' manipulations in the laboratory).

In the year 1989, the Department of Biotechnology (DBT), the Ministry of Science and Technology, and the Government of India prepared guidelines, procedures, and recommendations with regard to safety aspects, which emphasised that the safety regulations and their implementation in India for recombinant DNA research will be based on the 'report of the Recombinant DNA Advisory Committee' of the DBT.

The set of requirements for the import of semen/embryos has been laid down by the Government of India, and FAO recommendations for the movement of embryos should be made obligatory in all laboratories/institutions carrying out work on frozen semen and embryo transfer. The patho-biological aspects of embryo transfer relevant to Indian conditions should be carried out at the Indian Veterinary Research Institute (IVRI), and it is mandatory for all frozen semen laboratories/centres to establish a semen microbiology laboratory for screening as well as identifying viral, bacterial, and protozoal diseases. For specific typing, IVRI may be referred to.

Reference

WOAH, 2022. World Organisation for Animal Health. https://www.woah.org

Food-borne Infections and Intoxications 20

Abstract

'Healthy food—healthy man.' Sometimes, attractive, good-looking food is not healthy. It may contain pathogens or microbial toxins, and consumers fall sick (food poisoning) after consuming such food. The investigation of food poisoning should be comprehensive, beginning from the incriminating food item, tracing back through the kitchen (from the receipt of food ingredients through the processing steps to serving), and then to the chain of supply of the suspected ingredient (wholesale to retail to consumer, packaging, cold chain, mode of transportation, and time). Investigations may extend beyond the state where the outbreak occurred. Reverse tracing may lead the investigator to farms and examine farming systems that may reveal the use of untreated water for irrigation. The genome sequencing of food- poisoning-causing agents enables establishing the cause of sporadic cases and the tracing of the entry of pathogens into food or its ingredients to transmission through the trade route. This facilitates the stoppage of supply and the recall of contaminated food or ingredients.

The infection in food producing animals can be controlled by good animal management practices, excretion load and consequential contamination of soil and animal produce (harvest) can be eliminated or at least reduced to a minimal. Hygienic post-harvest processing further reduces/eliminates any escaping pathogens. Retailing and catering premises may also adopt Hazard Analysis Critical Control Points (HACCP).

Each pathogen has specific characteristics. The circumstances/conditions leading to contamination and persistence in food, survival through processing, infecting dose and virulence factors differ. These have been dealt with under the discussion on specific agents causing food poisoning.

K. G. Narayan et al., *Veterinary Public Health & Epidemiology*, https://doi.org/10.1007/978-981-19-7800-5_20

Everyone enjoys food. Processed food or even a meal may contain ingredients from multiple countries/continents. Food is global. Food chains may have been long wrapping up the planet. Thus, their safety depends upon international collaboration.

Food-borne infections and intoxications (diseases) are defined as diseases that result from the ingestion of contaminated or naturally hazardous food, animal source food (foods derived from animals, fish, and aquatic animals, including meat, milk, eggs, offal, fish and crustaceans), and produce such as fruits and vegetables sold fresh. The definition is expanded to include those transmitted through other routes, such as through water or direct contact with infected people or animals, if food plays an important role in disease transmission. Drivers/factors of re-emerging food-borne diseases (FBD) may be changing food preference, increasing demands and related changes in animal production systems including use of anti-microbials; animal density, international trade of animal feed, animals, animal produce, and products.

Outbreaks/epidemics of food-borne infections and intoxication apparently present the simplest form shoe-leather or cause effect epidemiology. It is not true. The condition has multi-etiologies and multiple vehicles originating commonly from terrestrial and aquatic animals or plants. Each causative agent has specific innate characteristics, which are influenced by a vast range of environments, through which it passes before entry to human hosts, wherein it begins the fight with innate resistance. Food consumed could be raw or processed. Source attribution is the most challenging.

Source attribution is the effort to quantify the number/proportion of sporadic human cases of a specific illness (e.g. food borne) to specific sources (food categories) and animal reservoirs. Data collected through integrated surveillance systems of humans, food, and animals comply with these requirements.

Veterinary public health epidemiologists have most of the knowledge on animal production systems, comparative pathology, diagnostic methods, food processing, and HACCP. They understand and follow the chain in marketing, processing, and hygiene in the kitchen and catering.

Multiple factors influence food-borne diseases.

20.1 Population, Pathogen, and Food and Its Production, Processing, and Trade

Population: growth, composition (susceptible groups like young, old, and immunocompromised), occupation (animal farmers, slaughter men, etc.), spatial distribution (urban and its periphery), etc. influence the quantity and quality of food production (raw, partially and fully cooked, food on wheels and food joints). Affluence increases demands for exotic food and pets.

20.1.1 Food Preference: Raw or Lightly Cooked Dishes (Examples) and the Farming System

Streptococcus equi infection related mostly to consumption of raw pork preparations (e.g. *tiet canh)* among slaughterhouse workers, pig breeders, butchers were high in Thailand compared to the Netherlands; the difference related to farming system.

Ke-jang is a raw crab soaked in soy sauce, which is popular in *the Republic of Korea*; raw drunken crabs and raw grass carp in China and raw fish (*lab-pla* and *plasom)* in Thailand are considered delicacies and attract tourists. However, these are dangerous causes of *trematodiases.*

Salmonella survives on intact tomatoes and jalapeno peppers and grows well at 12 and 21°°C on intact cilantro and chopped vegetables, like chopped jalapeno peppers (which are Mexican food 'salsa' ingredients).

Pathogens: susceptibility and adaptation to environmental conditions, like sunlight, temperature, and moisture, and the capacity to change/mutate, including acquiring anti-microbial resistance and/or virulence factors, are characteristics of pathogens influencing the attainment of an infective dose/infectious stage (Fig. 20.1).

Salmonella, *Campylobacter*, and *Vibrio cholerae* are capable of entering into dormancy (viable but not culturable) and of surviving under adverse aquatic environments without losing pathogenicity. Food animals and humans are reservoirs or carriers of pathogens that are passed on from their poops to the environment, e.g. in the soil, wherein these may persist (e.g. spores) or lie latent or dormant (e.g. *Salmonella*), undergo development (e.g. certain parasites), or even multiply (e.g. certain bacteria and parasites). The ingestion of these in an infectious dose directly or with water or food (vehicles of infection) will cause disease. A low infective dose can be ingested by a mechanical vehicle, like water, e.g. *Vibrio cholerae*. A heavy infective dose requires the multiplication of pathogens in the vehicle, and contaminated food provides this.

Clostridium perfringens form spores that survive in chunks of beef, pork, or turkey during storage in the freezer (−20 °C) or refrigerator (−4 °C) for long (3–6 months). Heating at 100°C for $\geq$30 to 120 min reduces the count by one log. It can survive salt and nitrite in the concentration used in meat products. It can multiply fast between 10 °C and 54 °C (post-cooking holding) because its doubling time is short. As much as 10^6 to 10^7 counts per gram are attained without any obnoxious change in food.

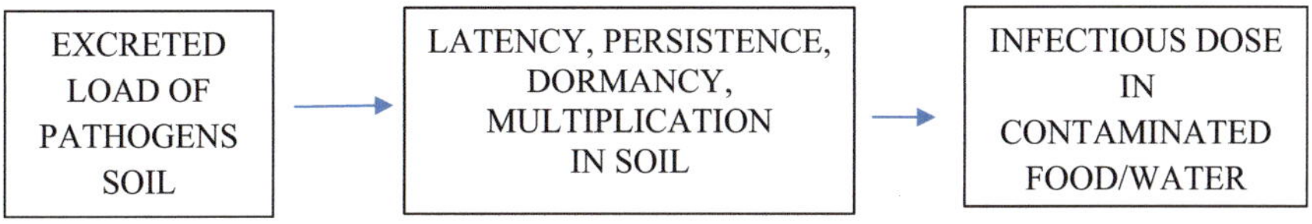

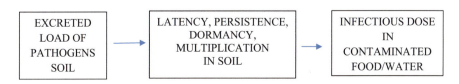

Fig. 20.1 Pathogens' journey to infectious stage/infective dose

Large meats (like roasted turkey or lamb) are commonly incriminated; consequentially number exposed/eating contaminated meat is large.

Spores of *Clostridium botulinum* are the most resistant of bacterial spores, requires commercial canning is heated at 121 °C for 3 min'. Botulinum toxin is destroyed by heating at >85 °C for >5 min.

Thermal-resistant enterotoxins of *Staphylococcus aureus* remain active after heating food even after the death of the bacteria.

In short, food-poisoning pathogens should be evaluated for innate characteristics, like infective dose, doubling time, growth temperature, resistance to heat, low temperature, and survival in sodium chloride, nitrite, acid, and food preservatives.

20.2 Source of Pathogens: Food Animal Production (Farming) System; Processing and Trade

Zoonotic food-borne-infection-causing agents are mostly found in live food animals and fresh meat. The journey of pathogens from farm to fork is depicted in Fig. 20.2. Farm management greatly influences the quality of produce from farm animals. In turn, it affects domestic and international trade and, finally, consumers' health. In 1881, some European countries banned the import of pork from the USA for fear of trichinae-infected pork. Trichinoscopy was advocated but not implemented. Portugal and other importing countries insisted on the inspection of pork carcasses and certificates of freedom from *T. spiralis*. On trichinoscopy, 3/482 carcasses were found positive. Reverse tracing revealed extremely poor hygienic conditions in 1/35 farms supplying pigs. Dead pigs were fed to pigs, allowing the perpetuation of *T. spiralis* infection on the farms.

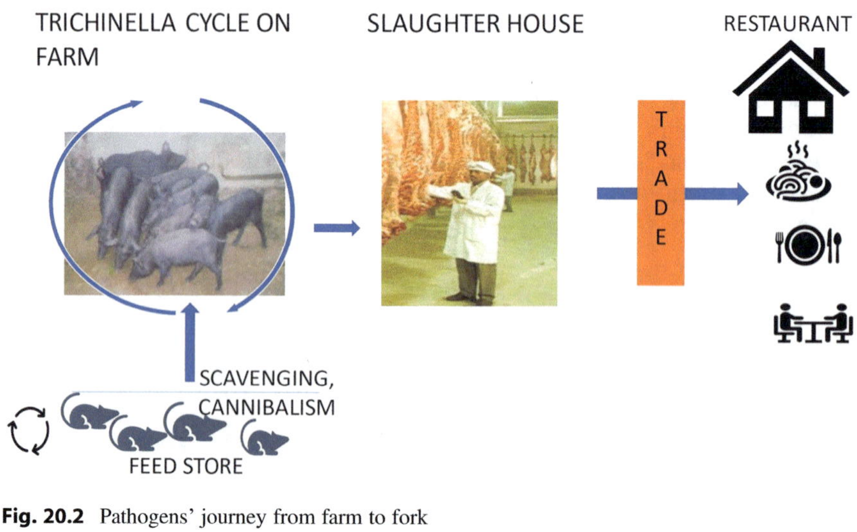

Fig. 20.2 Pathogens' journey from farm to fork

Food-borne bacterial pathogens, like *Salmonella*, cause asymptomatic or silent infection. *Salmonella* and other enteric pathogens spread endogenously to other tissues. This endogenous spread is accentuated by stress, e.g. transport to slaughterhouses or mismanaged grow out/lairage. Stress also increases the rate of the excretion of pathogens, resulting in pre-slaughter horizontal spread among pigs in lorries and lairage.

In the past, increased reports of human salmonellosis due to a serotype that was consistently found frequent in a particular brand of sausage were investigated. Two of the slaughterhouses that supplied pork to the identified brand of sausage manufacturer flouted the regulation. Pigs were allowed to stay in the lairage for an indefinite period and slaughtered as per the demand of the market. This resulted in the building up of *nidii* of the same *Salmonella* serotype in lairage, which were detected among pigs (silent spreader) and samples from slaughterhouses and carcasses.

Such silent spread is dangerous and is detected only by a laboratory examination of samples from on-line slaughter or of carcasses at the end of the slaughter. The detection of pathogens in a well-managed slaughterhouse and pig/poultry processing plant reflects a prevailing infection in the farms of origin of slaughtered animals.

Abattoirs and processing plants function as laboratories, and results (data) help in mapping the reverse tracing of infection.

Live animal or bird markets in some countries combine all processes but possibly without adequate intervention and inspection. Biswas et al. (2017) used live-bird markets (LBMs) with intervention (10) and without (22) to elucidate the incidence of zoonotic avian influenza viruses (AIVs) H5, H7, and H9 in Bangladesh. Specimens representing a chain of operational areas, poultry holding cages, slaughter areas, water used for meat processing, stall floors, and market floors were examined every month for 5 months in 2013. The incidence rates of AIV, H5, H7, and H9 per Live bird markets (LBMs)-month at risk were 0.194, 0.031, 0, and 0.175, respectively. *It was concluded that in absence of robust active surveillance of AIV affecting poultry in South Asian countries, this determined (a) the prevalence of AIV (b) contamination with H9 was higher than H5 and (c) there was no significant difference between the 'intervention and its absence'.*

Chicks may get infected at two levels: (a) from breeder flocks vertically and (b) in hatcheries through 'pseudo-vertical' transmission from externally contaminated eggs or pre-existing resident contaminants or through cross-contamination.

Eggs are more commonly associated with outbreaks and sporadic cases (i.e. diffuse outbreaks). Whole genome sequence of bacterial isolates should be authenicate. Eggs are contaminated internally also (vertical transmission), unlike poultry meat, and are not required to be stored in the refrigerator. Raw pooled eggs are used as ingredients in various food products. Eggs are expected to be more frequent vehicles of outbreaks, including diffuse outbreaks, compared to poultry meat.

Salmonellae are excreted in faeces and spread horizontally. *S.* Gallinarum and *S.* Pullorum are passed in eggs by infected hens vertically. *Salmonella*-infected/contaminated eggs follow the trade routes, finally reaching the consumers (Fig. 20.3).

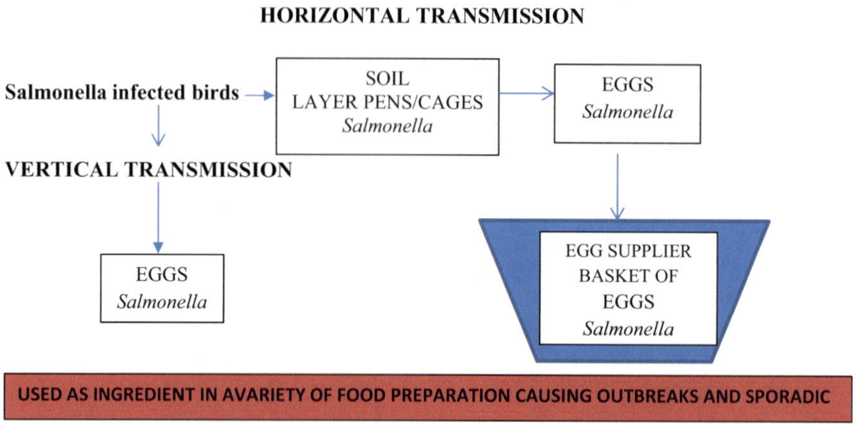

Fig. 20.3 Pathogens' journey from farms through trade routes of food to consumers

20.3 Causes

Animal source food and produce are large sources of FBD and illnesses. These accounted for 82% of disability-adjusted life years (DALYs) in the Netherlands and 51% of deaths in the USA.

20.3.1 FB Parasitic Disease Burden

The global burden of *toxoplasmosis (>1/3) and giardiasis (>1/10)* is high. *Cysticercosis* and *echinococcosis* cause serious illness. The global burden of food-borne parasitic diseases is around 18 million DALYs. These infections are cryptosporidiosis, amoebiasis, cystic echinococcosis, alveolar echinococcosis, ascariasis, trichuriasis (whipworm), toxoplasmosis, food-borne trematodiasis, and cysticercosis (Grace 2015).

Toxoplasma gondii: food-borne transmission is probably the main mode of transmission to humans, who ingest the tissue cysts (bradyzoites) and tachyzoites of *T. gondii* in meat and milk, respectively. Sporulated oocysts in the environment can contaminate fresh produce, shellfish, and water to infect humans after consumption. Finally, it was concluded that food-borne transmission accounted for 40–60% of toxoplasma infections, and a major source was meat (EFSA 2018).

Food-borne cryptococcosis is associated with the ingestion of fresh produce, e.g. fruits, vegetables and herbs, fruit and vegetable juice, molluscan shellfish, milk and dairy products, and meat contaminated during production and processing. Globally, 25 outbreaks were reported from 1984 to 2017, and the European Food Safety Authority (EFSA) received 53 reports between 2005 and 2016. Of the 23 EU/EEA countries that did report data on cryptosporidiosis, 13 reported only

0–10 cases in 2015 compared with the average reporting rate of 3.1 cases per 100,000 population. The UK reported over half of all cases (EFSA 2018).

Clonorchiasis, opisthorchiasis, paragonimiasis, and fascioliasis amounted to 200,000 cases, 7000 deaths, and 2.0 million DALYs (WHO 2021, 8 August).

20.3.2 Parasites

- Amoebiasis
- Ascariasis
- Angiostrongyliasis
- Anisakiasis
- *Cyclospora cayetanensis*
- Capillariasis
- Cryptosporidiosis
- Sarcocystosis
- Toxoplasmosis
- Ancylostomiasis
- Dioctophymiasis
- Echinostomiasis
- Trichinosis
- Trichuriasis
- Metagonimiasis
- Cystic echinococcosis
- Alveolar echinococcosis
- Cysticercosis
- Hydatidosis
- Clonorchiasis
- Diphyllobothriasis
- Fascioliasis
- Opisthorchiasis
- Paragonimiasis
- Taeniasis

Microbial pathogens cause most of the FBD burden in developed countries, manifesting in the form of intestinal (20–40%) and non-intestinal diseases. Grace (2015) estimated that 10% of the DALYs due to diarrhoeal diseases occurring in lower-middle-income countries (LMICs), corresponding to 9.0 million DALYs, were due to viruses and bacteria. The non-intestinal health impacts were considered equal and suggested an additional 9.0 million DALY burden.

20.3.3 Viruses

- Rotavirus.
- Astrovirus.
- Enterovirus.
- Adenovirus.
- Hepatitis A.
- Hepatitis E.
- Norovirus.
- Poliovirus.

  Prion (bovine spongiform encephalopathy (BSE))

20.3.4 Bacteria

- Anthrax.
- Aeromonas.
- *Bacillus cereus.*
- Botulism.
- Brucellosis.
- *Clostridium perfringens.*
- Campylobacteriosis.
- Diphtheria.
- *Escherichia coli.*
- Erysipelothricosis.
- Leptospirosis.
- Listeriosis.
- *Pseudoterranova* spp.
- *Plesiomonas shigelloides.*
- Q fever.
- Salmonellosis.
- Shigellosis.
- Streptococcosis.
- Staphylococcosis.
- Tuberculosis.
- *V. parahaemolyticus.*
- *Vibrio*, incl cholera.
- *V. vulnificus.*
- Yersiniosis.

Fungal toxins: aflatoxins are naturally occurring, toxic metabolites produced by some species of the *Aspergillus.* Maize, groundnuts, dairy products, and fermented traditional food may contain aflatoxin. Chronic exposure causes liver cancer. The condition of hepatitis B cases worsens with aflatoxin ingestion. Nearly 2/3 of aflatoxin-liver cancer cases have been detected in hepatitis-positive people.

Southeast Asia, China, and sub-Saharan Africa are high aflatoxin areas, and the estimated burden is 1.6 million DALYs. The latter two areas host 17% (88,400 cases) of aflatoxin-related hepatocellular carcinomas.

Chemicals in food include metals, pesticides, growth promoters, chemicals added to food during processing, chemicals added to adulterate food, dioxins, and toxins produced by cooking (polycyclic aromatic hydrocarbons and acrylamides). Knowledge about DALYs is not available.

20.4 Classes of Food and the Respective Common Pathogens

- Aquatic animals, fish, and seafood: *Aeromonas*, *Plesiomonas shigelloides*, *C. botulinum* type E, *Pseudoterranova* spp., *Vibrio* (*V. vulnificus*, *V. parahaemolyticus*, *V. cholerae*), *Capillaria philippinensis*, *Diphyllobothrium latum*, *Clonorchis sinensis*, *Opisthorchis*, *Paragonimus*, *Echinostoma revolutum*, and *Angiostrongylus cantonensis.*
- Vegetables, fruits, sprouts, and salads: *B. cereus*, *C. botulinum*, *E. coli*, *Salmonella*, *Listeria monocytogenes*, *Shigella*, *Fasciola*, *and Fasciolopsis buskii*—aquatic vegetation, water chestnut.
- Milk and dairy products: *Brucella* spp., *L. monocytogenes*, *Streptococcus pyogenes*, and *Staphylococcus aureus.*
- Meat and meat products: *C. perfringens*, *Salmonella* spp., *Streptococcus suis*, *S. pyogenes*, *Staphylococcus aureus*, botulinum, toxoplasmosis, sarcocystosis, trichinellosis, *Taenia solium* (cysticercosis), and *T. saginata.*

  Contaminated water and its use in any food (ready to eat without heating, such as salads, lettuce, etc.): amoebiasis, balantidiasis, giardiasis, and cryptosporidiosis.

Food-borne diseases may be classified as infection, toxi-infection, and intoxication. Bacteria/viruses ingested with contaminated food set up the infection. The pathogen invades tissues and organs to cause disease. In the case of toxi-infection, the toxin is produced in situ after invasion, e.g. endotoxins by Gram-negative bacteria and enterotoxin by *C. perfringens.* Intoxication is caused when food consumed carries already-formed toxins.

The incubation is generally short.

Important fish-borne intoxications are described below in brief.

20.5 Important Fish-Borne Intoxication

20.5.1 Ciguatera Poisoning

Most common marine toxin infection caused by ciguatoxins in Caribbean Sea, Indian and Pacific oceans, sometimes in Florida and Hawaii. Ciguatoxin is found in >400 species of reef fish. The export of reef fish may cause toxicity in regions beyond these geographical bounds.

Ciguatera fish toxin poisoning is caused by eating ciguatoxic fishes, commonly reef fish whose flesh has the toxin. Two common toxins are ciguatoxin and maitotoxin (produced by dinoflagellates, *Gambierdiscus toxicus*, and *Ostreopsis lenticularis*). These grow in and around coral reefs in tropical and subtropical waters. Other toxins produced by *Gambierdiscus toxicus* are gambieric acid, scaritoxin, and palytoxin.

Herbivorous fish eats dinoflagellates. These are predated by larger carnivorous fish, moray eel, barracuda, amberjack, sea bass, and sturgeon. Toxins get concentrated during this food chain. The toxin is tasteless and has no smell. Detection is not possible, and it survives conventional cooking. The toxin causes gastrointestinal, cardiovascular, and neurological symptoms.

The incubation period (IP) is minutes to 6 h, sometimes 48 h, depending upon sensitivity.

Victims report abdominal pain, nausea, vomiting, and watery diarrhoea. Neurological symptoms begin as sensitivity to hot and cold, paresthesia and numbness are experienced beginning from lips and oral mucosa to limbs; pruritis on palm and sole, arthralgia, myalgia. Tingling of extremities, a sensation of 'pricking by pins and needles' exacerbated by movement of air over skin, photophobia, and perception of flashing lights were experienced by a victim couple (Winter 2009). Severe cases report hypotension, slow heartbeats, dizziness, ataxia, lethargy, seizures, and coma. On the other hand, acute symptoms last for around 8–10 h, diarrhoea for about 4 days, and neurological symptoms for weeks to months but 20 years in extreme cases as well as long disability. Fatality is $<1\%$. Global annual cases range between 10,000 and 50,000.

The toxin is likely to be transmitted through breastfeeding and sex with a person suffering from ciguatera poisoning.

History of fish eating, i.e. the same fish preparation eaten by more people reporting sickness, helps diagnosis. Testing of remains of fish eaten confirm "infection"

20.5.2 Palytoxin

Palytoxin is synthesised by marine zoanthids (corals), e.g. *Palythoa* spp., *Zoanthus* spp., and *Ostreopsis dinoflagellates*. It is also found in sponges, mussels, starfish, and others like triggerfish, filefish, parrotfish, mackerel, and crabs living close to dinoflagellates by process of biomagnification. Eating triggerfish, filefish, parrotfish, mackerel, and crabs may cause toxicity. Aquarium hobbyists can get this while incorrectly handling corals, *Palythoa* spp., or those exposed to certain algae blooms. It is thermostable and survives boiling.

Palytoxin is a vasoconstrictor, a potent tumour promoter, and extremely toxic to mammals. It affects all types of cells. It targets sodium-potassium pump proteins and destroys ion gradients, which are essential for life.

Ingestion, inhalation, and skin exposure are routes of entry. The symptoms depend upon the route of entry and the amount. The incubation period ranges between 6 and 8 h after inhalation or skin exposure, and the duration of illness is 1–2 days. The following are the symptoms based on routes of entry:

- Skin exposure: reddening of the skin, rashes, swelling, numbness/tingling, and myalgia.
- Entry through the eye: irritation of the eye, conjunctivitis, and sensitivity to light.
- Inhalation: fever >38°C, headache, sore throat, runny nose, cough, chest pain, difficulty of breathing, and rapid heart rate.
- Ingestion: abdominal pain, cramp, vomiting, diarrhoea, bitter/metallic taste, tingling, impaired sensation, lethargy, slow heart rate, kidney failure, muscle spasm, myalgia, tremor, cyanosis, and breathlessness. It may also lead to death due to cardiac arrest caused by myocardial injury. Rhabdomyolysis is the common severe complication of palytoxin poisoning.

Deaths have been reported after the ingestion of palytoxin-containing crab and blue stripe herring, as well as near-fatal experiences after eating smoked fish and parrotfish (https://en.wikipedia.org/wiki/Palytoxin).

20.5.3 Tetrodotoxin (TTX)

The Tetraodontiformes order includes puffer fish, porcupine fish, sunfish, and triggerfish, in which this potent neurotoxin is found. The toxin has been named after this order of fish. Tetrodotoxin is found also in several animals, including blue-ringed octopus, rough-skinned newts, and moon snails. The toxin is produced by symbiotic or infecting bacteria, such as *Pseudomonas* spp., *Micrococcus* spp., *Acinetobacter* spp., *Aeromonas* spp., and *Vibrio* spp., and bioaccumulates in fish and animals.

The neurotoxin blocks the sodium channels in the nerve cell membrane, blocking the passage of sodium ions into the neurons. As a result, the passage of the message for muscle contraction after stimulation is blocked. The metazoans use this toxin to ward off predation.

The median lethal dose (MLD_{50}) of TTX in mice is 334 microgram/kg, more lethal than potassium cyanide. The modes of exposure to this toxin are ingestion, inhalation, injection, and through abraded skin (contact).

The ingestion of fish (e.g. pufferfish) causes poisoning. Toxin is found in the organs of fish, e.g. liver. The amount of toxin is enough to cause paralysis of the diaphragm and respiratory muscles, leading to death.

The incubation period is 10–30 min up to 4 h. Fatal cases have shorter incubation periods.

Neurological symptoms begin as paraesthesia of the lips and oral mucosa. Patients feel numbness of the limbs, ataxia, cramps, seizures, dysphagia, slurred speech, hyper-salivation, somnolence, flaccid respiratory muscles, incoordination, tremor, paralysis, breathing difficulty, and hypotension. Gastrointestinal symptoms are severe abdominal pain, nausea, vomiting, diarrhoea, and death due to respiratory failure in 4–6 h. Some patients may even enter into a coma. The first day, i.e. 24 h, is critical; if the patient survives, the chances of recovery without any sequelae are great.

The death rate is up to 60%.

20.6 Burden of FBDs

Food-borne illnesses are an important cause of diarrhoeal diseases, which are most common. Food-borne diseases accounted for 10% cases, 660 million illnesses, 420,000 deaths, and a loss of 33 million healthy life years in 2010. Annually, 550 million people, including 220 children <5 years, fall ill due to this illness (WHO 2018). The EU Food Safety Authority and EU Centers for Disease Control and Prevention (CDC) reported a total of 4786 food-borne outbreaks, including waterborne outbreaks. The most common agent was *Salmonella*. One out of six outbreaks was due to *S. enterica* serotype enteritidis. *Salmonella*-contaminated eggs/food combination continued to be the highest risk (EFSA-EUCDC 2017). FBDs give rise to 48 million cases, 128,000 hospitalisations, and 3000 deaths every year in the USA (www.fda.gov).

The world is a mix of low-income, middle-income, and developed countries. Low-income economies are defined as those with a gross national income (GNI) per capita of $1045 or less in 2014, and middle-income economies are those with a GNI per capita of more than $1045 but less than $12,736 (World Bank).

The full burden of food-borne diseases (FBD) in low- and middle-income countries is not known, and the principal causes are biological hazards and fresh, perishable foods sold in informal markets. Livestock, fish products, and other produce as well as the lengthening and broadening of value chains are potential risks of FBDs. Intervention is limited.

Grace cites a FAO report—'. . . there are no technically or economically viable alternatives to intensive production for providing the bulk of the livestock food supply for growing cities'—and suggests that '*concern for food safety and standard rachet should not affect the farmers and street food sellers.* The informal sector offers better prices to both farmers and consumers.'

Intensive farming has been associated with the emergence of new human diseases, including swine influenza in Mexico, salmonellosis in the 1980s (caused by *Salmonella enteritidis* phage type 4), 'mad cow disease' in the UK, and Nipah virus in Malaysia. It is alleged that it has led to deforestation and climate change. Training of farmers and street food sellers is required.

20.7 How to Mitigate

Safety concern: Grace (2015) cites food safety concerns in Vietnam. Media reports on pig diseases led many to stop consuming pork or switch to safer meat—chicken. Similarly, in Kenya, people demanded a certificate of freedom from Rift Valley fever during the outbreak and shifted to the consumption of chicken from ruminant meat. Food safety concerns affect trade in the form of rejection and bans. The UK suffered a huge loss due to bans on export, between March 1996 and 2 May 2006, of cattle and bovine products after mad cow was detected. The culling of birds due to bird flu outbreaks affects the economy, small farmers, and livelihood.

In the absence of a 'monitoring system', the prevalence/incidence of zoonoses in man and animals as well as the trend are unknown. A major problem is the absence of a 'legal mandate' (Vrbova et al. 2009). The collection and reporting of animal diseases and zoonotic diseases in animals, particularly wildlife, are not legally mandated to the same extent as in humans.

20.8 Mitigation Approaches and Methods

If the infection in food-producing animals is controlled by good animal management practices, excretion load and the consequential contamination of the soil and animal produce (harvest) will be eliminated or at least reduced to a minimum. Hygienic post-harvest processing will further reduce/eliminate any escaping pathogens.

Of the food-borne pathogens, there has been a large decline in *Salmonella* and *Campylobacter in the EU and US* due to vigorous control in poultry farming.

Food-borne pathogens may or may not show any signs or symptoms in infected food animals or birds. Those showing clinical signs and symptoms are separated and find no place in the human food chain, eliminated at ante-mortem meat inspection, or even earlier. Some infections are detected during post-mortem inspection, e.g. cysticercosis, trichinellosis, tuberculosis, etc., and decisions are taken accordingly.

A healthy human population, safe drinking water, and sewage treatment should eliminate the initial human source of contamination.

20.8.1 FAO Food Chain Crisis-Intelligence and Coordination Unit (FCC-ICU)

The FCC-ICU developed an integrated forecasting approach to predict FCC threats having a high impact on food and nutrition security and livelihoods. The FCC INTEGRATED FORECASTING APPROACH alerts, three months in advance, on (1) the likelihood of introduction from another country and spread and (2) the likelihood of re-emergence within a country (Food-Chain-Crisis@fao.org; www.fao.org/food-chain-crisis.(FAO 2016). Intensifying the food production system, expanding global trade, and changing agro-ecological conditions pose a risk of the emergence and spread of trans-boundary animal diseases and a threat to the food chain.

20.8.2 Harmonised Inspection

It is evident that to protect people from food-borne zoonoses, a harmonised inspection is required. The European Food Safety Authority suggested this based on an 'epidemiological indicator' (2011b). An epidemiological indicator is defined as the prevalence or incidence of hazards (identified) at a certain stage of the food chain or an indirect measure of the hazard (such as audits) that correlates to a human health risk caused by the hazard.

For example, food-borne hazards posed by pigs and pork are *Salmonella*, *Yersinia enterocolitica*, *Toxoplasma gondii*, *Trichinella*, cysticercus (*Taenia solium*), and mycobacteria. The food chain, the spread of pathogens, and its frequency are considered by the 'risk manager'. In the EU, 10–20% of all human salmonellosis are attributed to pigs and pig meat (EFSA 2010). Salmonellae are selected as a harmonised epidemiological indicator (HEI). Other pathogens may be added, e.g. salmonellae and cysticercosis (*T. solium*).

If an inspection detects salmonella in the food chain, targeted measures are taken (see the chapter on VPH).

Risk management regularly reviews and makes experience-based amendment to assure safety.

20.8.3 FoodNet

The Foodborne Diseases Active Surveillance Network, USA (Henao et al. 2015), contributes towards food safety and the prevention of illnesses. It conducts population-based surveillance at ten sites in the USA and laboratory confirmation of nine bacterial and parasitic pathogens transmitted through food. It

- Conducts epidemiological studies/monitors trends in enteric illnesses, identifies their sources, and implements special studies.
- Contributes to the establishment of reliable, active population-based surveillance of enteric diseases.
- Conducts epidemiological studies to determine risks and protective factors of sporadic enteric infections.

20.8.4 HACCP (Hazard Analysis Critical Control Points)

This is a system to recognise, identify, and mitigate the risk-causing health hazard. It has been adopted by many nations and the World Trade Organization for the management of the food safety in food business and trade.

It has seven principles and steps:

1. Conduct a hazard analysis.
2. Determine the critical control points (CCPs).

3. Establish critical limits.
4. Establish monitoring procedures.
5. Establish corrective actions.
6. Establish verification procedures.
7. Establish record keeping and documentation procedures.

The likely route of food-borne pathogens begins with animals. The pathogens proceed through the levels of harvest, retail, and food processing. Retailing and catering premises may also adopt HACCP.

If infections in food-producing animals are controlled by good animal management practices, excretion load and the consequential contamination of soil and animal produce (harvest) will be eliminated or at least reduced to a minimum. Hygienic post-harvest processing will further reduce/eliminate any escaping pathogens.

In a situation where HACCP is not applicable, an alternate approach could be **specific prerequisite programme and activities** (PRP/A), which include cleaning and disinfection of the food processing environment (FPE), water control, t/T (time and Treatment) control, and product information and consumer awareness.

Routine monitoring programmes for the agent should be designed following a risk-based approach and should be regularly revised based on trend analyses.

FPE monitoring is a key activity in the frozen vegetable industry.

Risk and Risk-Reducing Measures

- Biosecurity, rodent control, limiting the access of pets, birds, and other farm animals.
- Feed—freedom of feed from *Salmonella*.
- Comfortable (prefers short distance/time) and hygienic transport.
- Sanitation in lairage and slaughterhouses.
- Adequate cooking.

References

Biswas PK, GiasuddinM CP, Barua H, Debnath NC, Yamage M (2017) Incidence of contamination of live bird markets in Bangladesh with influenza a virus and subtypes H5, H7 and H9. Transbound Emerg Dis:1–9

EFSA assesses risk of salmonella from pig meat EFSA In FOCUS—Food, issue 07 July 2010, p 3

EFSA-ECDC (2017) The European Union summary report on trends and sources of zoonoses, zoonotic agents and food-borne outbreaks in 2016. EFSA J 15(12):e05077

EFSA (2018) Public health risks associated with food-borne parasites. EFSA J 16(12):5495

FAO (2016) Food-Chain-Crisis@fao.org; www.fao.org/food-chain-crisis

Grace D (2015) Food safety in developing countries: an overview. https://doi.org/10.12774/eod_er.oct2015.graced

Henao OL, Jones TF, Vugia DJ, Griffin PM, Foodborne Diseases Active Surveillance Network (FoodNet) Workgroup (2015) Foodborne diseases active surveillance network-2 decades of achievements, 1996–2015. Emerg Infect Dis 21(9):1529–1536

Vrbova L, Stephen C, Kasman N, Boehnke R, DoyleWaters M et al (2009) Systematic review of surveillance systems for emerging zoonotic diseases. National Collaborating Centre for Environmental Health. Available at: http://www.ncceh.ca/en/contracted_reviews/zoonoses_surveillance

Winter FD (2009) Ciguatera poisoning: an unwelcome vacation experience. Proc (Bayl Univ Med Cent) 22(2):142–143

WHO (2018) Salmonella (non-typhoidal) https://www.who.int/news-room/fact-sheets/detail/salmonella-(non-typhoidal)

WHO (2021) https://www.who.int/news-room/fact-sheets/detail/foodborne-trematode-infections

Food-borne Disease Outbreak Investigation 21

Investigation of a suspected food-borne disease (FBD) is important. A single case of suspected botulism is a public health emergency because it can signal an outbreak.

Two important steps to establish the cause of food-borne outbreaks are

1. Food-borne disease outbreak investigation.
2. Source attribution.

The methods are

- Case-control studies (including a systematic review).
- Analysis of data from outbreaks.
- Subtyping: this identifies the reservoir, prioritises intervention level (production), and reduces chances of cross-contamination and spread. It is data intensive and demands collections of representative samples and isolations; transmission pathways from reservoirs to humans are not known.
- Comparative risk assessment: this accounts for different transmission routes for the same reservoir (e.g. toxoplasmosis). Limitation includes few or lack of data.
- Expert knowledge elicitation: it is useful when data are lacking. It allows attribution to main transmission routes. Conclusions are based on expert judgement, which may be misinformed or biased.

Food-Borne Disease—Outbreak, Cluster, Epidemic, Sporadic

A disease caused by the consumption of food is a 'food-borne disease', which may be toxic or infectious.

Cluster, outbreak, and epidemic are often used interchangeably. However, 'cluster' describes a group of cases linked by time or place with no identified common food or source. FBD outbreak refers to two or more cases resulting from the ingestion of a common food. FBD epidemic involves a large number of people

K. G. Narayan et al., *Veterinary Public Health & Epidemiology*,
https://doi.org/10.1007/978-981-19-7800-5_21

over a wide geographic area. A case that cannot be linked epidemiologically to other cases of the same illness is a sporadic case (WHO 2008).

FBD is detected from data sources, such as the public, media, primary health providers/health care workers, food service facilities, or surveillance—laboratories/disease notification, etc.

The objective of an investigation is primarily to prevent the recurrence of such outbreaks. The immediate purpose is to control ongoing outbreaks(s) by detecting the implicated food and the risk factors related to the host, agent, and environment, such as those contributing to the contamination, growth, survival, etc. of the agent.

21.1 Example

21.1.1 Preliminary Assessment of the Situation

Collection of data/information to: *(i) validate the outbreak, (ii) identify cluster/cohort for interview to obtain clear picture, (iii) samples to collect for laboratory tests, and (iv) circumstances:*

Cases reported nausea, vomiting, and diarrhoea 4 to 11 h after eating in a Chinese restaurant (A). The menu consisted of sweet and sour soup, fried rice, noodles, paneer Manchurian, chicken Manchurian, and veg Manchurian. The clinical specimens collected were stool, vomit, and specimens of each of the leftover food items.

In-Depth Interviews

The lunch party, which consisted of a gathering of about 70+ people, was organised on 5 April 2020 and began around 11:00 a.m. Others participating were helpers, drivers, and neighbours.

Four cases reported to a hospital (H) in city X with symptoms of nausea and vomiting by 4:30 p.m. By 10 to 11 p.m., 11 more were admitted; they complained of vomiting, abdominal pain, and diarrhoea.

Commonalities were (a) symptoms, (b) the restaurant, and (c) Chinese food.

Formulation of preliminary hypotheses: the outbreak is associated with food, and the incriminated food item may be any from the menu.

Descriptive Epidemiology

Definition of confirmed and probable cases: those (*persons' age/sex,* etc.) suffering from nausea, vomiting, and diarrhoea (*clinical and/or lab criteria*) and had taken Chinese food at restaurant A (*place*) on 4, 5, and 6 April (*time*) were considered 'possible' cases, and those who took Chinese food on the fifth were 'probable' cases until the completion of the investigation. Add lab confirmation for 'confirmed' cases.

Information is obtained from the cases on the time of exposure, place, and person's exposure for identifying those at risk of becoming ill and formulating

Table 21.1 Summary of data on cases reporting to hospital H in city X

ID	Name	Age	Sex	Symptom				Specimen			IP
				Onset/ date, time	N	V	D	Food	Vomit	Stool	Hours
1	AK	23	M	5/4/ 20, 16:30	+	+	–	*B. Cere us* was grown (+) From the specimen of fried rice	+		4.30
2	BK	21	M	Do	+	+	–		+		4.30
3	MK	20	F	Do	+	+	–		+		4.30
4	KK	20	F	Do	+	+	+		–	+	4.30
5	CJ	42	M	5/4/ 20, 20:00	+	+	+		+	+	8.00
6	CH	35	F	Do, 20:15	+	+	+			+	8.15
7	SS	27	M	Do, 20:20			+			+	8.20
8	RK	25	M	Do, 21:00		+	+			+	9.00
9	SK	26	F	Do, 21:00	+	+	+				9.00
10	MS	41	F	Do, 21:15	+	+	+		+	+	9.15
11	MN	40	F	Do, 21:30	+	+	+				9.20
12	NN	30	F	Do, 21:30		+	+				9.20
13	GK	16	M	Do, 22:00	+	+	+			+	10.00
14	JS	11	M	Do, 22:00			+				10.00
15	TN	12	F	Do, 22:00	+	+	+				10.00
Patients not related to FBD outbreak being treated for other illnesses serve as CONTROL											
1	A	21	M		–	–	–			–	
2	B	23	F		–	–	–			–	
3	C	30	F		–	–	–			+	
4	D	12	M		–	–	–			–	
5	E	13	M		–	–	–			–	
6	F	40	F		–	–	–			–	

Symptoms: *N* nausea, *V* vomiting, *D* diarrhoea

hypothesis about the vehicle/exposure. Analysis follows. The immediate and initial steps required are cancelling ‘orders of home delivery’ and recalling those on their way to delivery. Data were collated and tabulated (Table 21.1).

Active Search
Eleven (11) cases could be contacted. They did not report to the hospital and were treated at their respective homes. No specimen could be available for laboratory examination. The frequency of signs and symptoms were depicted in Table 21.2.

Incubation Period and Duration of Illness
Cases were reported beginning at 12:00 noon. The incubation period ranged from a minimum of four and a half hours to a maximum of 10 h (Fig. 21.1). Roughly, the duration of the illness in the first seven cases was 24–28 h.

Review of the Data of the Public Health/Food Inspection Laboratory
Independent of any outbreak, samples of stool from diarrhoeic patients are examined for diarrhoea-causing agents. Weekly reports of (a) gastroenteritis in March and the first week of April and (b) the isolation of *Bacillus cereus* in the same period are plotted. Figure 21.2a, b present the epidemic curve.

The redline curve in Fig. 22.2b is for the isolation of *B. cereus*. The peak of the isolation of *B. cereus* coincided with the epidemic peak of gastroenteritis.

The *B. cereus* epidemic curve (restaurant A, city X) is in conformity with the common source of infection.

The epidemic curve is drawn by showing the number of cases on the *y-axis* and the time of the onset of the illness on the *x-axis*. Food-borne disease outbreak is a

Table 21.2 Frequency of signs and symptoms

Signs and symptoms	Number of cases	Frequency (%)
Nausea	11	73
Vomiting	13	87
Diarrhoea	14	93

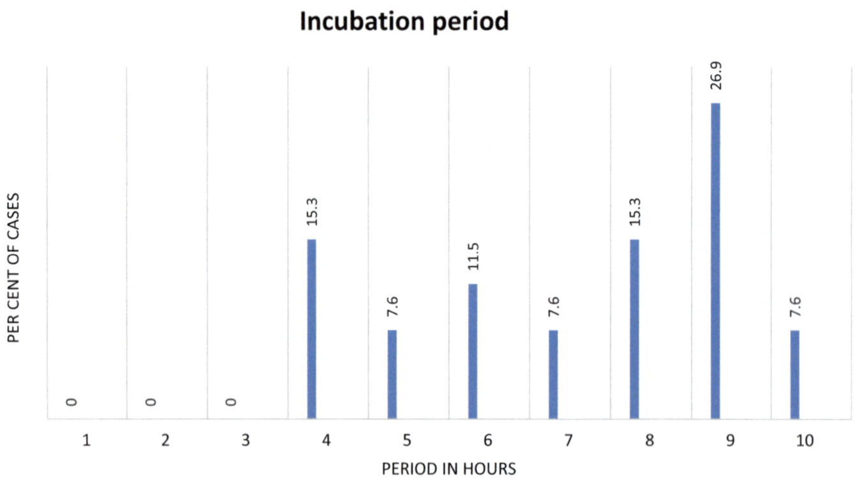

Fig. 21.1 Incubation period

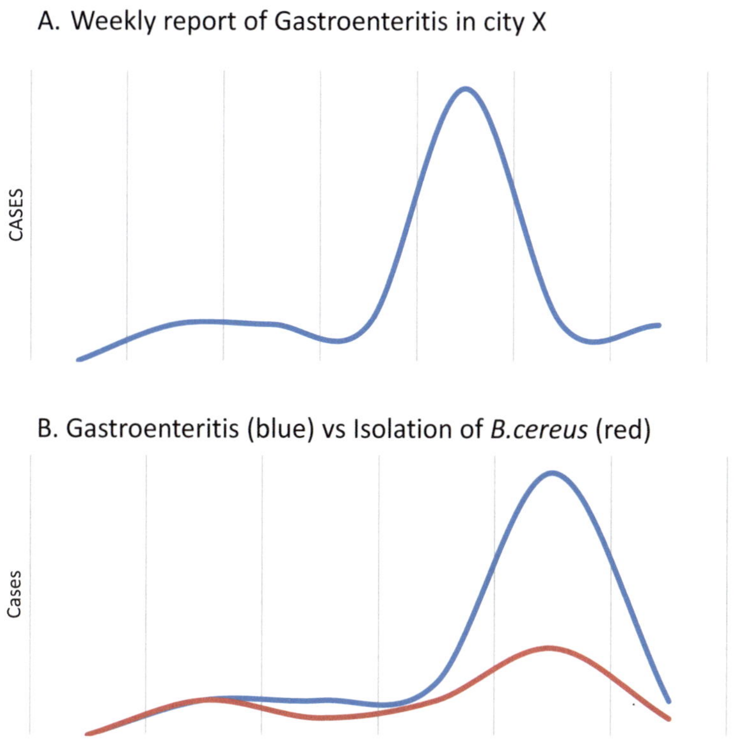

Fig. 21.2 Epidemic curve (outbreak in the first week of April 2020)

common source (i.e. food being the common/single source of the pathogen). The cases may report (i) at one point (point source), at several points in time (intermittent common source; see Fig. 21.3), or (iii) over a continuous period (continuous common source).

Report on Specimens Sent to the Laboratory

B. cereus was grown from stool (7), vomitus (5), and fried rice. Two cases had both vomitus and stool specimens positive for the bacteria.

21.1.2 Epidemiological Analysis

Two ways to determine the hypothesised risk factor (item of food linked to FBD) are (a) a retrospective cohort study and (b) a case-control study.

21.1.2.1 Hypothesis Testing by Retrospective Cohort Study

The hypothesis should address the source of the agent, the mode of vehicle transmission, and the specific exposure that caused the disease.

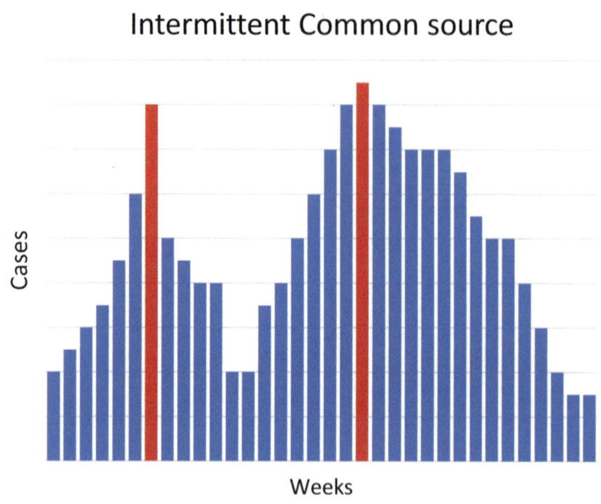

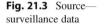

Fig. 21.3 Source—surveillance data

Table 21.3 Cohort study (interviewed = 80, those meeting the definition of case = 60)

	Those who ate food items			Those who did not eat		
Food items served	Ill	Total	Attack rate (%)	Ill	Total	Attack rate (%)
Sweet and sour soup	14	50	28	10	30	33.3
Fried rice	50	58	86.2	2	20	10
Noodles	22	30	66.6	6	50	12
Paneer Manchurian	18	35	51.4	23	45	51.1
Chicken Manchurian	22	45	48.8	14	35	40
Veg Manchurian	20	54	37.0	6	25	24

FBD investigation is a retrospective study, and two cohorts, of those exposed (i.e. consumed an item from the menu) and not exposed (did not consume), are made. Disease incidence in both is compared.

Tables 21.3 and 21.4 below calculate the attack rate for fried rice and the relative risk, respectively. From the tabulated data, the fried rice with the highest attack rate is most likely the vehicle of infection. The relative risk (*RR*) is calculated by dividing the attack rate in those who consumed fried rice (exposed) by the attack rate in those who did not consume fried rice (not exposed); i.e., 86.2/10 = 8.6, which means the risk associated with eating fried rice was 8.6. The attributable risk (*AR*) is calculated by subtracting the attack rate in those not exposed from the attack rate in the exposed; i.e., 86.2 − 10 = 76.2, which means the attribution of fried rice in producing disease is 76.2. The *RR* and *AR* values are the maximum for fried rice in comparison with the other food items served.

21.1.2.2 Hypothesis Testing by Retrospective Case-Control Study

Table 21.5 is related to a case-control study, and Table 21.6 depicts how the odds ratio is estimated. Cases make up one cohort. Who should make up a control cohort?

Table 21.4 Relative risk

	Ill	Well	Total	Attack rate (%)
Ate fried rice	50	10	60	86.2
Did not eat fried rice	2	18	20	10
Total	52	28	80	–

Table 21.5 Case-control (calculation of the odds ratio)

	Cases = 60[a]		Control = 65[b]		Odds ratio
Food items	Ate[a]	Did not eat	Ate	Did not eat	
Sweet and sour soup	14	10	14	41	4.1
Fried rice	50	10	12	53	22.0
Noodles	22	16	18	47	3.5
Paneer Manchurian	18	23	17	48	2.2
Chicken Manchurian	22	14	23	42	2.8
Veg Manchurian	20	6	20	31	5.1

[a]Met the definition of *cases* (data from Table 21.1)
[b]Helpers, drivers, and relatives of the participants as *control*

Table 21.6 Odds ratio

	Cases	Control	Total
Ate fried rice	50 (*a*)	12 (*b*)	58 (*a* + *b*)
Did not eat fried rice	10 (*c*)	53 (*d*)	55 (*c* + *d*)
Total	60 (*a* + *c*)	65 (*b* + *d*)	113 (*a* + *b* + *c* + *d*)

They should be those *not suffering from the disease* under investigation and provide information/data on exposure:

- A random sample of the population in the case of a community outbreak.
- Patients of the hospital/clinics where cases are admitted/treated.
- Neighbours of cases.
- Friends and family members of cases.
- *People who attended/participated in the party but did not fall ill (used in this example).*
- Those who ate at the implicated food service facility during the time of exposure but did not fall ill.

The number of control matters for statistical calculation. Generally, one control/case should suffice in outbreaks where cases are 50 or more. For outbreaks with <50 cases, controls should be more, maybe two to four/case.

21.1.2.3 Distribution of Exposure

The distribution of exposure among *cases* and a group of 'healthy individuals' (*control*) is compared. The questionnaire for control is the same for cases and controls. The details of clinical illness may not pertain to the controls.

From Table 21.6, the odds ratio can be calculated by using the formula:

$$a \times d/b \times c = 50 \times 53/12 \times 10 = 2650/120 = 22.0$$

Therefore, eating contaminated fried rice had a risk factor of 22.0. Fried rice was associated with food-borne disease.

21.1.2.4 Comments

Bacillus cereus appears to have caused the food-borne disease.

B. cereus is a spore-forming ubiquitous bacterium. It grows in temperatures between 8 °C and 55 °C (optimum 28–37 °C), pH 4.3–9.3, and water activity (aw) >0.92. Spores survive freezing, drying, and moderate heating. It produces cereulide, an emetic toxin. Diarrhoeal toxins may be produced in food or in the intestines. The infective dose is > 10,000 per gram of food; lower numbers may produce sufficient cereulide to induce vomiting.

Common food items associated with B. cereus poisoning are boiled or fried rice, spices, dried.

food, milk, dairy products, vegetable dishes, and sauces. The incubation period for the emetic syndrome is short, 1–6 h, and for diarrhoeal symptoms 8–16 h.

21.1.3 Environmental Investigation

After establishing a food-borne disease outbreak, investigation may be extended to trace the source and mode of contamination and the processing failures leading to the survival and/or multiplication of pathogens in food. Then suggest appropriate interventions.

Primary contamination or the contamination of raw food generally causes multiple outbreaks at different sites simultaneously, e.g. *Salmonella* infection of broiler breeder farms and *C. perfringens* contamination of whole turkey or beef cuts.

21.1.4 Source Attribution

A hypothetical situation: Overall, 102 gastroenteritis cases from four municipal areas of city X were reported between May 2015 and the end of January 2016. Additional 23 historical cases were added between 2014 December and January 2016. Surveillance data on reported gastroenteritis cases were plotted against time in weeks (Fig. 21.3).

Investigation revealed that diarrhoeic cases were (the peak in particular) epidemiologically linked to ready-to-eat preparations containing eggs. The public health laboratory identified *Salmonella* in stool samples of ill individuals and in ready-to-eat food preparations made through a conventional bacterial culture system. The *Salmonella* serotyping centre identified the serotype *S.* Enteritidis.

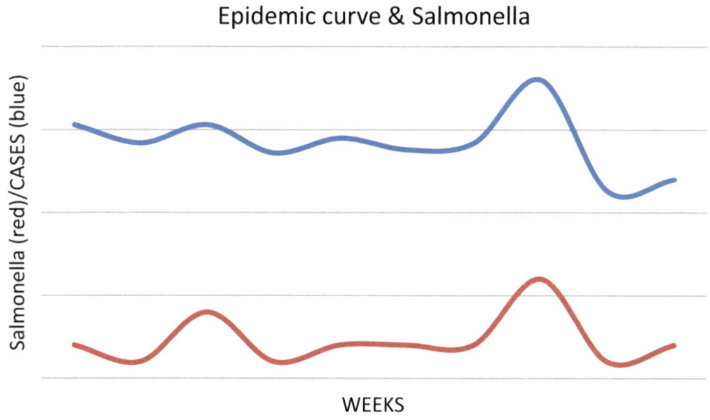

Fig. 21.4 *Salmonella* linked to epidemic

Coincidence of peaks of *Salmonella* isolations and cases (Fig. 21.4) established the cause of illness. Isolates from ready-to-eat preparations were genetically closely related to human isolates. Whole genome sequencing (WGS) is used to trace the source of contaminated eggs through the trade chain and to the poultry farm.

These strongly suggested that cases were part of an intermittent common source outbreak.

21.1.4.1 Illustrative Example (Source: https://www.cdc.gov/salmonella/newport-07-20/index.html)

An outbreak of salmonellosis occurred between June 19 and 11 Septemeber 2020. A total number of 1127 cases with seven hospitalisations were spread over 48 states of the USA. The age of ill individuals ranged from <1 to 102 years (median 41); 58% were female. Ninety-one per cent reported they had eaten onion and its prepation a week before falling ill; 66%, 63%, and 53% had eaten red, white, and yellow onions, respectively; and most had taken more than one type. Whole genome sequencing of *Salmonella* isolates showed that isolates from ill close genetic relatedness indicating a common source of infection. PulseNet system identified the illnesses that were part of the common source. Investigation was jointly carried out by the Centers for Disease Control and Prevention (CDC), public health regulatory officials of several states, the Food and Drug Administration (FDA), and Canada, and they found *S.* Newport was the cause and red onions the source. Trace back idtentified that Thomson international Inc. had supplied the red onion. White onions could also be the source as all the three had been harvested together.

Whole genome sequencing (WGS) and metagenomics are very useful for outbreak investigation, source attribution, and the risk assessment of food-borne pathogens. WGS is the most discrete way of identifying a bacterial strain. Food-borne investigation, source attribution, and also hazard identification are made precise. Targeted risk assessment and mitigation are made possible. Sporadic cases scattered geographically and associated with different food products can be linked to a common point source outbreak, facilitating epidemiological investigation and decoding transmission pathways.

21.1.5 Process of Linking a Case to an Outbreak

The first cluster consists of people who had their sample tested positive for bacteria and the bacteria had the deoxyribonucleic acid (DNA) fingerprint. Epidemiologists seek commonality through questionnaires/interviews of ill individuals and/or caregivers. Did they eat/purchase the same food from the same shop or the same brand? Those in the cluster involved and not involved may also be questioned. The suspected food is identified. Samples of suspected food are tested, and WGS is done. WGS or the DNA fingerprint of the bacteria (a) isolated from the food (b) ill people should match. When two or more people eating the same food are getting ill with the same illness, it is an outbreak.

21.1.5.1 Assessing the Level of Exposure/Dose-Responses

If the enquiry is made on the frequency of (how often?) and quantity of a food item is taken, and the contamination persists, it may be possible to establish a dose-response of infection.

Reference

World Health Organization (2008) Foodborne Disease Outbreaks: Guidelines for Investigation and Control. ISBN 978 92 4 154722 2 (NLM classification: WC 260)

Foodborne Viral Infections 22

In 2007, foodborne viruses were second most common, after salmonella, cause of foodborne outbreaks reported to European Food Safety authority (EFSA). Increasing viral foodborne outbreaks is attributable to (a) improved diagnostic and reporting (b) increased trade of fresh and frozen foods. Viruses do not multiply in foods during storage and processing. Foods act as vehicle only. Initial level of contamination or further addition of virus during processing cause infection. Those implicated in food and waterborne infections are Hepatitis A, Hepatitis E, Norwalk, Nipah, Adeno-, Astro-, Entero- and rota viruses and about one third of cases of food poisoning in developed countries. In the US, more than 50% of cases are viral, and noroviruses are the most common foodborne illness, causing 57% of outbreaks in 2004.

Three basic sources are animals, human and food handlers. Foodborne viruses of animals' origin (reservoir) are Nipah, Hepatitis E and SARS-Corona, infecting through milk, meat and saliva. The frequency is relatively low. Human (reservoir) originating viruses are Norwalk, Hepatitis E and Hepatitis A. Irrigation and sewage pollution is the route and occurrence is frequent. Food handlers, their hand and also others, transmit these viruses through faecal-oral route.

22.1 Norovirus (NoV)

22.1.1 The Virus

Norwalk virus named in 1972 has a history—Norwalk agent (Norwalk, Ohio USA) was associated with outbreak of acute gastroenteritis among children of an elementary school in 1968. Earlier in 1936, it occurred in Denmark, hence called Roskildesyge or Roskilde illness, winter vomiting bug, winter vomiting disease, stomach flu, viral gastroenteritis, Synonyms—Norwalk agent, Norwalk -like virus, small round-structured viruses (SRSVs), Spencer flu, Snow Mountain virus.

K. G. Narayan et al., *Veterinary Public Health & Epidemiology*,
https://doi.org/10.1007/978-981-19-7800-5_22

Of the five genera of calciviruses (family *Calciviridae*), NoV and sapoviruses only are known to cause human illness, gastroenteritis, while the animal viruses can cause a range of different clinical syndromes, including oral lesions, systemic disease with haemorrhagic syndromes, upper respiratory tract infections and others. There is an anecdotal zoonotic infection with vesiviruses (from rhesus macaques). NoV have been detected in pigs, cattle, mice, cats, dogs, and sheep, and sapoviruses in pigs.

The virus belongs to the genus noroviruses, family *Calciviridae* and is single stranded, positive sense RNA non-enveloped. NoV can be divided into distinct genogroups, based on phylogenetic analyses of the capsid protein. There are seven genogroups, GI-VII further divided into genetic clusters (genotypes). The two common genotypes are GI and GII. GI includes Norwalk, Desert Shield and Southampton viruses. GII viruses named after places—Bristol, Lordsdale, Toronto, Mexico, Hawaii, Snow Mountain. Genogroup, genotype 4 (GII.4) account for most adult gastroenteritis around the world.

Viruses of GI, GII and GIV are known to infect humans. GII viruses have additionally been detected in pigs, and GIV viruses have been detected in a lion cub and a dog. GIII viruses infect cattle and sheep, and GV viruses infect mice. Recombination between viruses from different genogroups is rare, suggesting that this constitutes a species level in taxonomy.

22.1.2 Prevalence

Norwalk virus is a common cause, nearly 50%, of all foodborne disease. Norwalk virus causes 200,000 deaths and 685 million cases globally every year in both developing and developed countries. The gastroenteritis occurs usually in winter, hence named winter vomiting bug. It affects most those under the age of 5 years causing 50,000 deaths in developing countries. It is a prominent cause of illness in Europe, the USA, Australia, Hong Kong and Japan.

22.1.3 Transmission

Norwalk virus is highly infective and contagious. Less than 20 virus particles (may be as low as five virus particles) can cause infection. Infected human shed NoV in the stool and vomit in huge quantity (10^8 to 10^{11} RNA copies of GI and GII per gram). Norwalk virus transmission follows faecal-oral route. Shedding in stool lasts for 3–4 weeks. Vomiting is projectile, virus gets aerosolised and spreads.

Vomit and toilet flush aerosolize the virus which can be transmitted also by breathing. Direct transmission, person to person occurs in 62–84% of all reported outbreaks, the rest is indirect through contaminated food and water. Areas near vomiting episode get contaminated and virus is likely to persist there even after cleaning to cause infection. Investigation into an outbreak among 126 diners revealed the distribution of cases among the diners sitting on six tables around the site of vomit on the floor that was cleaned. Of 52 reporting ill, 90% shared the table one of whom had vomited and was sick. Of the diners sitting on the adjacent table and on the other side of the restaurant also reported sick, rates were 70% and 25%, respectively. The US Centers for Disease Control and Prevention (CDC) report attributed outbreaks to person-to person, foodborne and waterborne.

Community acquired NoV caused gastroenteritis was detected in 11% of cases in The Netherlands, and 7% in the UK. NoV is the prominent cause of illness throughout EU, USA, Australia, Hong Kong and Japan. Doyle et al. (2009) reported 257 outbreaks in 39/67 counties of Florida—44% were lab-confirmed, genogroup GII of norovirus accounted for 93%. More outbreaks occurred in long-term care facilities, but only 10% were foodborne. Norovirus was persistent and widespread in the US. Noroviral along with *V. parahemolyticus* caused infection after consumption of raw seafood in Spain in 2005 (Sala et al. 2009). Study between 2007 and 2009 of diarrhoeal cases in Kolkata, India (Nataraju et al. 2011) detected norovirus infection mostly in children <2 years old. Infection associated with mild degree of dehydration occurred throughout the year. NVGII strains were sequenced. Clusters of GII.4 NoV followed by GII.13 and GII.6 were observed. Evidence of its occurrence across the world are mounting.

The illness is commonly known as 'winter vomiting disease'. It has followed seasonality in the US and parts of Australia. Other synonyms are—stomach flu, gastric flu, cruise ship virus (causing outbreak among vacationers on ship). It commonly occurs in institutional settings such as nursing homes and hospitals. Outbreaks occur as food (contaminated shellfish, rasp berries) and waterborne. It spreads by person-to-person and indirectly as environmental contaminant—fomites on carpets, toilet seats or door handles. Person-to-person transmission is the most common in the EU. This makes it difficult to factor out how much of the problem is to be assigned 'foodborne' (Verhoef et al. 2011).

22.1.4 Source

The source of contaminated water was varied—municipal supply, wells, lake, ice machine and recreational. Shellfish and salad ingredients (heated under 75°C) are common sources, picking up the virus at source or during handling. Outbreaks often involve large number of people. The Canadian CFIA Food Control Agency reported an outbreak (March-August 2017) in which 700 were ill. Contaminated frozen raspberry was the cause

NoV is likely to persist on vegetable crops after irrigation with contaminated sewage, on fresh produce under conditions of storage in house and for at least the period between purchase and consumption

22.1.5 Symptoms

Incubation period varies between 12–48 h. Fever, headache, non-bloody diarrhoea, vomiting and stomach pain are the common symptoms. Patients recover in 1 to 3 or 5 days. The virus affects small intestines. The illness is usually mild and self-limiting. Watery diarrhoea is the most commonly reported symptom, followed by vomiting, abdominal pain, cramps, nausea and fever. It affects all age group but more common in young children (<5 years) and the elderly. The disease may be severe, causes dehydration and sometimes long convalescence or mortality among co-morbid, young and elderly.

Computed tomography of abdomen revealed thickening of wall and enhancement of duodenum, jejunum and ileum and loops filled with water. Study of duodenal biopsies suggested a combination of events leading to diarrhoea. Epithelial barrier dysfunction, increased epithelial apoptosis, increased anion secretion and reduction of tight junctional proteins.

Protective immunity is absent. Chronic NoV infection occurs.

22.1.6 Surveillance

Routine harmonised surveillance, detection in food commodities and molecular typing should be done. Burden at the level of population can/should be estimated if incidence of illness, foodborne infection impact and also asymptomatic, pre- and post-symptomatic shedders are studied. Health care providers are expected to report outbreaks of acute gastroenteritis. The National Norovirus laboratory surveillance, CaliciNet and Norovirus Sentinel Testing and Tracking and National Outbreak Reporting System follow standard reporting and surveillance of norovirus infection in the US. NoroSurv uses standardised protocol for dual typing (Polymerase and Capsid) of suspected strains from hospitalised children under 5 years.

Decontamination as a means to prevent foodborne infection is recommended. Generally, washing reduces microbial load by 1–2 logs from fresh produce, depending on food.

References

Doyle TJ, Stark L, Hammond R, Hopkins RS (2009) Outbreaks of Noroviral gastroenteritis in Florida, 2006-2007. Epidemiol Infect 137:617–625

EFSA (2007) EFSA Panel on Biological Hazards (BIOHAZ) European Food Safety Authority (EFSA), Parma, Italy Scientific Opinion on an update on the present knowledge on the occurrence and control of foodborne viruses

Nataraju SM, Pativada M, Chatterjee D, Nayak MK, Ganesh B et al (2011) Molecular epidemiology of norovirus infections in children and adults: sequence analysis of region C indicates genetic diversity of NVGII strains in Kolkata, India. Epidemiol Infect 2011(139):910–918

Sala MR, Arias C, Dominguez A, Bartolome R, Muntada JM (2009) Foodborne outbreak of gastroenteritis due to norovirus and vibrio haemolyticus. Epidemiol Infect 2009(137):626–629

Verhoef L, Kouyos RD, Vennema H, Kroneman A, Siebenga J et al (2011) An integrated approach to identifying international foodborne norovirus outbreaks. Emerg Infect Dis 17:412–418

Hepatitis Viruses 23

Illness with episodes of jaundice described by Hippocrates 400 years ago probably corresponded to viral hepatitis. Two separate disease entities—'infectious' and 'serum' hepatitis were identified during early 1940s. Since 1965, five major aetiological agents—Hepatitis A, B, C, D and E have been identified. The terms 'infectious' and 'serum' indicate modes of transmission—the former is 'faecal-oral' route causing 'enteric' form, and the latter is 'parenterally' transmitted. The enteric form is caused by types A and E and are food and/or waterborne.

23.1 Hepatitis A Virus (HAV)

23.1.1 Virus

The etiological agent of hepatitis A is the hepatitis A virus (HAV) which belongs to genus *Hepatovirus* within family *Picornaviridae.* Phylogenetic study suggests rodent origin of hepatitis A virus. It is relatively stable virus. The capsid provides special capacity to survive extracorporeal for long periods in external environment during journey through faecal-oral route of transmission.

It has a non-enveloped icosahedral capsid of about 30 nm diameter containing a positive ssRNA genome. Genetic diversity occurs in the capsid coding region and is used for molecular typing. The VP1X2A junction between capsid and non-structural region is the most used genomic region for typing worldwide. There are six genotypes, with >15% nucleotide divergence. Genotypes I (IA and IB), II (IIA and IIB) and III are human origin and genotypes IV, V and VI are of simian origin. Genotype III has been isolated from human and owl monkeys. Most human isolates are genotype I, particularly IA.

HAV is a single antigenic serotype.

K. G. Narayan et al., *Veterinary Public Health & Epidemiology*,
https://doi.org/10.1007/978-981-19-7800-5_23

23.1.2 Reservoir

Human and other vertebrates are natural hosts. The virus multiplies in the liver, excreted in bile and then shed in stool. Viral shedding may begin even before the symptoms appear. The number may be as high as 10^{11} genome copies/g faeces after two weeks of infection and shedding may last for four more weeks. The infective dose is estimated at 10–100 virus particles.

HAV is a highly stable virus, able to persist for extended times in the environment, such as contaminated fomites, sanitary paper, sanitary tile and latex gloves.

23.1.3 Source

Foods that are most likely to get contaminated at the pre-harvest level are involved. Examples are bivalve molluscs—oysters, clams, mussels; salad crops, such as lettuce, green onions and other greens, and soft fruits, such as raspberries and strawberries. Source of infection has not been identified in most cases. The most significant outbreak of HAV infection occurred in Shanghai, China, in 1988, which caused almost 300,000 cases by consumption of clams harvested from a sewage-polluted area (Halliday et al. 1991). Raw oyster was involved in an earlier outbreak in Sweden

Risks include poor hygiene and sanitation, unsafe food and water, man sex with man (MSM) and persons who inject drugs (PSWID) and travel

23.1.4 Survival of Virus

HAV survived at pH 1 up to 5 h, in faeces after drying for 30 days under conditions simulating environment. Faecal contaminated surface, such as steel could transfer the virus from a minimum of 4 hours to 60 days, moisture favoured survival

Under normal storage conditions, the virus survives the period from purchase to consumption. Viruses do not multiply in foods during storage or processing. Hence survival and methods of reducing (decontamination) to below infective dose should be considered. HAV survive for several weeks in shellfish, several days in fresh water, 48 days in river water, >12 weeks in ground water and 60 days in tap water at various temperature. Survival period varied with the surface of fruits and vegetables; as observed, it was longest on cantaloupe than on bell pepper and lettuce at low humidity.

23.1.5 Transmission

Infection occurs per os, after eating contaminated food or drinking contaminated water. Transmission also occurs by close contact with infected person. Infected children often without symptom may spread directly. Other modes of transmission are active homosexuality in men and parenteral.

23.1.6 Distribution

Hepatitis A caused 1.4 million deaths/year (*Global Health Sector Strategy on Viral Hepatitis, 2016–2021*). It accounted for 0.5% of all deaths (7134) due to hepatitis in 2016 (WHO 2020). A total of 12,474 hepatitis A cases were reported in 2018 in the US, although the estimate number was close to 24,900. Outbreaks through person-to-person spread have been occurring since 2016 causing >32,000 cases, mostly among MSM and PSWIDs (https://www.cdc.gov/hepatitis/hav/afaq.htm).

It is most frequent foodborne infection. Illness occurs sporadically; outbreaks of food and waterborne are explosive in nature, as the Shanghai epidemic in 1988 that affected 300,000 people; cyclic recurrence caused prolonged suffering to communities (Halliday et al. 1991); occurs in poor sanitation and overcrowding areas. Distribution is closely related with the socioeconomic development—low in developed and high in underdeveloped countries.

Economic and social consequences in communities are significant because recovery may take weeks and months. The food establishments identified with *Hepatovirus* A incidents suffer substantially. The infection leaves a permanent immunity. Severe infections are rare among adults in endemic areas. Most infections in endemic areas occur in children early in life. In low endemic areas, most infections are observed in adult as a result of exposures during travel to endemic areas to contaminated water, food and risky sexual practices. Severe to fatal illness may result.

Shift to intermediate to low prevalence is observed in many countries. The Mediterranean basin as a whole should no longer be considered as an endemic area. Likewise, in several Asian and American countries a shift from high to moderate endemic has as well been described.

23.1.7 Symptoms

The virus enters through the oropharyngeal or intestinal epithelia, carried by blood to liver where it multiplies in hepatocytes and Kupfer cells. Entry to cells is by endocytosis and exit after replication by lysis and viroporins. The virus is secreted in bile and released in faeces in large number 11 days prior to appearance of symptoms or IgM antibodies. Alanine transferase released from virus-damaged liver cells and observed as increased level in blood,

The symptoms appear 15 to 50 days (IP average 28 days) after infection. There is high and long-lasting viremia. The duration of illness is usually 2 months. Prolonged duration or relapse may occur. Occasionally, fulminant hepatitis may occur in patients with underlying chronic liver disease. Acute liver failure may occur in old people.

Early symptoms are flu like, 80% adults show typical symptoms of hepatitis, majority of children asymptomatic. About 10–15% show recurrence during 6 months after initial infection.

Duration is 2 months, some case can be for 6 months.

Fatigue, fever, anorexia, nausea, abdominal discomfort, jaundice—yellowish white skin, yellow eyes, urine is amber coloured, diarrhoea, tool clay colour.

Other symptoms may be lymphadenitis, pancreatitis, red blood aplasia, joint pain.

23.1.8 Diagnosis

- HAV specific -IgM is detected 1–2 weeks after infection and persist for 14 weeks. IgG in serum indicates that acute phase of illness has ended. Vaccination also induces IgG antibodies.
- RT-PCR to detect the *Hepatovirus* A- RNA.

23.1.9 Treatment

No treatment, but it is essential to keep patient under comfort and maintain nutrition and fluid.

23.1.10 Prevention

Decontamination methods: Heating to an internal temperature of 85–90 °C for 90 s and 60 s destroyed the virus in molluscs and cockle meat, respectively. Boiling and not steaming for 3 min was effective. UV at mW s/cm^2 reduced HAV by 4.3 log in lettuce. Chlorine at 20 ppm reduced HAV by 1.7 log in strawberry, tomatoes and lettuce. Depuration of mussels caused marked reduction of HAV.

Vaccination is effective in preventing infection and illness. Inactivated *Hepatovirus* A and live attenuated vaccines are available. Children, 1–2 years and above, and those at risk should receive vaccine. First dose protects for one year beginning 2–4 weeks after injection. The booster/second injection is given 6–-12 months later protects for over 20 years. Vaccination has drastically reduced hepatitis A in some countries, such as in the US. According to WHO (2020), 34 countries were planning in May 2019 to introduce vaccination of children in specific risk groups.

Health education: Education and awareness on personal hygiene, sewage treatment and disposal, water sanitation, hygienic practices and food safety.

References

Halliday ML, Kang LY, Zhou TK, Hu MD, Pan QC et al (1991) An epidemic of hepatitis A attributable to the ingestion of raw clams in Shanghai, China. J Infect Dis 164:852–859

WHO (2020) Hepatitis A (27 July 2020) https://www.who.int/news-room/fact-sheets/detail/hepatitis-a

Hepatitis E Virus (HEV) 24

HEV belongs to family *Hepeviridae*. The two genera are *Orthohepevirus* and *Piscihepevirus*. All mammalian and avian isolates belong to the former. The cut-throat trout HEV belongs to the latter. Hepatitis E virus caused epidemic in 1955 in New Delhi. Four epidemics of jaundice occurred during 1978–82 in Kashmir. It was caused by Non-A, Non-B hepatitis virus (Khuroo et al. 2016). There were 52,000 patients and 1700 deaths, many were pregnant women. The virus isolated in 1983 by scientists investigating an outbreak in Afghanistan is hepatitis E.

24.1 Distribution

HEV occurs the world over, most commonly in East and Southeast Asia. According to Aggarwal and Jameel (2008), about two billion have been exposed worldwide. Southeast Asia, central, east and west Africa are hyperendemic and epidemics occur. Over 50% deaths occur in East and South Asia. East Asia accounts for 20–50% acute hepatitis cases and 10–50% seroprevalence. South Asia reports variable scale of cases and prevalence (Nan and Zhang 2016). Endemic zone includes Middle East, some regions of South Asia, South America. Thirty percent to 70% sporadic cases occurred in endemic areas. Sporadic zone comprises developed countries like France, Germany, the UK and other European countries wherein autochthonous HEV hepatitis is increasingly reported, caused largely by HEV3 and HEV4. Outbreaks have not been reported in developed countries like the USA, Japan and Europe and are considered low or non-endemic areas. Egypt presents a different pattern. Most cases are young; pregnant women manifest mild to no symptom and seroprevalence resembles HAV; possibly HEV1 subtype not affecting Asian population prevails in Egypt (Khuroo et al. 2016).

WHO estimates 20.0 million infections and 3.3 million cases per year, 44,000 deaths in 2015 accounting for 3.3% of mortality due to viral hepatitis (https://www.who.int/news-room/fact-sheets/detail/hepatitis-e). In European Union/EFA >21,000

K. G. Narayan et al., *Veterinary Public Health & Epidemiology*,
https://doi.org/10.1007/978-981-19-7800-5_24

acute clinical cases with 28 fatalities and an overall tenfold increase in the reported cases were reported over the last 10 years. France, Germany and the UK accounted for 80% of cases (8 June 2017; doi: 10.2903/j.efsa.2017.4886).

24.2 Virus

It is a member of genus *Orthohepevirus* and is positive sense, ssRNA non-enveloped. There is a single serotype. There are four species, A, B, C and D and eight (1–8) genotypes. All earlier recognised HEV genotypes 1–4 that infect human fall under *Orthohepevirus* A.

The genotype 1 is found in subtropical countries of Asia and Africa, and genotype 2 in Mexico, Nigeria and Chad. These two genotypes, restricted to human caused large epidemics in developing countries with poor sanitation. The strains under genotypes 3 and 4 are highly diverse and infected human (Table 24.1), pigs, wild boar, deer and other species of animals and caused sporadic cases in developing and industrialised countries.

HEV is an emerging foodborne illness involving animal products, pork pies, liver paste, wild boar, deer, under-cooked or raw pork, home-made sausages, raw pig liver sausage, porcine liver and meat (in general), unpasteurised milk, shellfish and ethnic foods.

The virus is stable in acid and mild alkaline condition, for 1 h at 56 °C in infected pig liver homogenate. It is susceptible to chlorine.

24.3 Reservoir

Potential zoonotic reservoirs are domestic pigs and wild boars, some species of deer and farm rabbits. HEV4, HEV5 and HEV6 have been detected in wild boar. HEV3 has been found in wild boar in Japan and European countries, and in Sika/Yezo deer (*Cervus nippon*) from Japan and red deer (*Cervus elaphus*) from The Netherlands. Isolation of virus from dromedaries from the Middle East, named DcHEV represents

Table 24.1 Zoonotic HEV genotypes (Nan and Zhang 2016)

Orthohepevirus A genotypes	Natural host	Human infection	Geographic distribution
1	Human	Yes	Asia, Africa
2	Human	Yes	Mexico, Africa
3	Human, pig, rabbit, deer, mongoose, wild boar	Yes	Industrialised countries
4	Human, pig, yak, wild boar	Yes	China, India, Indonesia, Vietnam Japan, France, Spain, Italy
5	Wild boar	Unknown	
6	Wild boar	Unknown	
7	Camel	Yes	Middle East

HEV7 and has recently been confirmed in a liver transplant patient who frequently consumed camel milk and meat, confirming zoonotic potential. Parboiled fish or liver (a treat in some countries) may cause outbreak of hepatitis E. Raw liver from supermarkets, molluscs from water bodies polluted with infected pig dung and Corsican Figatelli sausages are often infected with HEV (Khuroo et al. 2016).

HEV related viruses have been isolated from chicken and rats, but zoonotic potential is not yet established. Serological related agents have been suggested in cattle, horses and some pet animals. Eating uncooked wild boar and deer meat has caused infection. Other potential reservoirs are bandicoot rat, black rat and Asian house shrew (https://en.wikipedia.org/wiki/Hepatitis_E).

The infection is acquired early in life of pigs and is common in farmed pigs. HEV multiplies in liver, lymph nodes, small intestine and colon of pigs. Pigs are infected with HEV3 and HEV4. Infection occurs in pigs of 8–12 weeks old, when the maternal antibodies decline. Pigs do not show any symptoms. Most pigs show viraemia at the age of 3 months and faecal shedding of virus between 10–16 weeks of age. Some continue shedding even after 22 weeks of age. Seroconversion is seen between 14–17 weeks of age. Some pigs' liver has been HEV RNA positive.

24.4 Source

Overflowing sewage contaminating drinking water exposes large number of people generally during rainy season and resulting large scale outbreaks in endemic areas in Asian and African countries. Faecal contamination of water caused outbreaks. Low and middle-income countries with limited access to sanitised water, poor hygiene, and weak health service commonly reported outbreaks. Sporadic occurrence is occasionally observed in areas with better sanitation and safe drinking water supply. Most cases are zoonotic (genotype 3) related with ingestion of undercooked animal meat, particularly liver and pork. HEV is reported sporadically from France, The Netherlands, Spain, Hungary, the UK, Denmark, Norway (Teo 2009). It is notifiable in Germany and France where more autochthonous cases are observed. Pigs as source of infection: Widen et al. (2011) observed that isolates of HEV from farmed pigs and wild boars from same county in Sweden were related, suggesting endemicity. Serological studies, anti-HEV antibodies, detected large number in both endemic and industrialised countries

24.5 Routes of transmission

Faecal excretion of virus occurs for two weeks, occasionally up to 52 days in human. Transmission: (a) faecal-oral transmission (contamination of drinking water), (b) foodborne transmission, (c) transmission by transfusion of infected blood products, and (d) vertical (materno-fetal) transmission (Aggarwal and Naik 2009) and (e) direct contact with animals (may lead to seropositivity, not necessarily diseases). The faecal-oral route is most common

According to Lewis et al. (2010), persons with autochthonous HEV infection were on average older than the general population and predominantly male in Europe. Zoonotic transmission seemed possible, and person-to-person transmission was too inefficient to cause clinical disease. Probably multiple routes of transmission operated

Zoonotic transmission is evidenced by detection of ubiquitous infection in domestic pigs, goat and sheep. HEV4 is common in domestic pigs in India. HEV1 causes both sporadic and epidemic hepatitis; Zoonotic transmission is India is insignificant.

Heavy monsoon, flood causing stagnation and reverse flow in waterways contaminating drinking water, overflowing sewage and sewage polluting through seeping pipes lead to waterborne transmission of HEP. Person-to-person transmission is considered in epidemics which evidence of common source (water/food) is absent. Its role in HEV outbreaks is insignificant. Khuroo et al. (2016) followed 36 pregnant women infected with hepatitis E. Severity of disease in mother mirrored in vertically transmitted infection in foetuses/neonates.

24.6 Symptom

Most infection is asymptomatic. Generally, acute hepatitis E is common in older men. High risk group include pregnancy, those who drink alcohol (large quantity), suffering with liver disease and chronic hepatitis. Chronic infections last for weeks and then resolve. Those with immune deficiency/weakness like cases of organ transplant and infected with genotypes 3 and 4 suffer with chronic hepatitis, liver fibrosis and prolonged viraemia. Case fatality rate among young adults is 0.5–3%.

The incubation period varies between 2 and 10 weeks, average of 40 days. Cases occur in age group 15–40 and infected children are asymptomatic or manifest mild without jaundice and thus pass unnoticed. Symptoms are indistinguishable from other forms of viral hepatitis. Anorexia, jaundice, enlarged liver, abdominal tenderness and pain and nausea are common. Some cases may be fulminant, with hepatic failure in 43%. Death occurs in 51.9% of hepatic failure cases. Case fatality rate is low, except among pregnant women. Hepatitis E is mostly self-limiting.

The development of illness may be monitored. Nausea, fatigue and jaundice are prodromal symptoms that appear for short period. Viral RNA appears in stool and blood during incubation period. IgM and IgG are detectable just before the appearance of symptoms. Increased level of aminotransferase level is part of symptom. The duration of illness is 1–6 weeks. Recovery is accompanied with disappearance of virus and IgM from blood. Post recovery patient has high serum IgG and shedding of virus in stool continues.

Pregnant women, in second and third trimester suffer with severe form of illness leading to liver failure and 20–25% death due to HEV genotypes 1 and 2. Illness caused preterm delivery, abortions, still birth and neonatal death. HEV can also replicate in placenta, stomach, small intestine, spleen, kidneys, neurological tissues, besides liver. Kumar et al. (2014) reported 49% acute viral hepatitis and 75% fulminant hepatic failure in pregnant women in one area.

HEV has been the cause of pathological changes in other organs such as acute pancreatitis, glomerulonephritis, severe thrombocytopenia, aplastic anaemia, auto-immune thyroiditis, cryoglobulinemia (at low temperature antibodies react inappropriately) and neurological complications such as brachial neuropathy, peripheral neuropathy, encephalitis, Guillain-Barre syndrome.

24.7 Diagnosis

- Serological detection of IgM, rapid tests are available.
- RT-PCR on stool and blood samples to detect viral RNA.

24.8 Treatment

No specific treatment except patients' needs to be cared for comfort, maintenance of nutrition and fluid. Drugs like paracetamol and acetaminophen to check vomiting should not be given. Severe (fulminant) cases, pregnant women and immunodeficient (transplant) patients need hospitalisation.

24.9 Prevention

Same as for HAV.

Chinese vaccine, Hepatitis E – 239 is a recombinant subunit vaccine claimed to be protective. It has not been approved for routine vaccination and for use in other countries.

References

Aggarwal R, Jameel S (2008) Hepatitis E vaccine. Hepatol Int 2:308–315

Aggarwal R, Naik S (2009) Epidemiology of hepatitis E: current status. J Gastroenterol Hepatol 24: 1484–1493

EFSA BIOHAZ Panel (EFSA Panel on Biological Hazards), Ricci A, Allende A, Bolton D, Chemaly M et al (2017) Scientific Opinion on the public health risks associated with hepatitis E virus (HEV) as a food-borne pathogen. EFSA J 15(7):4886, 89 pp

Khuroo MS, Khuroo MS, Khuroo NS, Hepatitis E (2016) Discovery, global impact, control and cure. World J Gastroenterol 22(31):7030–7045

Kumar A, Devi SG, Kar P, Agarwal S, Husain SA et al (2014) Association of cytokines in hepatitis E with pregnancy outcome. Cytokine 65:95–104

Lewis HC, Wichmann O, Duizer E (2010) Transmission routes and risk factors for autochthonous hepatitis E virus infection in Europe: a systematic review. Epidemiol Infect 138:145–166

Nan Y, Zhang Y-J (2016) Molecular Biology and Infection of Hepatitis E Virus. Front Microbiol 7: 1419

Teo CG (2009) Much meat, much malady: changing perceptions of the epidemiology of hepatitis E. Clin Microbiol Infect 16:24–32

Rotavirus 25

Rotavirus is associated with gastroenteritis in animals and has been isolated from many species of domesticated and wild mammals and birds. Infection of livestock, cattle, swine and horses causes significant economic loss. Furthermore, interspecies transmission offers opportunity for re-assortment between human and animal rotaviruses. Domestic animals, cattle, swine, dogs and cats contribute to genetic diversity of rotaviruses found in human.

25.1 Aetiology

Rotavirus is a genus in the family of *Reoviridae* with the characteristic wheel-like appearance seen under electron microscope. It has no envelop. The capsid has three protein layers, inner, middle and outer. Inner capsid has 11 double stranded viral RNA segments; each segment encodes specific viral proteins. The virus has six structural (VP)—VP1, VP2, VP3, VP4, VP6 and VP7, and six non-structural proteins (NSP)—NSP1, NSP2, NSP3, NSP4, NSP5 and NSP6. Rotaviruses are grouped based on group protein antigen VP6. The five rotavirus serogroups are: rotavirus A (RVA), RVB, RVC, RVD and RVE. Additional groups are RBF, RVG, RVH and RVI (of dogs).

Rotavirus groups can be distributed according to hosts:

The groups RVA, RVB, RVC and RVH cause acute gastroenteritis in human and animals. Group B rotavirus was detected in humans, cattle, sheep, pigs, does and rats. Group C rotavirus infects pigs, humans, cattle, dogs and ferrets. Group H rotavirus was detected in humans in China and Bangladesh and more recently, in pigs in Japan and Brazil. Group D rotavirus, RVE, RVF and RVG were only detected in animals. RVD, RVF and RVG exclusively affect birds. Group E rotavirus was detected only in pigs (Luchs and Timenetsky 2016).

The serogroup A is the most common cause of acute infectious diarrhoea in children, various domestic animals and avian species. It constitutes one of the major

K. G. Narayan et al., *Veterinary Public Health & Epidemiology*,
https://doi.org/10.1007/978-981-19-7800-5_25

causes of severe gastroenteritis in young children (2 years) and nearly all animals, whales, snakes, cows, pigs spread worldwide.

Rotavirus A accounts for most cases of contagious diarrhoea in developing countries. Rota B virus is endemic in China, responsible for adult diarrhoeal disease affecting all ages. Sewage contaminated drinking water is a common source. It is also reported in India. Rota C causes rare and sporadic cases in children often reported in families.

25.1.1 Classification of Group A Rotavirus (RVA)

Strains of RVA have been further classified based on immunological reactions and structure of the structural proteins VP7 and VP4. The VP4 strains are classified as ‘P’ genotypes (P refers to protease) and VP7 as ‘G’ genotypes (G refers to glycoprotein). There are 37 ‘P’ and 27 ‘G’ genotypes of RVA.

Another system of classifying RVA strains is based on complete nucleotide analysis (complete genome sequence). Genetic relationship between human and animal RVA is better defined.

Such classification is useful in epidemiological studies.

25.2 Epidemiology

Rotavirus A (RVA) affects human and animals of all ages. The infection is ubiquitous occurring worldwide and causing significant economic impact.

At the population level, infection is asymptomatic and mild because of repeated exposure from birth to old age and vaccination. Immunocompromised children may suffer with severe, prolonged and even fatal rotavirus gastroenteritis. Adults and older adults also get infection but mild to asymptomatic except those with comorbidity, some of whom may require hospitalisation. Those caring for young children in childcare settings stand at risk of getting infection.

Rotaviral infection can occur anytime during the year. Before the introduction of vaccination in 2006, the illness was more common in winter and spring in the USA. The peak of illness began during December in the southwest part and move to the northeast by April and May. The pattern of occurrence is biennial (every other year) and the rotavirus seasons are of shorter duration (https://www.cdc.gov/rotavirus/surveillance.html).

25.3 The Global Burden of Disease

Study measured thirteen aetiological agents including rotavirus causing diarrhoea for each age, sex, geographic location and year between 1990 to 2016. The findings are based on a cross-sectional study (Troeger et al. 2018).

Accordingly, rotavirus is the third important cause of mortality among children younger than 5 years accounting for 130,000 per year. Over 40% of children <5 years experienced rotavirus diarrhoea in 2016.

There were over 258 million episodes of diarrhoea among children <5 years. The incidence was 0.42 cases per child-years; range is 0.024 in South Korea to 1.63 in the Democratic Republic of Congo.

An estimated 128,500 of children <5 years globally died, most (104,733) of these deaths occurred in sub-Saharan Africa. Southeast Asia and South Asia also reported high mortality.

Rotavirus accounted for 30% of diarrhoeal deaths in children <5 years irrespective of space and sociodemographic index, such as 4.6% in Nicaragua, 64.2% in Democratic Republic of Congo (low income) and 51% in Denmark and 62.6% in Finland (high income). In the USA, the numbers of episodes were 59,300 and incidence of 29.4/1000 child-years.

Rotavirus appears ubiquitous among children <5 years. According to Alkali et al. (2015), childhood diarrhoea in Nigeria is estimated at 160,000 of all deaths in children less than 5 years of age per year and nearly 20% was due to rotavirus. They detected rotavirus A in 25.5% of 200 diarrhoeic children they studied in Sokoto state.

Rotavirus is the most common cause of severe diarrhoeal disease in infants and young children globally accounting for 2.0 million children hospitalisation each year for treatment of dehydration. It causes 453,000 deaths every year (https://www.who.int/westernpacific/health-topics/rotavirus-infections).

Risk factors include (a) age, 3–35 months, (b) settings such as kinder gardens, children day care and nursing homes for elderly, hospital (nosocomial) and season, (c) cool and dry seasons, winter and spring in the United States, and (d) occupation, adults engaged in childcare.

25.4 Transmission

The route of transmission is faecal-oral. Source may be contaminated water, food, towel, toys and surfaces. The virus is shed in faeces of infected human, 10^{11} virus particles per ml. Samples of urine and upper respiratory tract have been found positive for RVA. The infective dose is small, ca.100 plaque forming units. Transmission may also happen through person-to person contact, through fomites and respiratory droplets.

Transmission (Group A Rotavirus) follows 'faecal-oral' route, directly from person-to-person, or indirectly through fomites, contaminated objects such as toys, towel contaminated water and foods.

Rotaviruses cause highly contagious diarrhoea. The virus can be detected in stool between 2 days before appearance of symptoms to 10 days after symptoms lessen, the period of potential viral transmission and spread by hand to mouth. The virus on surfaces can remain infectious for months. Nosocomial infections occur. Other common settings are day care and nursing homes for elderly.

Sources of infection are contaminated foods and water; contaminated water supply may cause outbreak. Rotavirus A is associated with >90% of human infections, millions of cases occur in developing countries. During pre-vaccination period, the rate of hospitalisation was twice among boys than in girls. Hospitalisation is primarily due to dehydration.

Over 95% cases occur in the age group 3–5 years, most common in <3 years with peak incidence in children aged 4–36 months. Infection in neonates is generally asymptomatic possibly because of maternal antibodies. Symptomatic infection in neonates may be due to unusual strains. Adults show no symptoms, infection is detected serologically. In adolescent and adults, RVA causes sporadic outbreaks in closed environments such as hospital, and schools. RVA infection among elderly, immunocompromised, travellers or parents of sick child can occur.

RVA outbreaks tend to occur in the coldest and driest months in temperate climate and throughout the year in the tropics. Luchs and Timenetsky (2016) observed an increased incidence between May to September, the coldest and driest period in the central, south and southeast regions of Brazil and uniform distribution throughout the year in the north and northeast.

Surveillance and vaccination impacted the epidemiology of RVA. There appeared to be a shift in the age of infection to 6–10 years in Brazil and the Unites States. The infection season was delayed by 1–2 months in Brazil, Belgium and the United States.

25.5 Zoonotic Potential

Rotavirus infects young of many species of animals, cause diarrhoea (high morbidity and mortality) in domesticated (calves, piglets—economic loss to farmers) and wild animals. The interspecies transmission and subsequent gene re-assortment are important mechanisms driving the diversity of rotaviruses and enabling the emergence of new pathogenic strains.

The most prevalent strains of RVA in human the world over are the combinations G1P [8], G2P [4], G3P [8] and G4P [8]. According to Luchs and Timenetsky (2016), the strain G9P [8] is fifth among the most prevalent genotypes in humans and G12P [8] was recognised as an emergent genotype, expanding all over the world, including Brazil. The most frequently detected RVA strains in developed countries were G1P [8], G2P [4], G3P [8], G4P [8] and G9P [8]. Some uncommon strains detected in developing countries show wide regional variation.

Animal rotaviruses can infect human through direct and indirect transmission; one or more segments of RNA is/are contributed for re-assortment with human strains.

RVA strains circulate in animals. RVA transmission occurs among mammals and from mammals to birds; between rabbits and calves; calves are susceptible to RVA of simian, swine, leporid origin; bovine RVA are detected in dogs and cats. RVA are of most likely zoonotic pathogen. Complete genome sequence analysis revealed a close relationship between RVA human and canine strains. Some genotypes are common among both man and animals, such as the G3 (common in cats, dogs and equines), G5 (common in pigs and horses), G10 in cattle and G9 (common in pigs and sheep). The genotypes of swine, G4, G5, G6 and G8 have been found circulating in humans, calves and camels (Luchs and Timenetsky 2016). These suggest animals may be RVA reservoirs.

Mukherjee et al. (2013) detected unusual human G8P [4] strains of artiodactyle—origin were in stool samples of three to 14 months old children with acute diarrhoea in eastern India. Human rotavirus A strains with porcine and bovine characteristic have been reported from eastern and north-eastern India. The study suggested re-assortment between artiodactyls and ruminant-derived re-assortment human rotaviruses.

Eight genotype G4P [6] rotavirus A strains collected from children admitted to hospital in the pre-vaccination period in Hungary were studied. These strains were strikingly similar to porcine and porcine—derived human strains worldwide. Genetic relatedness to some common human RVA strains was also seen. These strains might have originated by independent zoonotic transmission, probably from pigs. Simultaneous surveillance of human and animal RVA should be made (Papp et al. 2013).

Intimate contact with animals and consumption of drinking water or foods contaminated with infected animals' faeces are likely the modes of transmission.

25.6 Pathogenesis

Diarrhoea results from a multiprong attack by rotavirus. The digestion and absorption are affected due to damage/destruction of enterocytes. Rotavirus targets apical cells lining villi of the upper two-thirds of small intestine, infects enterocytes, causes cell desquamation and loss of absorption leading to diarrhoea. Following cytolytic replication and release of new virus particles further enterocytes are invaded and virus is excreted with stool.

NSP4 protein is released from the basal side of infected enterocytes and acts as enterotoxin. The digestion of carbohydrates and absorption of nutrients are impaired and there is concomitant inhibition of water reabsorption. Rotavirus induces moderate net chloride secretion at the onset of diarrhoea (Lorrot and Vasseur 2007). Enterocytes secrete lactase, used for digestion of milk. Lactase deficiency causes milk intolerance. Rotavirus damages enterocytes casing milk intolerance and persistence of diarrhoea. There is a mild recurrence when milk is re-introduced in child's diet. The vomiting centre in the brain is stimulated by the activation of afferent vagal nerve by serotonin (5-hydroxytryptamine). Secretion of serotonin is stimulated by rotavirus infected enterochromaffin cells of the intestine.

Systemic infection and dissemination throughout the body are suggested. Few cases have neurologic manifestations ranging from seizures to lethal encephalitis.

Immune response: Infection induces both T and B response, and development of IgG, IgM and IgA antibodies; passively transferred, protects experimental animals. The titres of IgG in blood and of IgA in gut correlates with the protection. IgG is transferred transplacentally to protect neonates and may interfere vaccination programme. There is a rapid innate response to infection. Types I and III interferons and cytokines appear, recruit macrophages and killer cells to prevent replication of the virus.

25.7 Symptoms

Incubation period is 48 h. There is an abrupt onset. Asymptomatic infection to mild to severe watery diarrhoeal disease; incubation period (exposure to appearance of symptoms) is short, <2 days; fever ≥102 °F, abdominal pain, irritable, fatigue, followed by diarrhoea lasting 3–7 days. The stool, which contains blood or pus, is black or tarry. The profuse diarrhoea leads to dehydration, electrolyte imbalance and associated symptoms such as excessive thirst, dry mouth, little or no urination, weeping without tears and dizziness, which may require hospitalisation. There may be shock and death.

Alkali et al. (2015) observed that 33% children with rotavirus diarrhoea had vomiting, 13.8% had no vomition and in nearly half of the cases, vomiting preceded diarrhoea. Ninety percent of cases had vomiting as symptom within 1–2 days; only few had up to 7 days. Rotavirus was detected in 15.9%, 17.8% and 42.4% of children who suffered with none, mild and severe dehydration, respectively.

The duration of illness may be prolonged among immunocompromised and adult. Generally, the disease is self-limiting. The duration of symptoms lasts for 4–8 days. Gastroenteritis symptoms last for 9 days; overall 2–22 days have been recently reported.

25.8 Diagnosis

Laboratory test is necessary as clinical presentation is confounded with a number of infections such as enteropathogenic bacteria, toxigenic coli and enteric parasites, adenoviruses, caliciviruses and astrovirus.

The following tests are useful for confirmation, reliable surveillance and for appropriate antimicrobial therapy. Faecal specimen is preferred.

- Antigen capture ELISAs (commercial kits are available).
- Polyacrylamide gel electrophoresis and silver staining.
- Latex agglutination—less sensitive than EIA.
- RT-PCR for type-specific diagnosis.
- Sequence analysis.
- Electron microscopic examination.
- Rotavirus can be grown in Cell culture.

25.9 Control and Prevention

Since 2005, deaths from diarrhoea among children <5 years decreased by 45%, which is largely attributable to improvement in sanitation, quality of drinking water and reduction in childhood malnutrition.

25.10 Vaccination

High transmissibility makes control difficult. Wide coverage of vaccination should be the priority. Several countries adopted vaccination, leading to consequential reduction in rotavirus associated number of episodes, cases, outpatients, hospitalisation and deaths. Vaccinations are implemented in 95 countries as of April 2018. Rotavirus-associated hospitalisation is reduced to 49–89% within 2 years of implementation. This observation was based on a data from eight high-income and middle-income countries (Bányai et al. 2018). Troeger et al. (2018) showed alleviation of rotavirus associated diarrhoea among children less than 5 years in several countries that adopted vaccination, viz., Finland, Rwanda and Ghana. Rotavirus-associated mortality decreased by 48.2% between 1990 and 2016 in the US. In 2016, 27.8% of children <5 years were vaccinated. Vaccine averted more than 28,000 deaths, and the expanded use of vaccine in sub-Saharan Africa in particular could have prevented 20% of all deaths attributable to diarrhoea among children <5 years.

25.11 Treatment

No specific treatment; fluid therapy to make up for fluid loss and prevent dehydration. Probiotics—an appropriate *Lactobacillus* spp. reduces duration of diarrhoea.

Spasmolytic therapy in severe cases and specific oral immunoglobulins in neonates may be useful.

25.12 Prevention

The World Health Organization recommends improved sanitation and hygienic measures. Most handwash solutions are ineffective but important especially after changing child's diaper and helping to use the toilet. Indirect transmission through unclean touch of toys, utensils and foods occurs.

Faeces, vomit, cloth etc. should be disinfected. Seventy percent alcohol is recommended for surface disinfection.

Asymptomatic excretion of virus makes it difficult to identify and isolate the infected. Infected wards in a hospital may be closed. Cohort nursing in small groups may be practiced. Stables and cowsheds should be closed if animals are found infected.

WHO recommended vaccines are:

Rota Teq (RV 5)—oral administered on months two, four and six; not approved for older children.
Rotatrix (RV 1)—oral for infants at 2 months and 4 months.

First dose at the age of 15 weeks, all doses must be administered before the age of 8 months; not to be administered to children with history of intussusception. Vaccine protects against severe rotavirus illness and hospitalisation in 85–98% cases and 74–87% protection against rotavirus illness of any severity (https://www.cdc.gov/rotavirus/clinical.html).

Vaccine averted more than 28,000 deaths, and the expanded use of vaccine in sub-Saharan Africa in particular could have prevented 20% of all deaths attributable to diarrhoea among children <5 years (Troeger et al. 2018).

Neither vaccine nor first infection guarantees full protection from future infection. The second infection is generally mild than the first one.

Surveillance

- Monitor impact of vaccination (reduction of morbidity and mortality).
- Monitor possible emergence of rotavirus strains that might escape vaccination accounting for vaccination failure.
- Identify group/population inadequately covered by vaccination.

References

Alkali BR, Daneji AI, Magaji AA, Bilbis LS (2015) Clinical symptoms of Human Rotavirus Infection observed in Children in Sokoto, Nigeria. Adv Virol 2015:890957, 6 pages. https://doi.org/10.1155/2015/890957

Bányai K, Estes MK, Martella V, Parashar UD (2018) Viral gastroenteritis. Lancet 392(10142):175–186

Lorrot M, Vasseur M (2007) How do the rotavirus NSP4 and bacterial enterotoxins lead differently to diarrhea? Virol J 4:31. https://doi.org/10.1186/1743-422X-4-31

Luchs A, Timenetsky M d CST (2016) Group A rotavirus gastroenteritis: post-vaccine era, genotypes and zoonotic transmission. Einstein (Sao Paulo) 14(2):278–287

Mukherjee A, Mullick S, Deb AK, Panda S, Chawla-Sarkar M (2013) First report of human rotavirus G8P[4] gastroenteritis in India: evidence of ruminants-to-human zoonotic transmission. J Med Virol 85(3):537–545

Papp H, Borzák R, Farkas S, Kisfali P, Lengyel G et al (2013) Zoonotic transmission of reassortant porcine G4P[6] rotaviruses in Hungarian pediatric patients identified sporadically over a 15 year period. Infect Genet Evol 2013(19):71–80

Troeger C, Khalil IA, Rao PC et al (2018) Rotavirus vaccination and the global burden of rotavirus diarrhoea among children younger than 5 years. JAMA Pediatr 172(10):958–965

Bovine Spongiform Encephalitis (BSE)/Mad Cow Disease 26

BSE is a transmissible spongiform encephalitis (TSE) caused by prion protein. Transmissible spongiform encephalopathies (TSEs) are characterised by fatal neurodegenerative changes in the brain, abnormal behaviour and death affecting man and several species of animals (Table 26.1). TSEs or prion protein diseases are inherited and infectious. Familial TSE is linked to the mutation of prion protein gene, *prnp*.

Prions are unconventional transmissible infectious agents composed largely or exclusively of misfolded prion protein also called as scrapie-associated prion protein (PrPSc). PrPSc propagates. Conversion of normal cellular prion protein PrPC into abnormal prion protein PrPSc proceeds as a chain reaction. Aggregates of PrPSc proteins damage brain, causing characteristic signs and symptoms.

The variant of Creutzfeldt-Jakob disease (nv or vCJD) is infectious and foodborne bovine spongiform encephalopathy (BSE). The characteristic neurodegenerative changes are spongiform, vacuolation, gliosis and accumulation/deposition of abnormal proteinase K resistant isoform or scrapie isoform of the prion protein (PrP^{Sc}) of naturally occurring host-encoded protein PrPc in CNS and other organs.

Transmission experiments to human PrP transgenic mice or primates suggest that namely L-type atypical BSE, classical BSE in sheep, TME, CWD agents might have zoonotic potential. One study suggested efficient transmission of a natural sheep classical scrapie agent to primates (EFSA 2011).

Note: Vets are comparative pathologists. Hadlow, a vet observed that Scrapie and Kuru had similarities and this initiated studies. Kuru is transmissible to primates by ingestion and inoculation. Kuru, GSS and CJD were similar. While GSS was only familial, CJD was familial, sporadic and iatrogenic.

Kuru is considered a close relative of vCJD; seen among the fore people of Papua New Guinea and linked with mortuary feasting—eating the corpse (brain tissue) by family members as a mark of respect for the dead. This practice was stamped out in 1950s, and the Kuru cases petered out. The incubation period was estimated at

K. G. Narayan et al., *Veterinary Public Health & Epidemiology*,
https://doi.org/10.1007/978-981-19-7800-5_26

Table 26.1 TSEs of man and animals

Animal TSE	Species (Infective tissues)	Year	Human TSE	Year
Scrapie - classical and atypical[a]	Sheep and goats (CNS, lymphoreticular systems—high titre. Placenta, adrenal, nasal mucosa, lungs, pancreas, liver, thymus, bone marrow, alimentary tract—low titre)	1730 approx.	CJD (Creutzfeldt-Jakob Disease)	1920
Transmissible mink encephalopathy (TME)[a]	Mink (After replication in CNS and lymphoreticular tissues- low titre in liver, kidney, intestine, salivary glands)	1965	GSSS (Gerstmann-Straussler-Scheinker Syndrome)	1928
Chronic wasting disease (CWD)[a]	Elk	1980	Kuru	1957
Mad cow disease or bovine spongiform encephalopathy (strains: Classical BSE and Atypical H and L types)[a] Classical BSE in sheep[a]	Cattle (CNS in case of natural; CNS, ileum and bone marrow if oral infection) Greater Kudu (natural low titre, skin, conjunctiva, submandibular salivary gland, spleen, lungs)	1986	Fatal Familial Insomnia	1986
			vCJD (Variant or new variant CJD)	1996
Feline spongiform encephalopathy	Feline	1990	Sporadic Familial insomnia	1999

[a]Classical BSE is zoonotic

12 years, ranging from 5 to 56 years, ascribed to a gene variant responsible for resistance to prion disease.

26.1 CJD and vCJD

CJD may be sporadic, inherited or acquired (through infection), with sporadic form being the most common. Classical CJD affects 50 years or older. The incubation period is long (10–40 years), death occurs in 6–12 months once the symptoms appear. Annual incidence is about one per million. vCJD progresses rapidly—4.5 months is the median time from onset to death.

Sporadic or spontaneous—Classical CJD is caused by mutation in normal protein PrP of brain to abnormal PrP^{sc} [sc refers to scrapie—prototypical protein] that is resistant to proteinase and multiplies. More and more abnormal brain proteins form.

Hereditary—Familial classical CJD accounts for 10–15% and is considered 'genetically transmitted (genetic mutation of PrP)'. Cluster of cases appear in families.

Acquired—Infectious prions are acquired through various routes. Incidence of iatrogenic CJD is twice more than vCJD.

GENETIC susceptibility: vCJD patients were generally methionine or valine homogenous *PRNP genotype* at codon 129. Peden et al. (2004) reported a heterozygote at codon 129 of *PRNP.*

26.2 Routes of Infection

Vertical—A traditionally held opinion is that scrapie is also transmitted from mother to foetus. As the incubation period is long, it is difficult to differentiate this from postnatal laterally transmitted infection.

As observed, parenteral transmission, especially intraperitoneal, is very effective in laboratory animals. Infection is through damaged skin, mucosa such as tongue or vascular system—blood vessels. Infection is rapid and effective, particularly if the entry is through a tissue rich in nerves, such as tongue.

During surgery—PrP^{sc} may be introduced both through peripheral and CNS system. i/c inoculation led to spread to sensory nerves and neuromuscular junctions in tongue (tissues rich in nerves). Contaminated neuro-surgical instruments [PrP^{sc} being resistant to disinfection] could also be the source of infection. Corneal and dura tissue transplant- and blood transfusion-associated CJD are known.

Growth hormone and gonadotropins originating from cadaver caused CJD.

Ingestion—vCJD is linked to consumption of meat products of cattle suffering from mad cow disease.

Aerosol infection has been observed in mice (Aguzzi and Zhu 2012).

26.3 BSE and vCJD

26.3.1 Epidemiology

Bovine spongiform encephalopathy (BSE) is a progressive fatal neurological disorder of cattle. It is caused by an unusual transmissible protein called prion, a modified form of a normal protein. This modification transforms normal prion protein into a pathogen. BSE is one of TSE or prion protein diseases reported in different animals and human (Table 26.1) characterised by accumulation of prion in nervous tissues. Two forms are known, classical and sporadic (spontaneous appearance). Classical BSE is transmissible and caused by consumption of contaminated feed. The sporadic form was detected in aged cattle only on intensive surveillance in the early 2000s with no evidence of transmissibility. The incidence of both is negligible; estimate approaches zero case per million cattle (OIE 2018).

A rapidly progressive encephalopathy of cattle (Classical BSE) was identified in the UK in 1986 and lab-confirmed in 1987. It was probably present since 1970s. Outside the UK, it was recorded in some 25 countries, mainly in Europe, Asia, the Middle East and North America.

Meat cum bone meal (MBM) was the suggested source. Prion in scrapie—infected sheep tissue survived 'rendering process' to enter beef rearing system as bovine spongiform encephalitis (BSE) agent, flourished in tissues, in recycled bovine offal from sick animals and spread through 'bovine offal', 'animal feed' and 'fertiliser'. Infected bovine offal/animal feed was also implicated in new diseases of cats, ungulates and primates.

The time of appearance of the epidemic coincided with introduction of new rendering process—'continuous processing at lower temperature with solvent extraction'—in early 1980s that was ineffective on prion. The old 'organic solvent extraction with steam stripping typically applied to greaves after primary cooking' was abandoned. BSE prion is not destroyed even by cooking and 'well done' contaminated beef stuff remained infectious. Prion remains viable and infectious over 600 °C or 1100 °F. Only partial inactivation is achieved at 350 °C.

The British Diabetic Association in 1990 and the European Commission in 1991 expressed concern. Banning the use of offal of bovine from human food in 1989, from animal feed in 1991 and from fertiliser retarded the rate of appearance of mad cow disease in the UK and elsewhere in Europe. The United States did not import beef from the UK since mid-1980s. As a result, no BSE was reported.

In the United Kingdom, BSE epizootic peaked in January 1993 with about 1000 new cases per week. Cumulatively, by the end of 2015, over 184,500 cases of BSE were confirmed in the UK alone in >35,000 herds. British beef was banned in March 1996 due to mad cow disease. The annual numbers of BSE cases in the United Kingdom have dropped sharply from 14,562 in 1995 to two cases in 2015 (https://www.cdc.gov/prions/bse/about.html.).

Experts from the block of 25 Member States approved lifting up of the ban when mad cow cases fell below the threshold of 200/million animals and it was finally lifted on 1 May 2006.

BSE has caused death in 13 species of zoo animals. These are: Bovidae—nyala, greater kudu, gemsbok, Arabian oryx, scimitar-horned oryx, eland, American bison = 7; Felidae—cheetah, puma, ocelot, tiger, lion and Asian golden cat = 6. Of these, a non-domesticated bovine from Africa—the greater kudu (*Tragelaphus strepsiceros*), appears to be the most susceptible. The agent is most widely distributed. Detection in skin, conjunctiva and salivary gland, and infectivity has not previously been reported in any naturally occurring TSE (Cunningham et al. 2004).

26.3.2 Sources of Infection

In a mad cow, the level of PrP^{sc} is greatest in CNS and also found in lymph nodes, tonsils, spleen of animals showing clinical symptoms. Saliva, milk, blood and CSF from cattle infected with BSE are infectious (Okada et al. 2012).

- Highly infective: Brain, eyes, spinal cord, skull, vertebral column, tonsil, trigeminal ganglia, dorsal root ganglia, distal ileum of cow.
- Medium infective: Lymph node, proximal colon, spleen, dura mater, pineal gland, placenta, CSF, pituitary, adrenal.
- Low infective: Distal colon, nasal mucosa, peripheral nerves, bone marrow, liver, lungs, pancreas, thymus, blood, faeces and uterus.
- Minimal infectivity: Heart, kidney, mammary gland, milk, ovary, saliva, salivary gland, seminal vesicle, serum, skeletal muscle, testes, thyroid, bile, bone, connective tissues, hair skin, urine.

PrP^{sc} is resistant to heat and chemical processes of sterilisation and thus likely to enter the animal feed—meat cum bone meal. BSE is thus sustained through exposure to feed contaminated with infected bovine tissues.

Urine from patients of sCJDMM1 (common subtype of sporadic form) was not infectious or prion was <0.38 infectious units/ml of urine (Notari et al. 2012).

Scrapie is maintained by infected animals and contaminated environment. Scrapie is not considered transmissible to human, but small ruminants (sheep and goats) are susceptible to BSE. BSE has been identified in goats (Spiropoulos et al. 2011).

CWD prion persist (elk—*Cervuselaphus nelson* and mule deer—*Odocoileushemionus*) in paddock environment and transmission to mule deer has been observed for ~1.8 years in a paddock where infected deer died, and carcass decomposed; for 2.2 years in paddocks where infected deer resided.

Cattle are infected generally in the first year of life through consumption of contaminated feed containing products derived from ruminant, such as meat cum bone meal.

26.3.3 Aetiology

26.3.3.1 Prion: Properties

PrP is a product of *gene prnp* of 231–253 AA. A number of octapeptide repeat regions determines the size and the species differences.

PrP is a glycoprotein found primarily on nerve (cell body and synaptic vesicles of neurons) and immune cells and in low concentration on many cell types. It is metal binding. Binding with copper stimulates endocytosis. Intracellular PrP modifies other proteins such as antiapoptotic Bcl-2, several heat shock proteins, neuronal synapsin, and growth factor signal adapter Grb 2.

26.3.3.2 BSE- Prion Protein

Using Western immunoblot analysis of fragment of the pathological prion protein (PrP^{res}) resistant to proteinase K, the three types are *classical (C-BSE), L-BSE* and *H-BSE*, representing lower or higher molecular mass. The latter two have been identified during active surveillance. The incidence is low in old cattle. Seuberlich et al. (2012) described another type from BSE-infected cattle in Switzerland.

L-type BSE seems to have wider distribution in Europe, America, Canada and Japan. Experimental studies in primates and mice suggest that it presents a higher public health risk than the classical BSE agent. It caused neurological symptoms in experimental mouse lemurs (a primate) infected through oral and intra-cerebral routes (Mestre-Francés et al. 2012).

The classical type (C-BSE) is the only transmissible to human through contaminated meat causing vCJD.

However, experimental and observational studies suggest continued evolution. Masujin et al. (2016) passaged serially H-type BSE in a bovinised transgenic (TgBoPrP) mice. Thus, a novel prion emerged, BSE-SW (SW for short incubation of 14.8 ± 1.5 months and weight loss). Intracerebrally inoculated cattle showed early clinical signs of the disease after 11.5 and 12.5 months of inoculation. Symptoms began as disturbance, mild fear or anxiety, altered gait, sometimes low head carriage; progressing to leaning towards floor, resting heads against wall after 1–2 months. Ataxia of the hind limbs developed. Getting up was difficult near terminal stage. In the duration of 2–3 months, there was weight loss. Anorexia, nervousness or aggressions were absent. Visual, acoustic and tactile responses were intact.

The study suggests 'intra-species transmission of H-BSE in cattle allowed emergence of novel BSE strains'.

BASE (Bovine amyloidotic spongiform encephalopathy)—During extensive survey for BSE at a slaughterhouse in the EU, abnormal prion (Atypical BSE) positive cows without symptoms were detected in Europe and North America. Strains from Italy are referred to as bovine amyloidotic spongiform encephalopathy (BASE). It is suggested that BSE strains has its origin in BASE and there is a potential link with a subset of sporadic CJD.

Surveillance and ban should continue.

26.3.4 Pathogenesis

Prion (PrP) is a normal protein component of neurons involved in their development, function and protection preventing cell death. Rarely (1 in 10^6), PrP may turn into an abnormal conformation, PrP^{sc}. PrP with appropriate receptors are expressed in gut epithelium and spread through follicular dendritic cells to peripheral nerves and subsequently to CNS.

PrP mutations with additional copies of the metal binding octapeptide repeat have properties similar to PrP^{sc}. PrP^{sc} promotes conversion of PrP molecules to PrP^{sc}—accumulation in brain cause neuronal damages and spongiform. There is further accumulation of incompletely cleaved products of PrP^{sc} which appear because PrP^{sc}

is resistant to proteases, such as protein kinase and the incompletely cleaved products are less soluble and tend to aggregate.

PrP occurs in three forms—non-, mono- and diglycosylated. TSE prions differ in the degree and pattern of glycosylation. BSE and vCJD contain high levels of diglycosylated and low levels of monoglycosylatedPrP^{sc}. On the other hand, scrapie and iatrogenic CJD have high proportion of monoglycosylated to diglycosylatedPrP^{sc}. Glycosylation profile is reflected in neuropathology. Hosts' PrP genotype also influences glycosylation of PrP$^{sc.}$

Aguzzi and Zhu (2012) summarised the entry, peripheral replication, neuroinvasion and neurodegeneration. Prions reach CNS directly following intracerebral inoculation, or by aerosols through immune-independent pathways, through autonomic nerves.

Following ingestion, PrP^{sc} molecules are acted upon by digestive proteolytic enzymes in human or rumen microbial proteases in cattle. Incompletely cleaved product is bound to ferritin and transported across intestinal epithelia. Intracellular damage and modification of other proteins result. The metal bound PrP^{sc} are picked up by follicular dendritic cells (FDCs). Prions colonise and replicate in these cells distributed in tonsils, Peyer's patches in ileum, spleen and thymus. B cell derived LTs and TNF support development and maintenance of FDCs. Replication, accumulation, spread and transfer to sympathetic nerves are also facilitated by cytokines from B cells and/or chronic lymphocytic inflammation. Deposition takes place when PrP^{Sc} production exceeds clearance by microglia.

Holznagel et al. (2015) fed simians BSE prions that entered CNS via afferent neurons. These prefer to travel along sensory nerve fibres from guts to CNS entering at the level of lumbar spinal cord. They centrifugally spread to tonsils and spleen from the sites of initial CNS invasion at later stage of incubation period.

50% of gut and 12% of tonsil samples were found in carriers before the onset of clinical disease, suggesting gut as preferred samples in case of simians. Prevalence studies in humans use tonsillectomy and appendectomy. Accumulation of prion protein (PrP^{res}) resistant to protease lymphoreticular tissues is indicative of infection.

Accumulation sites are Peyer's patches of distal ileum in cattle, spinal cord, stem and higher areas of brain. It has been observed that after the infectious prion particles reach brain/CNS, they spread centrifugally to salivary glands through autonomic nervous system and saliva is infective. This has been observed in scrapie, BSE, and chronic wasting disease in deer. Saliva, milk, blood and CSF from cattle infected with BSE are infectious (Okada et al. 2012).

26.4 Signs and Symptoms of BSE

It affected 3–5 years old, commonly dairy cattle of almost all breeds. The incubation period is long—2.5–8 years and the course usually sub-acute to chronic. Animals, which are affected present progressive neurological signs.

An affected cow is anorexic, lethargic, stays away from herd and shows progressive behavioural changes (aggression or nervous) and neurological signs such as aggression, reacting to noise or touch, twitching, tremor and slowly becomes ataxic. The animal has difficulty in rising from lying position and presents poor coordination and abnormal posture. There is loss of weight and reduction in milk yield. Since no treatment is available, animals eventually die.

26.5 Public Health Significance: vCJD

vCJD/BSE may be considered a man-made epidemic. Feeding meat and bone meal (MBM) to cattle is a man's decision. Prion entered the food chain. It affected beef production, trade and economy, human health directly and life in many ways.

The ECDC (2017) reported differences from the epidemic of BSE/vCJD in the UK. Occurrence of the disease in Europe was delayed. It peaked in 2004 (1999 in the UK) with 11 incident cases. France had the maximum (27) cases (Table 26.2). Periods between peak of BSE and vCJD cases were around 8 years in the UK and 2 years in non-UK Europe. The median age of vCJD cases in the EU was younger (median age of onset 28 years, range 11–74), i.e. tended to affect younger ones. Duration of illness was 14 months (6–114).

Table 26.2 Variant CJD cases worldwide as of 2015

Country	Total no. of primary cases	Number alive: blood transfusion	Resident of UK > 6 months during 1980–1996
UK	174	03	177
France	27	–	01
Republic of Ireland	04	–	02
Italy	02	–	0
USA	04[a]	–	02
Canada	02	–	01
Saudi Arabia	01	–	0
Japan	01[b]	–	0
Netherlands	03	–	0
Portugal	02	–	0
Spain	05	–	0
Taiwan	01	–	1
Total	226	3(0)	184

Source: http://wwwnc.cdc.gov/eid/article/21/5/pdfs/14-2017.pdf and www.cjd.ed.ac.uk

[a]The third US patient with vCJD was born and raised in Saudi Arabia and has lived in the United States permanently since late 2005. It is suggested that the patient was infected most likely as a child while living in Saudi Arabia. The investigation of the fourth US patient did not support the patient's extended travel to European countries, including the UK or Saudi Arabia. It was confirmed that the case was a US citizen with birth outside the Americas and he was infected before moving to the US. This patient resided in Kuwait, Russia and Lebanon (http://wwwnc.cdc.gov/eid/article/21/5/pdfs/14-2017.pdf)

[b]The case from Japan had resided in the UK for 24 days in the period 1980–1996

Three modes of human infection are known: ingestion, blood transfusion and penetration through skin.

Three vCJD infection in recipients of blood transfusion have so far been observed. Peden et al. (2004) reported death of a patient of non-neurological disorder receiving blood transfusion 5 years earlier from a donor who developed vCJD, subsequently suggesting the presence of prion in blood in those infected with vCJD and risk associated with transfusion of blood and blood products. Manufacture of fractional products such as albumin was banned in the UK since 1999 to prevent the spread of secondary infections. Other countries instituted their own policies. For example, anyone who spent 6 months in a particular European country or 3 months in the UK from 1980–1996 were precluded from donating blood. Sperm donation is banned, although vCJD is not sexually transmitted and the risk is negligible.

26.5.1 Symptoms vCJD

vCJD or nvCJD killed 177 people in the UK and 52 elsewhere by June 2014 (Table 26.2). An estimated 460,000 and 482,000 BSE infected animals entered the food chain of man before control measures were introduced in 1989.

vCJD is an ataxic cerebellar form of CJD. It affects young age (Table 26.3). The incubation period was 6–8 years; it was 13 years in a study of French cases. The incubation period is not dependent on age, but highest susceptibility or exposure is in teenagers and young adults.

Table 26.3 Differences between more common sporadic CJD and vCJD (Belay et al. 2005)

Features	Common sporadic CJD	vCJD
Age at death	68 years; ~10% at <55 years	28 years; almost all died at age of <55 years
Manifestation	Late appearance of frank neurological signs; no diagnostic electroencephalographic pattern	Psychiatric at onset; presence of pulvinar signs in MRI in >75%
Incubation period	13 years	6.5 years
Median duration of illness	14 months	<6 months
Most striking early neurologic manifestation		Sensory symptoms (dysesthesia or paraesthesia). Other signs: dystonia, chorea and myoclonus, which commonly developed late
Reasonably accurate pre-mortem diagnosis		Tonsillar biopsy
Definitive diagnosis		Brain tissue on autopsy

Initially, there are non-specific psychiatric symptoms. Patients show a progressive anxiety, depression and behavioural changes. Nearly half the patients have altered perception and sensory distortion. Central and peripheral nervous system are affected and are reflected in rapidly progressive cerebellar ataxia, disrupted speech, difficulty in walking and picking things, involuntary rhythmic jerking movement that progresses into more severe tremor, dementia, paralysis, wasting, coma and finally generalised muscular rigidity with disappearance of tremor, total immobility and stoppage of speech.

Grznarova et al. (2020) reported one of the two cases of vCJD outside the UK associated with potential occupational exposure. The lady technician handled murine samples contaminated with BSE 7.5 years earlier (May, 2010). She punctured her thumb that bled while handling frozen sections of brain of a transgenic mouse that overexpressing prion protein of man having methionine at codon 129. The mice was infected with sheep adapted form of BSE.

26.5.2 Timeline

November 2017: Burning pain in right shoulder and neck worsened and extended to right half of body during subsequent 6 months.

November 2018: CSF normal. MRI—slight increase in the fluid-attenuated inversion recovery (FLAIR) signal in the caudates and thalami.

January 2019: Depression, anxious, impaired memory with visual hallucinations. Hypertonia on the right side of her body. CSF for 14-3-3 protein was negative.

March 2019: MRI—increased FLAIR signal in pulvinar and dorsomedial nuclei of thalami.

Nineteen months after the onset of symptoms patient died. Neuropathological examination, analysis of plasma and CSF confirmed vCJD. She tested negative for sporadic CJD. Patient was homozygous for methionine at codon 129 of the gene of prion protein with no mutation.

The ability of this strain to propagate through the peripheral route has been documented, and experimental studies with scrapie strains have shown that scarification and subcutaneous inoculation are effective routes.

26.6 Diagnosis

Cattle: Symptoms of mad cow disease are not diagnostic and there is no antemortem test.

Human vCJD:

Asymptomatic: Lymphoid and appendix tissues are useful to detect prion protein in asymptomatic vCJD cases, detectable up to 2 years before the appearance of clinical signs.

Suggesting signs: Psychiatric, persistent painful sensation; dementia and after >4 months appearance of any two of reduced coordination, hyper-reflexia, myoclonus, chorea, visual signs.

- Electroencephalography—no TSE-specific changes.
- Brain imaging is done to exclude other encephalopathies.
- CSF—elevated protein 14-3-3 is observed in neurodegenerative disorders including TSE.
- Tonsil biopsy.

After death (generally age < 55 years), histopathology takes 2–3 days to detect

- Characteristic spongiform lesions.
- Astrocytic gliosis, and.
- Prion associated plaques/fibrils, vacuoles.

26.6.1 Specific Tests and Methods

- Immunohistochemical (the gold test for TSE) takes 2–3 days—sections stained with antibodies to PrP protein.
- CSF test – currently used is 77% sensitive and 100% specific.
- Olfactory neurons test (Orru et al. 2014)—Olfactory neurons are connected directly to brain. These are collected by brushing inside the nose. These compared to CSF—test took half the time and had sensitivity of 97% and 100% specificity. The methods used were *PET* blot and semiquantitative Western immunoblot assay.
- Biochemical assay – Differential digestion with proteinase K of PrP and PrP^{sc} is the basis. Enzymatic digestion leaves PrP^{sc}, separated electrophoretically on SDS-PAGE, blotted on membrane and specific identification is made by conventional techniques like ELISA or Western Blot.
- Bioassay in mouse—Injection of brain tissue triturate into brain or periphery of test animal—usually mouse. Note IP, symptoms. Confirmation by other tests required. Time taken is several months. Sensitivity is dependent upon mouse strain used. Strains that have been used are: C57/BL6, RIII and VM.

Commercial test kits based on 'biochemical assay' are available. Results are available in 4–8 h. Test specimen is 0.35–0.5 g of obex (portion of medulla or brain stem just distal to cerebellum). For example, PrioStrip test (Prionics AG, Schlieren, Switzerland).

26.7 Treatment

Supportive; there is no specific treatment.

26.8 Prevention

Red meat, milk and milk products are considered safe. In principle, beef and its products should no longer carry risk since the European Community and individual European countries took measures to prevent the entry of potentially contaminated products in the food chain of man. Lifting ban on beef export from Britain further alleviates this fear.

According to Aguzzi and Zhu (2012), generating PrPC-deficient farm animals would provide prion-free biologicals of all kinds—cytokines, growth factors, therapeutic antibodies, meat, MBM, etc. PRNP knock out cattle and goats have been raised. How tasty would meat be is unknown.

26.9 Prevention and Control of BSE

OIE recommended effective strategy to prevent introduction of BSE and dealing with its occurrence. Important ones are: targeted surveillance of all clinical neurological diseases; reporting BSE; import restrictions on bovines and their products; removal of SRM during slaughter from human food and animal feed; safe disposal of animals suspected to be exposed to feed contaminated with prion.

Depending on the occurrence of BSE, OIE categorises a country/zone/compartment with 'controlled' and 'negligible' risk status.

Imposition of strict restrictions on import of live ruminants and their products from countries reporting existence of BSE.

The measures include regulations to stop recycling of mammalian protein into ruminant feed (some countries extended it to feed of all mammalian species); removal of head and vertebral column of cattle slaughtered before further processing; and prohibiting certain nervous system and visceral tissues for consumption by man.

Travelers need to be careful about such countries where BSE is present or likely to appear with safeguards not fully implemented.

Beef as such is not dangerous. Mechanically removed meat contaminated with nervous tissues is often added to precooked foods like sausages, hot dogs, canned beef products, beef stews and broths, meat pies—i.e. any product containing beef in a precooked and often unrecognisable form. Mechanically removed meat even after removal of vertebral column is not allowed for human use in the UK (consult The European Commission of Food Safety website for new information).

Feed ban prohibits most of the proteins including potentially BSE infectious tissues called 'specified risk materials' from all animal feeds, pet foods, fertilisers in the US and Canada. Removing SRM (brain, eyes, spinal cord, skull, vertebral column, tonsils and distal ileum) from the entire animal feed system addresses the risks associated with the potential contamination of cattle feed during production, distribution, storage and use (https://www.cdc.gov/prions/bse/feed-ban.html).

References

Aguzzi A, Zhu C (2012) Five Questions on Prion Diseases. PLoS Pathog 8(5):e1002651

Belay ED, Sejvar JJ, Shieh W-J, Wiersma ST, Zou W-Q, Gambetti P et al (2005) Variant Creutzfeldt-Jakob disease death, United States. Emerg Infect Dis 11(9):1351–1354

Cunningham AA, Kirkwood JK, Dawson M, Spencer YI, Green RB, Wells GAH (2004) Bovine spongiform encephalopathy infectivity in greater kudu (*Tragelaphusstrepsiceros*). Emerg Infect Dis 10(6):1044–1049

ECDC. Europe.EU (2017) Facts about variant Creutzfeldt-Jakob disease. https://www.ecdc.europa.eu/en/vcjd/facts

EFSA Panel on Biological Hazards (BIOHAZ) (2011) Joint Scientific Opinion on any possible epidemiological or molecular association between TSEs in animals and humans. EFSA J 9(1):1945

Grznarova K, Denouel A, Plu I, Bouaziz-Amar E, Seilhean D et al (2020) Variant Creutzfeldt–Jakob disease diagnosed 7.5 years after occupational exposure. N Engl J Med 383:83–85

Holznagel E, Yutzy B, Kruip C, Bierke P, Schulz-Schaeffer W, Lower J (2015) Foodborne-transmitted BSE prions ascend in afferent neurons to the simian CNS and spread to tonsils and spleen at a late stage of the incubation period. J Infect Dis 212(9):1459–1468

Masujin K, Okada H, Miyazawa K et al (2016) Emergence of a novel bovine spongiform encephalopathy (BSE) prion from an atypical H-type BSE. Sci Rep 6:22753

Mestre-Francés N, Nicot S, Rouland S, Biacabe A-G, Quadrio I et al (2012) Oral Transmission of L-type Bovine Spongiform Encephalopathy in Primate Model. Emerg Infect Dis 18(1):142–145

Notari S, Qing L, Pocchiari M, Dagdanova A, Hatcher K, Dogterom A et al (2012) Assessing prion infectivity of human urine in sporadic Creutzfeldt-Jakob Disease. Emerg Infect Dis 18(1):21–28

OIE (2018) OIE-WAHIDHome "Diseases" Bovine spongiform encephalopathy. Accessed 06 Oct 2018

Okada H, Murayama Y, Shimozaki N, Yoshioka M, Masujin K et al (2012) Prion in saliva of bovine spongiform encephalopathy– infected cattle. Emerg Infect Dis 18(12):291–292

Orru CD, Bongianni M, Tonoli G, Ferrari S et al (2014) A test for Creutzfeldt-Jakob disease using nasal brushings. N Engl J Med 371:519–529

Peden AH, Head MW, Ritchie DL, Bell JE, Ironside JW (2004) Preclinical vCJD after blood transfusion in a PRNP codon 129 heterozygous patient. Lancet 364(9433):527–529

Seuberlich T, Gsponer M, Drögemüller C, Polak MP, McCutcheon S et al (2012) Novel prion protein in BSE-affected cattle, Switzerland. Emerg Infect Dis 18(1):158–159

Spiropoulos J, Lockey R, Sallis RE, Terry LA, Thorne L (2011) Isolation of Prion with BSE Properties from Farmed Goat. Emerg Infect Dis 17(12):2253–2261

Viruses Occasionally Reported as Foodborne

27

SARS-CoV and avian influenza are low probability but high impact viruses. According to Lau et al. (2004), SARS corona virus spread in human population through the preparation and consumption of foods of animal origin, which probably got infection from another reservoir, possibly bats.

Avian influenza H5N1 virus has been cultivated from duck meat and human infection with duck blood has occurred (Tumpey et al. 2003). Although foodborne avian influenza virus infection is less likely, it cannot be ruled out. Nipah virus infection has been associated with pig/pork, fruit, 'toddy contaminated with bats' saliva and possibly urine'. Infection is also nosocomial. Tickborne encephalitis is associated with raw milk, butter, yoghurt and cheese.

27.1 Detection of Virus

Various reverse transcription-PCR (RT-PCR) assays have been designed to detect NoV, HAV and HEV in samples from clinical cases, environment, food and water. EIA has been developed but negative samples need to be tested by RT-PCR.

Genotyping is recommended for source/attribute determination.

Recovery of viruses from foods requires standardisation of method. Elution from fresh foods such as lettuce, onions etc. has to be done.

Time taken in detection of viruses on foods is important, particularly when foods are 'ready-to-eat'.

A recently developed technology claims to declare a sample positive and negative, time taken are 15 and 75 min, respectively. The technique is based on combination of 'isothermal DNA amplification and bioluminescence- detection generates light' (http://www.meatprocess.com/Safety-Legislation/Revolutionary-15-minute-pathogen-test-will-reduce-time-and-cost-3M?utm_source=copyright&utm_medium=OnSite&utm_campaign=copyright).

K. G. Narayan et al., *Veterinary Public Health & Epidemiology*,
https://doi.org/10.1007/978-981-19-7800-5_27

27.2 Sources

The common reservoirs/sources of foodborne viruses are sewage, irrigation water, animals and workers engaged in harvesting, processing, etc. Food workers' error—infected or carrier with poor personal hygiene, bare-hand contact and failure to wash hands properly may be responsible for contamination with NoV, HAV and *Salmonella*, especially in ready-to-eat food infections. Food may get contaminated during all stages of food supply chain, primarily during production and further during processing. Non-availability of data on these makes it difficult to assign risk to these factors. An investigation in Belgium revealed that food handlers, water, bivalve shellfish and raspberries were responsible for the outbreak in 42.5%, 27.5%, 17.55% and 10.0%, respectively (Baert et al. 2009)

27.3 Stability of Viruses and Processes of Decontamination

Viruses cannot grow in the food but survive. The infective dose may be as small as a single virus particle. This makes virus important foodborne hazard. Knowledge of their stability in the environment, processing of food and survival through the processing is essential. NoV and HAV are stable and persist in the environment and food. HAV persists on hands up to several hours, on surfaces several months, on fresh produce several days, on shellfish up to several weeks. NoV persists on surface up to 4–8 weeks, on fresh produce up to several days to months, several weeks on shellfish.

27.4 Effective Control Measure

Effective control measure begins as prevention of contamination, primarily (a) at the pre-harvest level for products such as bivalve molluscs, fresh produce for raw consumption such as lettuce and jalapeño; (b) at the harvest level such as manual handling—picking fresh fruits and vegetables; and (c) at the post-harvest level such as manual preparation of ready-to-eat foods.

27.4.1 Intervention Methods

Decontamination and preservation methods are useful intervention strategies.

Decontamination procedures may be water, hypochlorite, peroxyacetic acid, or electrolyse oxidising water.

Acidification

Preservation methods like heat, high hydrostatic pressure processing and irradiation.

While short time–high temperature (72 °C, 15 s) accomplished less than 1 log reduction for some enteroviruses, the conventional pasteurisation (63 °C—30 min/

70 °C—2 min) is needed to achieve more than a 3 log reduction. The required time-temperature combination depends on the food matrix and its physical-chemical conditions. Bivalve shellfish required additional/alternate methods (EFSA 2011).

References

Baert L, Uyttendaele M, Stals A, Van Coillie E, Dierick K et al (2009) Reported foodborne outbreaks due to noroviruses in Belgium: the link between food and patient investigation in an international context. Epidemiol Infect 137:316–325

EFSA Panel on Biological Hazards (BIOHAZ) (2011) Scientific opinion on an update on the present knowledge on the occurrence and control of foodborne viruses. EFSA J 9(7):2190. https://doi.org/10.2903/j.efsa.2011.2190

Lau SK, Woo PC, Wong BH, Tsoi HW, Woo GK et al (2004) Detection of severe acute respiratory syndrome (SARS) coronavirus nucleocapsidprotein in SARS patients by enzyme-linked immunosorbent assay. J Clin Microbiol 42:2884–2889

Tumpey TM, Suarez DL, Perkins LE, Senne DA, Lee J et al (2003) Evaluation of a high-pathogenicity H5N1 avian influenza A virus isolated from duck meat. Avian Dis 47:951–955

Foodborne Bacterial Infections 28

28.1 Salmonellosis

Salmonellosis is an infection and disease caused by any of the over 2600 serotypes of Salmonellae. Of the total global diarrhoeal diseases, about 25% are caused by *Salmonella*. The illness may be mild to life threatening depending on serotype and host factors. Antimicrobial resistant serotypes pose serious public health problem (WHO 2018).

Zoonotic Salmonellae cause millions of human salmonellosis and infections worldwide each year. Zoonotic, sporadic non-typhoidal salmonellosis reported in the European Union were 94,530 confirmed of 96,039 cases in 2016 in 28 Members States (Suffredini et al. 2019). In the USA, 1.35 million infections, 26,500 hospitalisation and 420 deaths occur every year (https://www.cdc.gov/salmonella/index.html).

According to Suffredini et al. (2019), a total of 3637 outbreaks of foodborne salmonellosis affecting 29,250 human cases were reported in the EU during 2014–2016. Epidemiological and microbiological investigations revealed strong evidence of association of vehicles in 753 outbreaks with total of 10,858 cases. The vehicles were: broiler meat and products in 46 outbreaks (550 cases); eggs and products in 296 outbreaks (3547 cases), meat and meat products in 32 outbreaks (566 cases); other/mixed/unspecified poultry meat and products thereof in 10 outbreaks (44 cases) and mixed foods in 65 outbreaks (1143 cases). *S.* Enteritidis was the most common serovar causing outbreaks and cases associated with broiler, egg and its products in the EU and were associated with international trade in eggs.

Other vehicles associated with foodborne outbreaks were pig meat and products in 55 outbreaks (1041 cases), bovine meat and products in 17 outbreaks (132 cases) and turkey meat and products in 5 outbreaks (297 cases).

K. G. Narayan et al., *Veterinary Public Health & Epidemiology*,
https://doi.org/10.1007/978-981-19-7800-5_28

28.2 Aetiology

There are two species—*S. enterica* and *S. bongori*. *S. enterica* has six subspecies that consist of 2600 serotypes. They are gram-negative rod-shaped bacteria in the family *Enterobacteriaceae*. Most are motile, facultative anaerobe and chemotrophs. The six subspecies are *S. e. enterica (serotype I), S. e. salamae (serotype II), S. e. arizonae (serotype IIIa), S. e. diarizonae (serotype IIIb), S. e. houtenae (serotype IV)* and *S. e. indica (serotype VI)*. Serotypes are differentiated based on the combination of somatic O- and flagellar H-antigens. *Salmonella enterica* subsp. *enterica serotype* Typhimurium or *Salmonellae* Typhimurium is the way to express. *Samonellae choleraesuis* was the first salmonella to be isolated and described.

Growing on triple sugar iron agar detects hydrogen sulphide + bacteria, most likely *Salmonella*. DNA extracted can be subjected to tests such as pulsed field-gel electrophoresis, genome sequence, multilocus sequence, real time polymerase chain reaction and for antibiotic resistance genes.

Salmonellae are facultative intracellular and classed as invasive, typhoidal and non-invasive, non-typhoidal. The latter are zoonotic, transmitted from 'animal to human then human to human' and invade gastrointestinal tract. In sub-Sahara, non-typhoidal can be invasive causing paratyphoid requiring immediate medical attention (https://en.wikipedia.org/wiki/Salmonella).

Host adapted salmonella affecting animals and birds and two others are tabulated (Table 28.1) as example.

Human infection with some serotypes adapted to animals, e.g. *S. enterica* serotype Dublin (adapted to cattle) and *S. enterica* serotype Cholerasuis (adapted to pigs) are invasive, severe and even life-threatening.

Table 28.1 Host adapted salmonella affecting, man, animals and birds

Serotypes[a]	O serogroup[b]	O antigens[c]	H-antigen Phase 1	H-antigen Phase 2	Adapted to host spp.
Dublin	9 (D1)	1,9,12 (Vi)	G, p	–	Cattle
Gallinarum-pullorum	9 (D1)	1,9,12	–	–	Avian
Typhi	9 (D1)	9,12 (Vi)	D	–	Human beings
Abortus ovis	4 (B)	4,12	C	1,6	Ovine
Abortus equi	4 (B)				Equine
Cholerae-suis	7 (C1)	6,7	C	C	Swine
Enteritidis	9 (D1)	1,9,12	G, m	[1,7]	Wide host range
Typhimurium	4 (B)	1,4[5],12	I	1,2	

[a] Serotypes of *S. enterica* subspecies *enterica* are named
[b] Some serogroups were designated by letters formerly and are indicated in parenthesis
[c] Somatic factors associated with phage conversion are underlined; [x]—antigen is not present in all strains of the serotypes

28.3 Epidemiology

The most common ***route*** of salmonella infection is per os, and the commonest ***cause*** is contaminated food, and the ***source*** is animal or human faeces ***spread*** by any and all types of foods—meat, poultry, eggs, milk, green vegetables and fruits. Transmission may also be direct contact with infected animals, pets and human. The spread of *Salmonella* followed foreign and domestic trade routes of animal feed, animal and poultry farms, processing plant and processed products.

Salmonella Generally, a small number of *Salmonella* serotypes of the total isolated in a given region and a defined period (e.g., five) are found responsible for most reported foodborne or zoonotic salmonellosis. New serotypes (in this region) may be imported with animals, tourists and animal feed. In subsequent years, other than these five serotypes may become most frequently reported.

Auxotrophic serotypes adapted to single host grow in minimal salt medium containing suitable growth factor(s). Auxotrophic strains of prototrophic serotypes (certain strains of Typhimurium) also occur.

Salmonellae grow well at body temperature. *S.* Typhimurium can grow at a minimum temperature of 6.2 °C and a maximum of 44 °C. These prefer to grow at neutral pH but can grow between 4 and 8 pH. Under certain special conditions, these may even proliferate slowly at <4.0 °C and survive at <4.0 pH. These are aerobic to facultative anaerobic. Most salmonellae are prototrophic and grow in media containing salts and a suitable source of carbon. The thermal reduction time at 57.0 °C is less than a minute. Yet their capacity to survive in the environment is great (Table 28.2).

Salmonellae are readily available in free living state and are omnipresent to infect a susceptible host at any time.

Source Wild, domestic, food animals, pets, turtles and reptiles are reservoirs (Table 28.3). Salmonellae may enter animal feed and human food chain from

Table 28.2 Survival of salmonellae in the environment

Objects	Survival in days
Earth and pasture	200
Sweepers' dust	300
Feeder pig barns, water dug outs (wet, warm conditions)	Months
Rodent faeces	148
Poultry faeces	9
Cattle faeces dried	1000
Egg shell	21–350
Dog faeces	84 (period observed)
Cloth	228

Table 28.3 Natural sources of salmonellae

Class	Sources
Molluscs	Oysters, clams, snails, slugs
Arthropods	Flies, fleas, cockroaches, ticks, mites, crayfish, lobsters, crabs and crustacean
Fish	Carp and other scavenger fish
Reptiles	Snakes, lizards, tortoise
Birds	Sparrows, starlings, doves, ducks, geese, swan, pheasants, turkeys, peafowl, Guinea fowl, crows, pigeons, partridges, rooks
Mammals	Rodents, mice, squirrel, grophers, dear, elk, moose, monkey, man, carnivores specially foxes, skunks, bears, hedgehogs
Pets, zoo-, lab-animals	Cats, dogs, sun fish, snakes, alligators, turtles, canaries, parakeets, parrots, chicks, ducklings, pigeons, Guinea pigs, hamsters, rabbits
Domestic animals	Swine, cattle, sheep, goats, equines, camels
Eatables	Water, ice, milk and its products, poultry and its products, eggs and its products, meat and its products, goat meat, baker products especially those containing eggs, coconut, fish, shellfish, fruits and vegetables
Animal feeds	Meat meal, poultry feed, meat cum bone meal, feather meal, fish meal, poultry offal meal, crushed bone flour, protein concentrate meal
Others	Sewage, abattoir drains

primary production and spread down to household kitchen or food-service establishment

Reservoirs—Food animals Analysis of retrospectively collected data in Europe showed the association of poultry, turkey and pig as reservoirs; subclassified according to the two most common serovars *S.* Enteritidis and *S.* Typhimurium monophasic. The relative risk with reservoirs is dynamic.

The human *Salmonella* cases could be traced to following reservoirs—11.2% to laying hens, 41.5% to pigs, 24.9% to broiler and 7.5% to turkeys.

S. Enteritidis accounted for 40.9%, 33.2% to pigs, 19.8% to layers and 6.1% to turkeys.

S. Typhimurium and its monophasic variant, the majority (87.2% of 0.48 million human cases and 91.5% of 0.45 million human cases, respectively) could be attributed to the pig reservoir. Only 1.67% and 0.46%, respectively, could be attributed to the laying hen reservoir.

The process of '*Infection → clinical disease → carrier state'* and also the reversal of carrier state to clinical disease due to stress or inter current infection appears to occur naturally.

Salmonellosis is a widely prevalent disease recorded in almost all countries. Dublin infection may be absent from many farms and sporadic in few. Stress may convert an asymptomatic infection into an overt illness. Stress of transport, drought, parturition and overcrowding may contribute to excretion of *Salmonella* and spread. A carrier animal may be converted to a florid diarrhoeic state leading to multiple cases and/or deaths and extensive environmental contamination. Nutritional deficiency (prolonged starvation, vitamin B deficiency) may cause severe outbreaks in endemic farms.

Isolation of a single serotype from such an outbreak strongly suggests a 'common exposure/origin' of the outbreak.

Studies on stocking density, group size, enriched cage or a combination of various factors providing better condition of life and thus ability to resist colonisation showed that high stocking densities can lead to stress, increase contact between animals and faeces and *Salmonella* transmission. Stress can induce immunosuppression that promotes spread and persistence of *Salmonella* within a flock.

Contaminated animal feed is another important determinant. Feeds of animal origin (such as bone cum meat meal, meat meal, fish meal) have been more common source than oil seed meal and grains of infection. Contaminated animal feed—rodent cycle in a farm feed store creates a natural nidus. This is true of non-host adapted serotypes. Pre-sterilising such animal feed component before feeding prevents infection.

Animal produce Eggs are more commonly associated with outbreaks and sporadic cases (i.e., diffuse outbreaks). WGS of isolates should authenticate. Eggs are also contaminated internally (vertical transmission) unlike poultry meat. Eggs are not required to be stored in refrigerator. Raw pooled eggs (content) are used as ingredients in various food products. Eggs are expected to be more frequent vehicle of outbreaks including diffuse compared to poultry meat.

Climate Factors that influence meat borne salmonellosis are climate (temperature and humidity) and consumer's preference for raw, partially cooked meat. Human and laying hen infection is increased during warmer months.

Cross contamination in kitchen back to the farm. WGS of isolates from different sources and outbreaks is helpful in establishing linkage.

28.4 Pathogenicity

Salmonellae are capable of (a) invading a variety of cells such as epithelial, M cells, macrophages and dendritic; (b) multiplying within phagocytes; and (c) surviving oxygen radicals and nitric oxide produced by the phagocytes. These invade blood stream and organs; secrete endotoxins, cause septic and hypovolemic life-threatening shock.

Septicaemic salmonellosis After entering the hosts' body, *Salmonella* is carried by lymphatics and lymph glands to blood supply to cause typhoid/enteric fever. In the septic form, these spread to other organs, spleen, liver, kidney and bone marrow and infect the tissues. Endotoxic pathology is caused by endotoxins acting upon vascular and nervous tissues. There is vascular permeability and blood vessels are flaccid

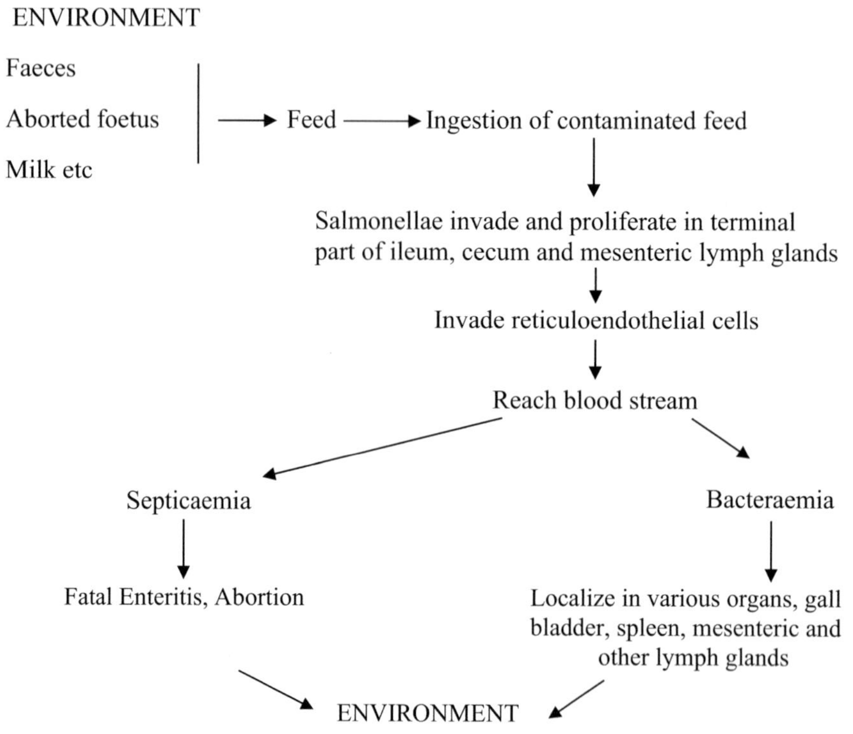

Fig. 28.1 Infection cycle and pathogenesis

resulting in decreased circulation, low blood pressure and may be hypovolemic shock. Shock may range from hypovolemic, mixed hypovolemic and septic or the serious septic shock. There is fluid and electrolyte loss, toxaemia and hypoxia may affect kidneys to cause oliguria and azotemia. Mortality may be high if not treated (Fig. 28.1).

'Bacteraemic salmonellosis' begins as a non-specific fever, showing symptoms such as pain in muscle, fatigue and weakness. Symptoms may subside. The infection may persist in latent form with deteriorating reticuloendothelial function for months and years. During bacteraemia, *Salmonella* may spread to any part of the body and localise to cause pathologies recognised depending on the organ/tissue as salmonellosis of urinary tract, CNS, bone, joints and soft tissues (Fig. 28.1).

Salmonellae pathogen cross intestinal cell wall barrier. The typhoidal and non-typhoidal serotypes adopt different paths for invasion.

The typhoidal serotypes prefer phagocytic cells and the trafficking CD18 positive immune cells to breach the intestinal barrier. These enter macrophages through pinocytosis. Spread in the host's body is by the mononuclear phagocytic system. Only a small number of salmonellae is required for infection.

The non-typhoidal serotypes prefer M cells of the wall of intestine to enter by endocytosis and initiate inflammation; disrupt the 'tight junction' between cells of intestinal wall. The affected intestinal cells fail to stop the flow of ions, water and immune cells into and out of the intestines. Diarrhoea is induced.

Salmonellae use virulence factors (effectors) for infection and invading hosts' cells and tissues. Type III secretory system (T3SS) is important and is used to manipulate innate and adaptive immunity during infection for colonisation of intestine, inflammation and diarrhoea. Injection of effectors into host's cell and uptake of salmonellae by nonphagocytic cells are facilitated by T3SS-1 resulting into massive efflux of electrolytes and water into intestine. Salmonellae reside and replicate in *Salmonella* containing vacuole (SCV), a membrane bound compartment of macrophages and nonphagocytic epithelial cells; the SCV is acidified stimulating T3SS-2 secretion required for survival and systemic spread. Zinc metalloproteinase effectors disrupt the specific arms of host's immune system. *S. Typhimurium* inhibits the innate immune system by binding the target cell phytic acid (IP6), serine/threonine acetyltransferase and the AvrA toxin injected by the SPI 1 type III secretory system.

28.4.1 Typhoidal and Non-typhoidal *Salmonella*

***Typhoidal* Salmonella** *S. typhi* and *S. paratyphi* A, B and C are strictly adapted to primates and human and cause systemic infection, typhoid, paratyphoid and foodborne infection and spread from human to human. They are invasive. In sub-Saharan Africa, non-typhoidal serotypes are invasive causing mostly gastroenteritis with potential to cause bacteraemia. It was reported in 2012 with isolations from blood of patients presenting fever and case fatality rate of 20–25%. It affected age group 2 months to 3 years. The invasive non-typhoidal *Salmonella* infection (iNTS) is caused by *S. enterica* Typhimurium and *S. enterica* Enteritidis. It is thought that iNTS originated in Congo Basin and the strain picked a resistance gene that made it resistant to chloramphenicol. The economic burden caused was high as expensive drugs had to be used. The susceptibility of the population was attributed to malnutrition, malaria and immune suppression, HIV. It is thought that the non-typhoidal serotypes are evolving to typhoid-like to be able to invade the host efficiently, suggested by the observation of diverse pathology such as hepatosplenomegaly, infection of respiratory tract than gastrointestinal tract.

Non-typhoidal serotypes are generally non-invasive. They are commonly associated with food poisoning. A set of ingested number of salmonellae survive (have evolve to tolerate) gastric acidity to reach intestine and multiply in tissues. Some others may be covered by oesophageal mucus and reach intestine. Dead *Salmonella* release endotoxins that cause inflammation, and gastrointestinal disorder appears by the end of incubation period (within hours of ingestion). It is self-limiting and resolves in a week.

28.5 Symptoms

Typhoid fever is a systemic disease prevalent in areas or countries with poor sanitation and low hygienic standards of drinking water. Travel to such areas is risky. Human adapted serotype, *Salmonellae typhi* is the cause.

Contaminated food and water, shellfish from sewage polluted areas, vegetables and fruits irrigated with untreated human sewage are common sources. Occasional direct faecal-oral and transmission/spread by flies from infectious agent (human excreta) to foods. Outbreaks occur if the common source of water supply or foods from food processing/service establishments are contaminated.

The onset of typhoid fever is gradual and prolong. There is fever, anorexia, malaise, headache, insomnia, constipation and abdominal symptoms. The liver and spleen are enlarged. There may be bradycardia and pneumonia. Complications occur by the third week in untreated cases—gastrointestinal and cerebral may prove fatal in 10–20% cases. Typhoid is fatal in children <4 years. *S. typhi* persists in biliary tract of about 2–5% of recovered cases. They are permanent carriers (https://www.who.int/ith /diseases/ typhoidfever/en/).

Non-typhoid illness manifests after an incubation period of 12–72 h in either mild or severe form. Contaminated food is the common source. The mild form presents as abdominal pain, nausea, vomiting and diarrhoea. The duration is 4–7days. Illness may resolve by itself; there is no specific treatment. Patient may require rehydration.

Severe cases show high fever, aches, short-term or chronic arthritis, headaches, lethargy, a rash and blood in the urine or stool. Some cases, especially those with weak immune systems such as infants, children <5 years old and persons with HIV or undergoing chemotherapy may end fatally. Possible sequelae: reactive arthritis, rheumatoid syndrome, cholecystitis, colitis, meningitis, myocarditis and pancreatitis.

28.6 Diagnosis

Traditional method of *Salmonella* identification is wet lab typing (bacterial culture and serotyping). Culture independent method is whole genome sequencing (WGS).

Stool and blood are the required specimens. There are three procedures:

- Culture—isolate the bacteria.
- Culture—independent detects genetic material.

Result is communicated to the doctor

- Reflex-culturing—culture-independent test positive specimen is cultured.

Isolate is serotyped and subjected to whole genome sequencing (WGS).

Serotyping and molecular characterization is useful in epidemiological studies (https://www.cdc.gov/salmonella/general/diagnosis-treatment.html).

PulseNet is a national network of public health and food regulatory agency laboratories coordinated by the U.S. CDC. It receives and maintains database. It includes local and state health departments, agricultural laboratories and federal agencies (CDC, the U.S. Department of Agriculture's Food Safety and Inspection Service, and the U.S. Food and Drug Administration). It shares data with participating health departments for comparing WGS profiles (PulseNet I PulseNet I CDC).

Source attribution Zoonotic salmonellae cause millions of human salmonellosis infections worldwide each year. Control and preventive strategies are based on information and data on source of salmonellae. Attempts are made to search association of human salmonellosis to animal reservoirs or to contaminated environment and relate environmental isolates to different animal reservoirs. Traditional method of *Salmonella* identification is wet lab typing (bacterial culture and serotyping). Culture independent method is whole genome sequencing (WGS).

Source attribution is the effort to quantify the number/proportion of sporadic human cases of a specific illness (e.g., foodborne) to specific sources (food categories) and animal reservoirs. Data collected through integrated surveillance systems of humans, food and animals complies with these requirements. A cluster of infections with the same or very similar WGS profiles is indicative of an outbreak. Finding the same profile in a food and cluster of human infection is suggestive of causal association of specific food source to illness.

In European Union zoonotic, sporadic non-typhoidal salmonellosis cases reported in 2016 were investigated (Koutsoumanis et al. 2019). The top 5 causative serovars were: *S.* Enteritidis (94.7%), *S.* Typhimurium (93.8%), 1,4,[5],12: i:- (monophasic), *S.* Typhimurium (93.3%), *S.* Infantis (92.4%) and *S.* Derby (95.6%). *S.* Enteritidis, *S.* Typhimurium, including monophasic *S.* Typhimurium caused 75.9% of the reported human cases with known country of origin of infection, of these, *S.* Enteritidis alone accounted for 57.1%. The route of spread of some zoonotic serovars was traced.

S. Enteritidis in particular contaminated hatching and table eggs internally and was consistently traced from breeders to broiler and to broiler meat. *S.* Typhimurium, *S.* Infantis, *S.* Kentucky and *S.* Senftenberg were traced back to breeders.

Faecal contamination of hatching eggs originating in hatchery is likely to bring wide range of serovars in flock of broilers. It was observed that *S.* Enteritidis infected chicken. Epithelial cells and lymphoid cells in the reproductive tract of chickens were invaded. Immune system was evaded in some. Intestinal infection was established in minority of birds which become super shedder.

28.7 Outbreaks

Outbreaks of *Salmonella* Infections Linked to Backyard Poultry (https://www.cdc.gov/salmonella/backyardpoultry-05-19/index.html).

Public Health officials of U.S. CDC investigated a 13 multistate outbreak linked to backyard poultry. This outbreak affected the largest number of people, 1134 sick from 49 states. The cases started reporting from January 1 and continued till 9 October 2019. They fell in age group <1 to 99 (median 34) with 21% of <5 years. Females (56%) were more than males. There were 2 deaths and 219 (30%) hospitalisation.

Epidemiological, laboratory investigation and traceback indicated that outbreak occurred due to contact a week before onset of illness (reported by 63% of 619) with chicks and ducklings from multiple hatcheries of backyard poultry.

Infection was caused by *Salmonella* serotypes Agona, Alachua, Altona, Anatum, Braenderup, Enteritidis, Infantis, Manhattan, Montevideo, Muenchen, Newport and Oranienburg. Antibiotic resistance tests revealed that strains were resistant to one or more of the nine antibiotics tested.

Safety measures: Birds look healthy but carry and shed salmonella. Wash hands with soap and water after handling poultry. Use hand sanitiser. Adults should supervise children following these. Children <5 years should not be allowed to touch/kiss/snuggle chicks and ducklings. Poultry and all activities related with them should be kept outside the house.

Foodborne salmonellosis mostly originates from domestic animals and poultry. A brief description of salmonellosis in animals and poultry is presented at the end.

28.8 Outbreaks of Foodborne Salmonellosis

28.8.1 Raw Fruits, Vegetables and Sprout as Sources of Human Salmonellosis

Raw fruits, vegetables and sprouts are potential sources of human salmonellosis. Of late, outbreaks have been traced to these. Wastewater re-use in irrigation of fruits and vegetables has been ascribed. Epidemiological studies—precisely three case-control studies—were reported by Behravesh et al. (2011). *Salmonella enterica* serotype Saintpaul outbreak occurred in 2008 in the US. The number of cases were 1500, 2 deaths and 21% hospitalisation. The outbreak strain was isolated from raw tomatoes, serrano and jalapeño pepper, and agricultural water. The odd ratio for eating raw tomatoes not linked to restaurant was 5.6 and for household having raw jalapeño pepper was 2.9. The Mexican style restaurant had an odd ratio of 4.6 where consumption of the three preparations—pico de gallo salsa (4.0), corn tortillas (2.3) and salsa (2.1) seemed to be responsible. Survival and growth of a mixture of strains of *Salmonella* in salsa and related major ingredients—were tomatoes, jalapeño peppers and cilantro mixed with intact and chopped vegetables held at 4, 12 and 21 °C for 7 days was observed by Ma et al. (2010). *Salmonella* survived on intact tomatoes, jalapeño peppers and grew well at 12 and 21 °C on intact cilantro and chopped vegetables—chopped jalapeño peppers most supportive.

28.8.2 Egg-Associated Outbreak (ECDC-EFSA 2017)

In 14 countries, outbreak occurred between 1 May 2016 and 24 February 2017 with peak in September 2016. There were 218 confirmed cases caused by 2 distinct clusters of WGS and 252 probable cases sharing *S.* Enteritidis phage type (PT) 8, multiple locus variable-number tandem analysis (MLVA) profiles 2-9-7-3-2 or 2-9-6-3-2. *Eleven of the confirmed cases had travelled to Poland during incubation period and likely affected the outbreak.* Epidemiological, microbiological and environmental investigation traced infection to eggs originating from three Polish packing centres, further traced to some egg laying farms where *S.* Enteritidis persisted.

S. Enteritidis phage type (PT) 14b caused a multi-country outbreak from March to November 2014. It was associated with contaminated eggs. It affected >400 cases from France, Luxembourg, Austria and the UK.

Hormansdorfer et al. (2017) re-evaluated combining the epidemiological data with molecular technique and retrospective traceback of the incriminated food across countries to its source at the farm and linking different parts of the outbreak to distinct premises of one large egg supplier.

The large Bavarian egg producer with four distinct premises (three in Bavaria + one in Czech Republic). WGS grouped the outbreak isolates of *S.* Enteritidis (PT) 14b in three related clades which could be linked to different premises of the egg producer. Study revealed that all notified 91 laboratory-confirmed cases of *S.* Enteritidis PT 14b from Bavaria were sporadic and unrelated with any outbreak.

Comments: *Salmonella enterica* ssp. *enterica* serovar Enteritidis (*S.* Enteritidis) is important zoonotic foodborne pathogen commonly found in the intestinal tract of both humans and animals.

Salmonellae commonly contaminate poultry meat and eggs. The EU introduced regulatory targets of reduction of *S.* Enteritidis and *S.* Typhimurium in adult laying hens and mandatory control programmes in 2009, which are regularly monitored. This has proven very effective. Of 34,757 flocks of laying hens, only 2.54% were positive for salmonellae in 2014 in the EU. *S.* Enteritidis was detected in 0.7% of all flocks.

Molecular techniques discriminate clonal members *of S.* Enteritidis. Phage typing or MLVA is low discriminatory technique useful for local and small outbreaks. WGS is high discriminatory technique. It is useful for large scale, cross border, long-lasting outbreaks, and makes distinct, unambiguous classification of isolates.

28.8.3 Outbreak (Brazil Nuts)

ECDC-EFSA (2020) reported 123 cases of *S.* Typhimurium ST19 and 1 of *S.* Anatum ST64 between 1 August 2019 and 20 October 2020. Most cases (60%)

occurred during March–April 2020; 53% were male, median age was 40 years. Highest number (84.6%) of *S.* Typhimurium ST19 cases and hospitalisation including two children <5 years were in the UK. There was no travel history. Thirty-six out of thirty-eight cases were from a single clonal population within the 5-SNP cluster genetically distinct from the majority of the *S.* Typhimurium isolates originating from humans and animals in the UK. At the following weeks, genetically closely related *S.* Typhimurium were isolated from Canada (1), France (14), the Netherlands (1) and Luxembourg (3). A case control study by Public Health England (PHE) in the UK indicated a nut product, Brazil nuts, as suspected vehicle of infection. Patients interviewed confirmed consumption of any type of nut products (96% of 50 interviewed), of Brazil nuts (61.9%) and bars/cereal bars (62.5%). Brazil nuts tested positive for *Salmonella* isolates matching the outbreak strains. Recall and withdrawal of nut products have been implemented.

28.8.4 Multi-Country Outbreak of *Salmonella* Agona

EFSA (2018) reported multi-country outbreak of *Salmonella* Agona infections possibly linked to ready-to-eat food. EFSA supporting publications 15 (7) first published on 31 July 2018.

Over all 147 cases from 5 European countries were reported, 122 since 1 January 2017 and 25 historical between 2014 and 2016. Most cases (129) were from the UK followed by (15) from Finland; the rest are from Denmark, Germany and Ireland. WGS identified 17 *S.* Agona from foods in the UK in 2018 which were genetically closely related to human isolates. Isolations showed distinct seasonal spring peaks. These strongly suggested that cases were part of intermittent common source outbreak. The contaminated food sampled in the UK was cucumber, during processing before/after washing, and ready-to-eat products containing cucumber. The cucumber originated in Spain. RTE containing contaminated cucumber was the cause, but the level of contamination is still being investigated.

RISK: Variety of foods, meats—pork, chicken, vegetables, sprouts; chicken nuggets, pot pies. Increased exposure—(1) travel (international travel), (2) owning pet birds and reptiles, (3) use of antacids to reduce stomach acidity allowing *Salmonella* passage to intestine, (4) recent use of antibiotics that can reduce the population of natural probiotics and (5) immune problems—sickle cell anaemia, malaria.

28.9 Control

Integrated control measures at primary production (broiler) and final production (meat) Complete integration of feeding and rearing (farm level) and processing (plant level), or partial integration means separate control measures at farm and plant levels. Both may be practiced. Generally, control measures are directed primarily to the top 10 prevalent serovars, although emerging serovars are also kept in mind (FAO and WHO 2009).

Control measures at the primary level aims at (a) raising *Salmonella*-free 'breeder flock', (b) all-in all-out production at the broiler farm to avoid any carry over during processing, (c) logistic slaughter planning scheduled to avoid pathogens being transferred from contaminated processing equipment to another flock and (d) satisfactory cleaning of transport crates. Good hygienic Practice (GHP) includes (a) scalding, de-feathering and evisceration; washing and chilling at processing plant and (b) handling at the levels of retail and consumer. Finally, decontamination methods, such as (a) 'chemical treatment'—chlorinated water, acidified sodium citrate, acetic or lactic acids as spray or dipping and (b) 'physical treatment'—freezing, crust freezing, heat, steam-ultrasound, steam or hot water spray, force air chilling and irradiation applied as per need.

Maintaining records and analysis of data will enable evaluating the effect of interventions applied. Action to prevent contamination at multiple steps from farm to dining table is required for which integrated efforts of food industry, regulatory agencies, food service, consumers and the public health authorities are essential.

28.10 Poultry, Pet and Domestic Animal Salmonellosis

28.10.1 Poultry Salmonellosis

Pullorum disease and fowl typhoid are the two *Salmonella* illnesses of birds. However, any *Salmonella* serovar can infect birds and they are transmitted through meat and eggs to human beings as foodborne salmonellosis.

28.10.1.1 Pullorum Disease

It is widely distributed in the world including India and affects domestic fowls, turkeys, quails, ducks, pigeons and sparrows. Most chicks die as dead-in-shell and within a day or 2 of hatching. There is no age resistance. It occurs in newly hatched chicks, age groups >3 weeks, seldom in >6 weeks. Males and light birds (e.g., Leg horns) are more resistant. Severe cold, overcrowding, unsanitary conditions and intercurrent infections such as aspergillosis, rickets favour infection. The case fatality rate may reach 50%, maximum in the first week, declining in the following weeks up to 4 weeks.

The disease is transmitted both vertically and horizontally. Possible sources of infections may be infected progeny during hatching or brooding, contaminated incubators, brooders, chick boxes, attendants and their clothing, feed, water, cannibalism and flies.

28.10.1.2 Signs and Symptoms

The infected eggs or the infection acquired during hatching in incubators manifest in dead-in-shell embryo, rapid spread of disease and death reaching peak in 7 days.

Infection acquired after hatching in brooders manifest in about 10 days (incubation period) and show lower mortality, maximum during third to fourth week. Chicks appear sleepy, huddled together with eyes closed, chirp continuously and are pot-bellied. Appetite is lost and urates are seen on vents sometimes.

In broilers, hock joints are markedly swollen. The birds are poorly developed and feathered.

Chicks dying in the first week of age show hardly any change except enlargement and streak of haemorrhage on surface of liver and congestion of lungs in some. The carcass of older chicks may present blood stained cheesy inspissated unabsorbed yolk and firm yellow cecal casts. Birds dying after a prolonged illness, typical white greyish, necrotic pinpoint spots are seen throughout liver, spleen, surface of heart, lungs and gizzards. Carcass of broilers shows gelatinous exudates in joints and necrotic lesions in myocardium and liver.

The infection acquired during pullet stage is localised and chronic. Adult birds show depression, loss of appetite, pale comb, diarrhoea followed by death in few days, resembling those seen in fowl typhoid. Post-mortem show characteristic lesion in ovary. Most of the ovules are mis-shaped, angular and attached with ovary through long stalks. The ovules may be cystic, greenish or brownish in colour. The contents of ovules may be blood stained, firm and cheesy or dark red or yellow. There may be unabsorbed and coagulated egg yolk. Detached ovules in peritoneum may cause peritonitis. Other lesions include thick pericardial sac containing opaque or coloured fluid or adherent to myocardium. In males, there may be abscess in testicles, myocarditis and pericarditis.

Most survivors become carriers. About 34.0% of eggs laid by carrier hens are infected (Chauhan and Roy 2000).

Fowl Typhoid (Gallinarum)

Turkeys, ducks, quails, pheasants, pea fowls, Guinea fowls are susceptible. The causative agent has also been isolated from birds such as partridge, pigeons and rooks. Although all ages of domestic fowl are susceptible, the disease is most common in pullets from 3 months to the age of lay, and maximum mortality occurs up to the age of 5 months. Outbreaks in chickens are rare. Disease is seen more in heavy birds and those maintained on free range.

Source of infection may be carrier birds, excreta, contaminated water and feed, animal attendant, carcass of diseased bird. The bacterium survives for 1–2 months in excreta, several months in the carcass and recovered from maggots feeding on it for 150 days in stagnant water in which the diseased bird carcass was thrown. Scavenger animals such as cats, dogs, rats can carry parts of carcass and spread infection. The mode of transmission is commonly horizontal but egg borne transmission is also possible. About 10–50% of eggs laid by carrier hens may carry the bacterium.

28.10.1.3 Signs and Symptoms

Fowl typhoid is a septicaemic disease. It occurs in acute, subacute and chronic forms. The incubation period is 4–6 days. The course of the disease is short in acute form, death occurring in 48 h with case fatality rate of 4–50%. Mortality declines in about 5 days. The course is 5–6 days in subacute form. Sporadic deaths occur in chronic form which are common in endemic areas.

The acute form of the disease is manifested as high temperature, accelerated respiration, loss of appetite, dejection, depression, watery yellow urates, foul smelling droppings, thirst, cyanosis of comb and wattles. Post-mortem shows birds in good flesh, congested and jaundiced. In acute cases, liver and spleen are enlarged and congested. The surface shows characteristic distinct greenish brown sheen (copper colour) on exposure to air for a short time. Changes in liver, lungs, gizzard and ovary are similar to those seen in Pullorum disease. In chronic cases, synovitis, arthritis, consolidation of lungs, nodular (grey lumpy nodules) or necrotic lesions on heart and in intestines may be seen.

28.10.1.4 Diagnosis

Tentative diagnosis is based on symptoms and lesions. Chick mortality in incubator or brooder and ovarian lesions are strongly suggestive.

28.10.1.5 Laboratory Diagnosis

Bacteriological culture, IFT and serodiagnosis may be done. The commonly used is slide agglutination test using Pullorum antigen to detect antibodies in the blood of test bird.

28.10.1.6 Control

Rapid whole blood agglutination test for screening; two consecutive tests must prove negative. In case of tube agglutination test, 1:40 is considered as the positive titre.

- Infected shedders are culled.
- Infection-free premises are used for shelter of treated birds.
- Useful disinfectants are 2.0% hot caustic soda, 2–3.0% formalin for floor and 1 in 1000 phenols for equipment.
- Infected litter should be incinerated.
- Poultry feed—pelleted should be preferred.
- Source of chicks should be Pullorum-tested Breeder Flock and declared free.

Probiotics—Bdellovibrio administered orally to *Salmonella* infected chicken reduced the latter by 90%; the birds grew well suggesting the therapeutic effect. The effect tapered after 48 h (Atterbury et al. 2011).

Vaccine—A live attenuated vaccine contains a rough strain 9R of *S*. Gallinarum. Birds of 9–10 weeks are vaccinated. Immunity wanes after 5–6 months, and this covers most part of the susceptible age. It is necessary to monitor for reinfection and carrier status by conducting whole blood agglutination test.

Sanitation of eggs and incubator. Collection, storage and setting of eggs should be careful and hygienic. Collection should be made frequently, three or more times a day. Storage should be in a vermin proof—nest litter preferably of wood shavings maintained clean by frequent renewal at 9–13 °C, RH 75%.

Fumigation of eggs soon after collection for 20 min with formalin—45.0 mL of formaldehyde (40%) added to 30 g of KMnO4 per m^3 of space in incubator or 10 g of paraformaldehyde when hotplate method is used. Eggs should be routinely fumigated before setting in hatchery or treated with germicide by dipping a wire basket containing eggs in germicidal solution for 15 min and hung dried before setting.

Dirty and cracked eggs should be culled.

28.10.2 Dog Salmonellosis

Pets such as dogs and cats can be infected by any of the serotypes of salmonellae. Acute enteritis is manifested as severe diarrhoea with septicaemia in puppies, kittens and also stressed adults (e.g., stress of concurrent disease). Pneumonia and abortion in pregnant dogs may be observed. Sometimes cats may also suffer with conjunctivitis.

An isolate from fatal acute haemorrhagic enteritis in an adult dog was identified as *S.* Ohio. Pups were experimentally infected with the isolate and followed (Choudhury et al. 1985).

After incubation period of 14 h to 3 days, fever (99.5–103 °F) and febrile symptoms appeared. Gastroenteritis developed in 36 h, beginning with semi solid and mucoid stool followed by frank blood and mucus in 3.5–5.5 days post infection. Death followed, earliest 4 days to a maximum of 17 days after infection. Rectal swab samples were positive for *S.* Ohio 3.5 days after infection. Post-mortem: Frank congestion and haemorrhagic intestinal mucosa, clotted blood in large intestine, enlarged and congested mesenteric lymph glands besides changes in liver and other organs were observed on post-mortem examination. Histopathology showed mucosal ulceration, denudation of villi, fibrinous membrane on mucosa, engorgement of capillaries and diapedesis in stomach and intestines. The submucosa was oedematous and blood vessels in submucosa and serosa were engorged with blood cells. Pathological changes were more severe in large intestine. Sloughed up villous mass and red cells were seen in the lumen.

This *Salmonella* serotype was found to survive in experimental pups' dried (moisture 11.4%) stool for 84 days (the period of observation). This information is important in explaining the spread of infection.

Dogs and cats share human environment. The social distance is short in case of pets. Healthy dogs and cats may be infected with salmonella and shed it intermittently in faeces for 12 weeks. Prevalence rate varied between 1–36% in dogs and 1–18% in cats. Transmission to human, especially infants is most likely.

Behravesh et al. (2010) reported human salmonellosis-linked to contaminated dry dog and cat food. The serotype involved was *S.* Schwarzengrund. The odd ratios observed were: recently purchased contaminated brand of pet dry food 6.9; cases—households 3.6, illness among infant case patients associated with feeding pets in kitchen, 4.4. Subsequent to this investigation, the authors isolated this serotype from acute diarrhoea in human beings.

28.10.3 Swine Salmonellosis

28.10.3.1 A. Septicaemia

S. Cholerae suis is the most common cause of pig salmonellosis. The disease is most common in pigs <4 months of age, occasionally market pigs or adult breeding stock. The following is based on our experience.

The age distribution of affected pigs in an outbreak that occurred during April and May (1980) at Ranchi, Bihar, India is given below (Table 28.4).

In this outbreak 140 pigs of breeds—Yorkshire, Landrace, Russian Charmukha and their crosses were affected. The morbidity rate was 72.8%, and case fatality rate was a little over 90%.

The incubation period is 24–48 h. The affected animals are anorexic, found huddled in a corner of stye. The temperature is high, 105–107 °F. Healthy pigs are found dead. Patches of dark red to purple on skin in ventral abdomen, ears, tail and extremities easily attract attention. There is subcutaneous petechiae, tremor, weakness and death. Diarrhoea appears on third to fourth day. The faeces are watery and yellow. Recovered pigs are carriers and also shedders for years. In the outbreak cited above, possibly a carrier pig introduced to the farm was responsible. Experimental infection reproduced the disease in pigs in 12–16 h. The characteristic skin lesions were observed on belly, base of ear and lower jaw. The post-mortem lesions were similar.

Post-mortem lesions are extensive. Spleen is enlarged and shows infarction. There is generalised serohaemorrhagic lymphadenitis and generalised petechial and ecchymotic haemorrhages on serosal surface, mucosa of larynx, urinary bladder and renal parenchyma. The liver is golden yellow and swollen, and the icterus is pronounced. The kidney shows red haemorrhagic spots giving an appearance of turkey egg.

Disseminated focal necrosis, hyaline capillary and venule thrombosis are seen on histopathological examination.

Differential diagnosis—Hog cholera, Acute erysipelas, Oedema disease, Coliform enteritis of weaning pigs, Mulberry heat disease, Streptococcosis, Haemolytic *E. coli* toxaemia.

28.10.3.2 B. Enteritis

The incubation period is 36 h. Faeces is foul smelling and contains sheds of gut mucosa and fibrinous exudates. The perineum of the sick pig is soiled. The animal is unthrifty, dehydrated and hairs are rough. The entire intestine is inflamed, and all functions are lost. Erosion and oedema of cecal mucosa occur 64 h after infection,

Table 28.4 Age distribution of fatal cases (Choudhury et al. 1980)

Age group	Mortality (in %)
0–56 days	61.9
56–240 (8 months)	90.9
240–365 (1 year)	35.3
Breedable (1 year and above)	38.4

necrotic membrane (thick wall of caseation over erosion) 96 h and sloughing of necrotising membrane 128 h after infection. Additionally, there may be pneumonia, hepatitis and encephalitis, and death in some cases may be due to asphyxia or pneumonia. Enlarged tonsils and lymph nodes in the cervical region cause asphyxia. Post-mortem reveals severe lesions in ileum, cecum and colon. There are large leathery discrete or confluent ulcers with adherent necrotic membrane. Intestinal wall is thickened, ileum is like a hose pipe. The spleen and draining lymph glands are enlarged. Lungs show consolidation and caseated nodules.

28.10.3.3 C. *Salmonella* Typhimurium Infection

Typhimurium salmonellosis in pigs is characterised by acute or chronic diarrhoea, dehydration, low appetite and fever affecting adults of purebred breeding herds and testing stations. The profuse diarrhoeic faeces may have mucus and blood in later stage. The spread in a herd is rapid. Morbidity is high, mortality is low. Diarrhoea occurs in two to three bouts—the first lasting for about 3 days. The course of the disease may last for several weeks. Death may be due to dehydration or hypokalaemia. There is focal or diffuse necrotic colitis. There are sharply delineated button ulcers. Lesions are seen in caecum, descending colon and rectum. The content of ileum is watery and yellow, the mucosa is red and rough. Ileocecal mesenteric lymph gland is greatly enlarged. Rectal stricture syndrome in feeder pigs is common sequelae. Histopathological examination shows necrosis of cryptal surface enterocytes. Necrosis may extend to muscularis mucosa, submucosa and lymphoid follicles.

Differential diagnosis—Swine dysentery, Necrotic enteritis, Rota- and Corona viruses, Postweaning colibacillosis, Coccidiosis are confounding conditions. However, clinical features in these have no similarity with clinical features of salmonellosis in weaned pigs.

Other manifestations are acute pneumonia, bronchopneumonia (similar to those seen in Pasteurellosis) and pleuropneumonia (similar to those seen in Actinobacillosis). Cutaneous lesions are similar to those described above.

Recovered animals become carriers and intermittent shedders. In experimental *S.* Typhimurium infection, the bacterium was isolated for the first 10 days daily from faeces, frequently for the next 4 months and following slaughter after 4 months from 39/45 pigs' faeces, caecum and mesenteric lymph nodes (Wilcock 1982). In natural cases, there is prolonged and sporadic shedding.

28.10.4 Bovine Salmonellosis

Four distinct forms are known—septicaemia, acute enteritis, subacute enteritis and chronic enteritis.

28.10.4.1 A. Septicaemia: *Salmonella* Dublin Infection

In newborn calves and foals (less than few weeks of age), the disease is characterised by high fever, 105–107 °F, profound depression, nervous incoordination and nystagmus. There is dyspnoea and death in 24–48 h. The case fatality rate may be 100%. Survivors suffer with severe enteritis, diarrhoea appearing 12–24 h after illness. Those surviving severe enteritis show residual effects such as arthritis and pneumonia. Experimental infection in calves of 6–7 weeks with *S.* Dublin resulted in fatal septicaemia showing acute necrotising pancreatitis. In 12–14 weeks-old calves, there was progressive fatal diarrhoea within 1 week (incubation period). The animals suffered a great fluid and weight loss. There is endarteritis resulting to gangrene of extremities such as tail, ears and limbs. The fetlock joint shows distinct normal skin above and swollen necrotic, cool, painless, dry or moist skin below. Animals go lame. The tip of ear is indurated. Possible sequelae are epiphyseal osteomyelitis of metaphyses, polysinovitis and arthritis. Meningoencepahlomyelitis and associated symptoms may also be observed.

28.10.4.2 B. Acute Enteritis

B. Acute enteritis—In new born calves, the common signs and symptoms are high temperature, 104–106 °F, anorexia, thirst, abdominal pain manifested as kicking at abdomen, rolling, crouching and groaning. The dung is putrid fluid and contains mucus, sometimes blood, fibrinous cast. There is dysentery with tenesmus. The heartbeat is rapid, respiration rapid and shallow and dyspnoea. The mucosa is congested. Animals manifest weight loss, weakness, recumbency and death in 2–5 days. The case fatality rate may be 75%. The course of the disease varies from 3 to 7 days. In calves older than 1 week, enteritis is common.

S. Dublin and *S.* Typhimurium cause per-acute enteritis in newborn kids. Natural cases are rare. Sheep and adult horses suffer with subacute enteritis.

Adult of all species suffer with pyrexia, anorexia, enteritis, toxaemia and severe dehydration. Abortion and hypoagalactia occur in pregnant cows. Abortion is common between 124 and 270 days of pregnancy. *S.* Dublin multiplies in placenta. Placenta is retained. There is foetal death, foetus may survive but live born calf dies. *S.* Dublin also causes chronic active mastitis.

28.10.4.3 C. Subacute Enteritis

C. Subacute enteritis—is generally manifested as mild fever (103–104 °F), anorexia and abortion. A few days later, diarrhoea in the form of soft faeces is observed. In some cases, dehydration may occur.

28.10.4.4 D. Chronic enteritis

D. Chronic enteritis—as observed in cattle and pigs is characterised by intermittent or persistent diarrhoea. The stool may contain spots of blood, mucus and fibrinous cast. There is anorexia, loss of weight, emaciation and low-grade intermittent fever 102 °F. When terminal part of rectum is affected in pigs, stricture develops. This may be observed by palpation only or on necropsy.

S. Typhimurium infection—This serotype may affect newborn calves or recently calved cow or small number of animals at a time. Abortion and retention of placenta are observed.

Differential diagnosis—Colibacillosis (enterotoxigenic and verotoxigenic *E. coli*), Paratuberculosis, *C. perfringens* types B and C enterotoxaemia, BVD, IBR, Coccidiosis, Cryptosporidiosis, Ostertagiasis, Winter dysentery, Copper deficiency (molybdenosis), Arsenic poisoning.

28.10.5 Sheep Salmonellosis

S. Abortus ovis causes fever and abortion. Sometimes ewes die after abortion. Many lambs born alive may die later. Mortality is high in lambs of few weeks age. In the others are seen enteritis, dehydration and toxaemia. Other known salmonellae affecting sheep and goats are *S*. Typhimurium, *S*. Dublin, *S*. Anataum and *S*. Montevideo.

28.10.6 Equine Salmonellosis

Carrier status in horses is common and long (about 14 months). Stressors such as post-surgery hospitalisation, oral use of certain antibiotics, transport especially through sales yard, feed and water deprivation followed by over feeding as may happen during transport, foaling, etc., precipitate infection and introduce and reintroduce salmonella. Stud farms get contaminated. Susceptible horses get infection. *S*. Typhimurium may cause (a) fatal septicaemia in foals of up to 2 days of age, (b) severe acute fulminant enteritis in adults manifested by pain, profuse diarrhoea, dehydration, weakness, depression and death in 24 h; the case fatality rate is high, almost 100%; leukopenia and neutropenia is characteristic, and (c) subacute enteritis in adults. The incubation period is 24 h as observed in experimental infections. Infected horses may also be asymptomatic carrier. Other common serotypes affecting horses are *S*. Anatum, *S*. Newport, *S*. Enteritidis and *S*. Arizonae.

28.11 Control of Salmonellosis in Domestic Animals

Salmonella infection in animals occurs in two ways, through association with an infected fellow animal (carrier/shedder) and contaminated animal feed. Fish meal and bone cum meat meal are the common components of animal feed. They are most likely contaminated with more than one serotypes of salmonella. The *S. cholerasuis* outbreak cited above was controlled after detecting *Salmonella* contamination in fish meal and introducing 'cooking' it before mixing with the pig feed. Animal contact in animal fare and markets, transport and trade spread salmonellosis.

References

Atterbury RJ, Hobley L, Till R, Lambert C et al (2011) Effects of orally administered *Bdellovibrio bacteriovorus* on the wellbeing and *Salmonella* colonization of young chicks. Appl Environ Microbiol 77(16):5794–5803

Behravesh CB, Ferraro A et al (2010) Human *Salmonella* infections linked to contaminated dry dog and cat food, 2006–2008. Pediatrics 126:477–483

Behravesh BC, Mody RK, Jungk J, Gaul L et al (2011) 2008 outbreak of Salmonella Saintpaul infections associated with raw produce. N Engl J Med 364(10):918–927

Chauhan HVS, Roy S (2000) Poultry diseases, diagnosis and treatment. New Age International (P) Ltd, New Delhi, pp 23–30

Choudhury SP, Singh SN, Narayan KG (1980) *Salmonella cholerae suis* infection in a pig farm. Indian J Anim Sci 52:910–915

Choudhury SP, Kalimuddin M, Prasad G, Verma BB, Narayan KG (1985) Observations on natural and experimental salmonellosis in dogs. J Diarrhoeal Dis Res 3(3):149–153. https://www.jstor.org/stable/23497937

ECDC-EFSA. European Centre for Disease Prevention and Control and European Food Safety Authority (2017) Multi-country outbreak of *Salmonella* Enteritidis phage type 8, MLVA type 2-9-7-3-2 and 2-9-6-3-2 infections, 7 March 2017. ECDC and EFSA: Stockholm and Parma; 2017

ECDC-EFSA. European Centre for Disease Prevention and Control, European Food Safety Authority (2020) Multi-country outbreak of *Salmonella* Typhimurium and *S.* Anatum infections linked to Brazil nuts – 21 October 2020

EFSA (2018) Multi-country outbreak of *Salmonella* Agona infections possibly linked to ready to eat food. EFSA, Parma, vol 15, no 7, pp 1–17

EFSA BIOHAZ Panel (EFSA Panel on Biological Hazards), Koutsoumanis K, Allende A, Alvarez-Ordóñez A, Bolton D, Bover-Cid S, Chemaly M, De Cesare A, Herman L, Hilbert F, Lindqvist R, Nauta M, Peixe L, Ru G, Simmons M, Skandamis P, Suffredini E, Dewulf J, Hald T, Michel V, Niskanen T, Ricci A, Snary E, Boelaert F, Messens W, Davies R (2019) Scientific opinion on the Salmonella control in poultry flocks and its public health impact. EFSA J 17(2):5596, 155 pp. https://doi.org/10.2903/j.efsa.2019.5596

FAO and WHO (2009) Microbiological risk assessment series 19. *Salmonella* and *Campylobacter* in chicken meat. Meeting Report—i1133e-S *Salmonella Campylobacter* pdf

Hormansdorfer S, Messelhausser U, Rampp A, Schonberger K, et al (2017) Re-evaluation of a 2014 multi-country European outbreak of *Salmonella* Enteritidis phage type 14b using recent epidemiological and molecular data. Eurosurveillance Weekly; 22

Ma L, Zhang G, Gerner-Smidt P, Tauxe RV, Doyle MP (2010) Survival and growth of *Salmonella* in salsa and related ingredients. J Food Prot 73(3):434–444

Suffredini E, Dewulf J, Hald T, Michel V, Niskanen T et al (2019) Scientific opinion on the *Salmonella* control in poultry flocks and its public health impact. EFSA J 17(2):5596

WHO (2018) Salmonella (non-typhoidal). https://www.who.int/news-room/fact-sheets/detail/salmonella-(non-typhoidal)

Wilcock BP (1982) Salmonellosis (Ch 42). In: Lehman AD, Glock RD, Mengeling WL et al (eds) Disease of swine, V edn. Iowa State University Press, Ames, pp 445–456

Escherichia coli 29

Pathogenic E. coli are responsible for variety of conditions—neonatal meningitis, gastroenteritis, urinary tract infections, hemolytic-uremic syndrome, peritonitis, pneumonia, mastitis and septicemia.

Escherichia coli is ubiquitous and also a multifaceted bacterium. It is useful in biological studies, especially in recombinant DNA technology, and has been used as vector for production of useful proteins, antigens, etc. It belongs to coliform groups of *Enterobacteriaceae*, genus *Escherichia.* It is said to be the first bacterium to colonise infant intestine (within 40 h of birth), adhering to mucosa of large intestine, protecting it against invading intestinal pathogens and producing healthful molecules, such as vitamin K, and may be used as probiotics. About 0.1% of gut flora are *E. coli* and transmission is thus faecal-oral. Its detection/presence in environmental specimens of water, salads, sprouts, kitchen wares, drinking water, etc. indicates faecal contamination.

There are six phylogenic (evolutionary history) groups. Whole genome sequence studies cluster them into five subspecies (A–E). But this is not related with pathology. Group A consists of all strains used in research. Group E includes a clade of strains of *E. coli* O157:H7. All enterohemolytic (EHEC) strains are not genetically related.

E. coli bacteria are genetically diverse, only 20% are common. Genetic transfer is horizontal through conjugation and transduction. This allows the spread of genetic material through the existing population. Transduction uses bacteriophage. The gene coding shiga toxin was transferred from *Shigella* to *E. coli* O157:H7 by bacteriophage.

E. coli is a gram-negative rod shaped non-sporing bacterium. It has peritrichous flagella and hence motile. It is facultative anaerobic growing at an optimal temperature of 37 °C, although some laboratory strains may grow at 49 °C. It takes 20 min for division in optimal growth conditions.

K. G. Narayan et al., *Veterinary Public Health & Epidemiology*,
https://doi.org/10.1007/978-981-19-7800-5_29

E. coli strains are commonly characterised by a combination of antigens: O (somatic lipopolysaccharide), H (flagellin) and K (capsular) such as O157:H7. There are about 190 serogroups.

O antigen consists of a combination of (a) a polymer of immunogenic repeating oligosaccharides, (b) phosphorylated nonrepeating oligosaccharides core and (c) lipid endotoxin. There are 0–1 to 0–181 somatic antigens with some like 031,047, 067... and 0174 to 0181 provisional; subtypes like 0128ab and 0128ac.

There are H1 to H56; exceptions H13 and H22 are not *E. coli*. Capsular or K-antigen is acidic polysaccharide, thick, mucus like surrounding cells and are K1 to K60. Based on molecular weight, there are three groups—KI 100 kDa, II <50 kDa (associated with extraintestinal diseases) and III is small group (in between kDA, e.g. K3, K10 and K54/K96).

29.1 Pathogenic *E. coli*

Pathogenic *E. coli* cause a variety of diseases in animals and birds—diarrhoea and septicaemia in newborn calves, acute mastitis in cows and colibacillosis. Along with lesser pathogens, it can cause inflammation in all animal tissues—pericarditis, peritonitis, peri-hepatitis, etc. It is a common cause of gastroenteritis and urinary tract infection in human. *E. coli* causes a number of pathologies affecting various organs, urinary tract via endogenous, wounds and frequently intestines via exogenous routes. Healthy cattle and other species are shedders—hence can infect human via food and water, direct human-to-human transmission also occurs.

In a meta-analysis of 73 studies and 18,068 isolates, Alizade et al. (2019) found the distribution of diarrhoeagenic *E. coli* (DEC) as: enterotoxic (ETEC) 16%; enteroaggregative EC 11%; enteropathogenic (EPEC) 11%; shiga toxin producing EC 9%, diffuse adherent EC 6% and enteroinvasive EC 4%. The prevalence in Iran was low. According to Nobili et al. (2017), verotoxic (VTEC) was fourth commonly reported zoonosis in the EU in 2015 with 5901 cases. Six serogroups, O157, O26, O103, O145, O111, and O104 VTEC are foodborne public health hazard. Contamination of meat in Italy during 2015–2016: 8.4% (21/250) of the samples were positive for *vtx* genes, 2% VTEC isolated—genetically diverse from raw ground beef, beef hamburger and beef carpaccio.

Source of pathogenic *E. coli* is human and animal excreta and all food and drinks contaminated with it. The transmission route is faecal-oral. Epidemiological investigations pin down to the use of manure as fertiliser or irrigating crops, sewage contaminated water and cross-contamination in kitchen as cause of foodborne infections. Common eatables that have or can cause infection include items that are eaten raw such as sprouts, cucumber, salads and uncooked/inadequately cooked items such as unpasteurised fruit juices, milk and meat. Flies and direct contact or even airborne infection may occur in animal rearing environment. Personal poor hygiene among those working with animals and birds is also a risk factor.

29.2 *E. coli* Associated with Food Poisoning/Gastroenteritis

29.2.1 Invasive *E. coli*

Invasive *E. coli* are present in large number in (a) an inflamed bowel tissue correlating with severity of inflammation; and (b) intestinal mucosa in cases of ulcerative colitis and Crohn's disease.

E. coli is a common food poisoning bacterium from consumption of unwashed vegetables or contaminated but not well-cooked meat. Young children, old and immunocompromised ones suffer severely. Some strains produce potentially lethal toxins.

Examples are: O157:H7, O104:H4, O121, O26, O103, O111, O145 and O104: H21. Some strains may be enterohaemorrhagic/EHEC (e.g., O157:H7) causing haemorrhagic diarrhoea or enteroaggregative (adhering and forming clumps) and also enterohaemorrhagic.

In the year 2006, clusters of cases of suspected *E. coli* infections were reported from as many as 26 states in the USA. A joint investigation and outbreak-control measures were undertaken by state public health officials, CDC and the FDA. Fifty-two percent of 183 ill had to be hospitalised, 16% had haemolytic-uremic syndrome (HUS) and 1 died on 26 September. Most reported the onset of illness from 19 August to 5 September. The traceback study revealed that 95% of the infected had eaten uncooked fresh spinach during the 10 days preceding the onset of illness. Spinach grown in three California counties was contaminated. The isolates of *E. coli* O157:H7 had matching pulsed–field gel electrophoresis (PFGE) patterns (Ongoing Multistate Outbreak of *Escherichia coli* serotype O157:H7 Infections Associated with Consumption of Fresh Spinach—United States, September 2006. MMWR. Sept. 26, 2006/55 (Dispatch) 1–2).

The strain O104:H4 caused major foodborne illness in Germany in 2011 as EHEC and HUS requiring medical emergency (EFSA/ECDC 2011: Joint Rapid Risk Assessment, Cluster of haemolytic uremic syndrome (HUS) in Bordeaux, France 29 June 2011 (http://ecdc.europa.eu/en/publications/Publications/2011 June29_RA_JOINT_EFSA_STEC_France.pdf) and 15 other countries in Europe and North America. More recently, another cluster of cases in the Bordeaux region of France, and a single case in Sweden, have been reported (https://www.euro.who.int/en/health-topics/disease-prevention/food-safety/outbreaks -of-e.-coli-o104h4-infection).

29.2.2 Shiga toxin-producing *E. coli* (STEC)

Shiga toxin-producing *E. coli* (STEC) can grow between 7 and 50 °C, pH 4.4 and in food with minimum water activity of 0.95. A thorough cooking wherein all parts of food reach a temperature of 70 °C destroys it. It is the common cause of severe foodborne infection, involving raw or undercooked ground meat products, raw milk, vegetables and sprouts (https://www.who.int/news-room/fact-sheets/detail/e-coli).

Shiga toxin producing (STEC) *E. coli* O121 caused an outbreak of severe food poisoning necessitating hospitalisation of 44% of patients. Nineteen persons distributed over 6 states of the USA were affected. The outbreak was traced to eating contaminated raw clover sprouts. Multistate Outbreaks of Shiga toxin-producing *Escherichia coli* O121 Infections Linked to Raw Clover Sprouts (Final Update Posted August 1, 2014 2:15 PM ET. http://www.cdc.gov/ecoli/2014/o121-05-14/index.html).

STEC O157:H7 caused an outbreak spread over four states of the USA in which as many as 58% of those ill had to be hospitalised. The suspected food was contaminated ground beef. The contaminated product was withdrawn from the market (Multistate Outbreak of Shiga toxin-producing *Escherichia coli* O157:H7 Infections Linked to Ground Beef) (http://www.cdc.gov/ecoli/2014/O157H7-05-14/index.html). In both the outbreaks, none suffered with HUS.

Other serotypes are frequently involved in sporadic cases and outbreaks.

E. coli strains classified according to the virulence factors:

1. Enteroaggregative or EAEC—are human strains causing diarrhoea without fever; possess fimbriae enabling to aggregate tissue culture cells in vitro; bind to intestinal mucosa, produce ST and haemolysin are non-invasive.
2. Enterohaemorrhagic or EHEC—inhabit intestine of human, cattle and goats; cause haemorrhagic diarrhoea without fever and can also cause HUS with sudden kidney failure. It possesses phage-encoded shiga toxin that causes intense inflammation, e.g. O157:H7.
3. Enteroinvasive or EIEC are human strains causing profuse diarrhoea and high fever similar to shigellosis.
4. Enteropathogenic or EPEC cause diarrhoea in human, dogs, cats, horse and rabbits. These strains use adhesins called intimin or binding to host cells and lack fimbriae. They possess virulence factors similar to *Shigella* and may also produce shiga toxin. They bind intestinal cells, efface and are moderately invasive. Shiga toxin producing *E. coli* (STEC) #O157:H7 is also called bioterrorist agent. They are toxic to Vero cells—Verotoxin producing; also cause bloody diarrhoea and hence called enterohaemorrhagic (EHEC), e.g. *E. coli* O104:H4. Other strains in the STEC group, such as O145, O26, O111, and O103 are sometimes called 'non-O157STEC' group and cause severe diarrhoea and haemolytic uremic syndrome and kidney failure. The identification of strains in this group is more complex.
5. Enterotoxigenic or ETEC cause enterotoxicity resulting to diarrhoea without fever in humans (common in children and travellers), and animals like sheep, goats, pigs, cattle, horses and dogs. These strains are non-invasive and use fimbriae for adhering to enterocytes. They produce enterotoxins. LT (heat labile) is the larger molecule similar in structure and function to cholera toxin. The smaller molecule, ST (heat stable) causes accumulation of cGMP in the target cells and consequent secretion of fluids and electrolytes.

29.3 Symptoms

Symptoms commonly appear after 1–3 days of exposure, and commonly last for 3–4 days, most recover only with supportive therapy without antibiotics and hospitalisation. Symptoms include profuse watery diarrhoea, abdominal cramp, fever, nausea—with/without vomiting. There is anorexia, chills, headache and myalgia. In some, recovery is slow, which may take up to 3 weeks. There may be post-diarrhoea haemolytic urinary syndrome. It may occur in any age group, but most commonly in young children under 5 years.

29.4 Extra-Intestinal Infections

E. coli infections in the extra-intestinal tissues may cause peritonitis and haemolytic uremic syndrome. Its spread outside the intestine to peritoneum may be through perforating ulcer, ruptured appendix or surgical error.

29.4.1 Uropathogenic *E. coli* (UPEC)

E. coli accounted for 80–90% of community acquired and 30–50% of nosocomially acquired UTIs. Recurrent UTIs (women reporting within 6 months of acute episode) were about 25%.

Based on a triplex PCR, *E. coli* strains fall into four phylogenetic groups, A, B1, B2 and D, and virulent extra-intestinal strains (ExPEC) belong to groups B2 and D. ExPEC strains from hospital were studied for virulence properties and microbial resistance—70.6% of the *E. coli* isolates from our patients also belonged to phylogenetic group B2 and D; B1 was least frequent—suggested prevalence of these in man and animals here (Allahabad, U.P and Mangalore, Karnataka). Isolates belonging to the four groups were equally associated with sepsis, those of groups B2 and D with UTI. Isolates from B2 caused persistent and severe infection responsible for relapses and death. These produced virulence factors like biofilm responsible for initial step, adherence to various cells or tissues and haemolysin (potent virulence factor). Antimicrobial resistance exhibited by strains mostly of groups A and B1 which produced beta lactamase. B2 isolates were susceptible.

Urinary tract infection (UTI) can possibly occur through unnatural sex. Such strains are called UPEC. Possible modes of entry of intestinal bacteria urogenital tract are wiping back to front after defecation or switching from anal to vaginal intercourse in females and anal intercourse in males. The bacterium may ascend through urethra, urinary bladder and even to kidneys and prostate gland in males. Almost all or 90% of UTI infection is caused by *E. coli*. As the urethra is short in females, the risk factor is 14× than in males, and UTI is more common. Pathogenic mechanisms may be as follows:

1. The pyelonephritis-pili of *E. coli* (fimbriae) bind to the urinary tract cells to colonise. The specific receptors are D-galactose-D-galactose moieties on the P blood-group antigen of erythrocytes and uroepithelial cells absent in some of the population and so they are not infected.
2. The toxin (alpha and beta haemolysins) destroys premature erythrocytes and UT cells. Kidney tubules get clogged and haemolytic uremic syndrome (HUS) results. Small blood clots may lodge in capillaries of various organs—brain, lungs, kidneys, legs and arms with consequential oedema in these tissues impeding their function. Lung and heart functions are affected and blood pressure increases.
3. *Dr.* family of adhesins of *E. coli* bind *Dr. blood group antigen (*Dr^a*)* found on decay accelerating factor on RBC and other cells and induce cellular extensions wrapping the bacteria and also activating several reactions to cause cystitis and pregnancy-associated pyelonephritis.
4. UPEC adopt mechanisms to evade natural defenses—complement system by forming IBC (Intra Bacterial Community).
5. The K-producing (capsular polysaccharide) *E. coli* generally affect the upper UTI and are protected from immune factors and antibiotics because of the biofilm they form.
6. Hematogenous/systemic *E. coli* infection is rare. The invading bacterium enters the kidney, bladder and ureter from the blood stream.

29.4.2 *E. coli* Neonatal meningitis

E. coli **neonatal meningitis** is a serious condition caused by strains having K1 antigen. The infection is picked by the newborn from the mother's vagina. Intestine is colonised. Bacteraemia occurs. The protective IgM antibodies cannot cross the placenta at this age. Further, the K1 antigen resembles the cerebral glycopeptides, and the body recognises it as a 'self-antigen' causing severe meningitis.

Some strains of *E. coli* produce genotoxic substance, colibactim that can promote tumorogenesis by harming DNA. It can happen only when mucosal barrier is broken due to some concurrent infection causing inflammation, and colibactim is injected to enterocytes.

29.5 Diagnosis

29.5.1 Bacterial Culture

Specimens, stool or suspected food, are inoculated on MacConkey or EMB agar. Pink colonies on MacConkey and black with greenish-black metallic sheen on EMB agar are selected for further characterisation. *E. coli* are lysin+, A/A/g+/H_2S- on Triple Sugar Iron (TSI) agar, indole and methyl red + and VP− (IMViC ++--).

Strains are tested for pathogenic properties by growing on mammalian cells. Agglutination test is done for serotyping.

29.5.2 DNA Fingerprinting (CDC PulseNet = Pulsed-Field Gel Electrophoresis (PFGE) Patterns)

DNA fingerprinting of *E. coli* O157 isolates from stool samples of diarrhoeic, non-diarrhoeic people but sharing same suspected contaminated food, water or animal are carried out and the pattern matched. Isolates with the same pattern are likely to have the same origin/source. Illness can be ascribed to the isolate. People sharing the common source can be delineated and further interviewed for detail investigation.

Time for laboratory diagnosis and fingerprinting—generally incubation period (time of eating to appearance of symptoms) varies between 1 and 3 days. Sample should be collected from the time the first symptoms appear until medical care is sought, 1–5 days. Laboratory diagnosis takes 1–3 days. Fingerprinting should take 1 day but depending on the labs, it may take 2–4 days; add 0–7 days shipping time.

29.6 Treatment

The basic approach is to replace loss of fluid and electrolytes. The commonly used antibiotics are fluoroquinolones. Antibiotics–susceptibility test provides selecting antibiotic of choice for treatment.

29.7 Prevention

Most important are personal hygiene such as frequent washing of hands, before and after cooking and before eating. Good hygienic practices in kitchen include avoiding cross-contamination (separating and separately handling raw and cooked foods), defrosting frozen foods on counter, keeping foods including left-over frozen or refrigerated.

References

Alizade H, Teshnizi SH, Azad M, Shojae S, Gouklani H, Davoodian P, Ghanbarpour R (2019) An overview of diarrhoeagenic *Escherchia coli* in Iran: a systematic review and meta-analysis. J Res Med Sci 24:23

Nobili G, Franconieri I, La Bella G, Basanisi MG, Salandra GL (2017) Prevalence of verocytoxigenic *Escherichia coli* strains isolated from raw beef in southern Italy. Int J Food Microbiol 257:201–205

Klebsiella spp. 30

Klebsiella are potential cause of outbreaks of nosocomial bronchopneumonia, septicaemia and urinary tract infection and that too with antibiotics resistant strains. It accounts for a significant proportion of all nosocomial infection. Mortality is high even with optimal therapy. Prognosis is worse for old age, diabetes and immunodeficiency. Residual impaired lung function is observed in survivors who take months for recovery. The convergence of virulence and resistance genes may potentially result in the emergence of invasive *K. pneumoniae* infections, which may be non-treatable. It colonises the mucosa of respiratory and gastro-intestinal tract of patients in hospital. Factors such as comorbidities, compromised immune status and exposure to multiple antibiotics help colonisation and the development of drug resistance.

30.1 *K. pneumoniae*

A bacterium (Friendlander's bacillus) isolated from lungs of person who died of pneumonia by Karl Friendlander in 1882 was named *Klebsiella pneumoniae* in 1886. It is a member of family *Enterobacteriaceae. Klebsiella* are non-motile, diplobacillary form in vivo and rods with rounded ends. These can use citrate and glucose as source of carbon and ammonia for nitrogen for growth at pH 7.2, 35–37 °C. *Klebsiella oxytoca* (earlier *K. oxytocum*) produces indole, is positive to Voges-Proskauer reaction and causes liquifaction of gelatine apart from other features of *Klebsiella* species.

They form capsule (K antigen)/surrounded by slime and has lipopolysaccharide (O) antigen coat used for serological identification. They are ubiquitous, found in man, animals, soil and water.

Common pathogenic species are *K. pneumoniae, K. oxytoca and K. variicola.* The first two are associated with a number of pathologies reported in community and hospital settings. *K. pneumoniae* colonises well in the hospital environment—carpet,

K. G. Narayan et al., *Veterinary Public Health & Epidemiology*,
https://doi.org/10.1007/978-981-19-7800-5_30

sink, flower, skin of patients and hospital staff. *K. oxytoca* is a nitrogen fixer and found on a variety of plants, common on banana and sugarcane. It commonly infects young, old and those being treated for cancer, often in hospital setting. *K. variicola* causes bovine mastitis and also infects human. Many hospital isolates are drug resistant.

30.2 Pathogenic Factors

Hosts' response to infection is cellular in the form of polymorphonuclear granulocytes phagocytosing the invading bacteria. Serum complement proteins are bactericidal. In case of *K. pneumoniae* infection, neutrophil myeloperoxidase and lipopolysaccharide-binding proteins and alternate pathway of complement activation are active. However, *K. pneumoniae* is equipped with pathogenic factors. The four pathogenic factors are Capsular (K antigen-78); Adherence factor, Lipopolysaccharides (LPS, O antigens =9) and Siderophores.

1. K antigens protect from opsonophagocytosis and killing by serum. K1 and K2 are more virulent than others.
2. Adhesins located on fimbriae are responsible for haemagglutination. These are fimbrialadhesin types 1 and 3, the former (D-mannose-sensitive haemagglutination) is expressed by 80% of strains and common in clinical than environmental isolates. The latter causes D-mannose-resistant haemagglutination. There are non-fimbrial adhesins also, e.g. 29 kDa adhesin 'CF29K' and the novel fimbrial adhesin 'KPF-28'. They enable *Klebsiella* to adhere to the intestinal and carcinoma cells.
3. Lipopolysaccharide (LPS) protects against complement-mediated killing. O1 is most common which is associated with extensive necrosis of tissue.
4. Siderophores act as iron-scavenging systems. Iron-chelating compounds with high-affinity are secreted and after they have collected Fe-ions, are taken up. Four to six such iron-repressible outer membrane proteins are produced by *K. pneumoniae* during infection, e.g. enterochelin, aerobactin, yersiniabactin. Some isolates of *K. pneumoniae* from urine and blood of hospitalised patients in Munich secreted yersiniabactin.

30.2.1 Virulent and Hypervirulent Lineages (Dorman et al. 2018)

Siderophores, fimbriae, LPS and extra-cellular polysaccharide capsule production by isolates of *K. pneumoniae* make these virulent. The majority of the hyper virulent isolates of *K. pneumoniae* represent capsule types K1 and K2 strains. Excessive capsule production is strongly associated with hypervirulence in *K. pneumoniae.*

The ~200-kb virulence plasmid *K. pneumoniae* is also associated with hypervirulent phenotype, encodes siderophores such as aerobactin and salmochelin and regulators positive for biosynthesis of capsule. Hypervirulent lineage in clinical setting is a matter of concern, because these infect (a) even the immunocompetent hosts, (b) metastasise and (c) cause infection in unusual sites.

Drug resistance: *Beta-lactamase hydrolyses beta-lactum ring in antibiotics. ESBLs hydrolyse oxyiminocephalosporins. Third generation cephalosporins are made ineffective. Carbapenems (imipenem, meropenem, and ertapenem) became the option for treatment for ESBL. Carbapenem resistant Enterobacteriaceae emerged. K. pneumoniae is the most common.*

K. pneumoniae is one of the ESKAPE pathogens (six nosocomial pathogens exhibiting multidrug resistance and virulence are *Enterococcus faecium, Staphylococcus aureus, K. pneumoniae, Acinetobacter baumannii, Pseudomonas aeruginosa* and *Enterobacter* spp.) which are MDR and of serious public health concern. These MDR pathogens are *Enterococcus faecium, Staphylococcus aureus, Klebsiella pneumoniae, Acinetobacter baumannii, Pseudomonas aeruginosa* and *Enterobacter* species. Genes responsible for enzymes that inactivate antibiotics/drugs are located on mobile genetic element with potential for transfer to other bacteria.

Epidemiological studies of ESKAPE pathogens, particularly *K. pneumoniae* are desired to elucidate the development of drug resistance and virulence, and transmission pathways between human, animal, food and the environment.

MDR *K. pneumoniae* in animals is challenging because (a) they are difficult to treat, (b) animal host reservoir, (c) spread through animal produce and (c) spread of resistance to other bacteria through plasmid.

30.3 Epidemiology

Originating from the intestines of human and animal reservoirs, *K. pneumoniae* has ubiquitous distribution. In the hospital setting, the patients' gastrointestinal tract and hands of hospital staff are the important source. It is almost similar in veterinary hospital settings. The bacterium is carried to foods from the source and/or also from a number of sources during handling. Infection/pneumonia may be more common than actually diagnosed, especially in community setting.

K. pneumoniae is widely distributed in nature, soil, water, vegetation and a variety of domestic and wild mammals and insects and isolated from foods. It is pathogenic to man and animals. It causes pneumonia, epidemic metritis and cervicitis in mares and septicaemia in foals; pneumonia, mastitis and even deaths in bovines. Its prevalence is increasing in animals, especially dairy herds and food chains. Infection in animals, zoonotic and foodborne significance are least studied.

Wareth and Neubauer (2021) reviewed *K. pneumoniae* prevalence in Germany in farm and companion animals, dogs, cats, rabbits, guinea pigs, and mice, skin of chicken broiler and defeathering machine, pet, captured and zoo birds, falconry birds, zoo—snakes, free living reptiles, amphibians in health and disease.

30.4 Animals

Klebsiella pneumoniae in farm and companion animals (Germany).

Clinical specimens of companion and farm animals, i.e. dogs, cats, horses, rabbits, rats, chicken and pigs yielded *K. pneumoniae*. Of the mucosa-associated bacteria isolated from pigs, 84% were *K. pneumoniae.* Isolates from samples of soft tissues from infections of urinary, respiratory and the genital tracts, wounds of dogs, cats and horses were MDR carbapenemase and ESBL producing; suggested that MDR strains of *K. pneumoniae* were associated with pathologies. ESBL producing *K. pneumoniae* subsp. *Pneumoniae* was extensively prevalent, recovered from veterinary clinics in 27/30 different towns. Five clonally related isolates of *K. pneumoniae* from dogs in the same veterinary clinic between June and October 2012 co-expressed *bla* CTX-M-15 type ESBL, and harboured quinolone resistance genes, which were plasmid-mediated, suggest colonisation/prevalence in veterinary hospital setting. The clonal group carrying *bla* CTX-M-15 was the most predominant type and interestingly considered highly prevalent zoonotic agent. The possibility of spread and transfer of MDR genes between human and animal population is evidenced by the observation of isolates from animal and human sharing PMQR and OXA-48 genes (Wareth and Neubauer 2021). There is evidence of contamination and spread through animal carriers between various clinics.

Studies on clinical specimen from dogs and cats in Japan revealed that MDR ESBL-*K. pneumoniae* are spreading directly and indirectly (Harada et al. 2016).

30.5 Environment

Klebsiella pneumoniae can be present in a wide range of environment such as soil, water and vegetation. Dust around pig farm, moth flies around hospital and wastewater treatment plants were positive for *K. pneumoniae,* often MDR. Recently, evaluation of dissemination of resistance to antibiotic by effluents of wastewater treatment plant (WWTP) in Germany with different catchment areas showed that the daily discharge of *K. pneumoniae* in food-producing WWTP effluents was higher in comparison to communal and hospital-impacted WWTP effluents.

30.6 Food

Klebsiella pneumoniae is a member of *Enterobcteriaceae* but does not belong to classic foodborne bacterial pathogens and often missed and unsuspected to have contaminated foods, for example meat products. Yet it has often been found to contaminate retail meat and poultry products.

Almost half of retail chicken, turkey and pork products in the USA tested positive for *K. pneumoniae*, a common cause of gastrointestinal illness, the first indication that the bacterium may be a significant foodborne pathogen.

A study made by Davis et al. (2015) suggested that consumers can be exposed to potentially dangerous *Klebsiella* from contaminated meat. Samples of turkey, chicken and pork products sold in nine grocery stores in Flagstaff, Arizona were analysed in 2012. Urine and blood samples were taken from Flagstaff area patients in 2011 and 2012. Of the 508 meat products, 47% harboured *Klebsiella*—and many strains were antibiotic resistant. Of the 1728 positive cultures from patients, 10% were *Klebsiella*, including drug-resistant strains. Whole genome sequencing revealed that isolate pairs from the meat and from patients were nearly identical. In vivo virulence test (subcutaneous mouse model) that measures sepsis, illness and lethality was also done. A close genetic relatedness between isolates from clinical specimens and meats suggested that retail meats were the potential source of human infection. The strains were virulent. Antibiotic resistance reflected their use in production of food animals. The authors concluded 'Now we have another drug-resistant pathogen in the food supply, underscoring the public health concern regarding antibiotic use in food animal production'.

Wareth and Neubauer (2021) reported prevalence in foods in Germany where strains of MDR *K. pneumoniae* were found in rocket salad and mung bean sprouts. In 2016, from a German mastitis milk, a *K. pneumoniae* strain was isolated. Retail raw sea foods sampled between 2015 and 2016 consisted of white leg shrimp, black tiger shrimp, blue mussels, venus clams, razor shells, and cockles, most harvested abroad. From black tiger shrimps, 13 ESBL and AmpC-producing *K. pneumoniae* were isolated.

30.7 Human

Klebsiella pneumoniae is an opportunistic pathogen of human and animal (companion and domestic animals such as horses and cows). It is a part of normal flora of mouth, nose and intestine of human and animals. It colonises intestines including those of humans, causes gut diseases. It has the potentiality to infect other organs and causes a range of diseases—from wound infection to pneumonia, meningitis, osteomyelitis, cystitis, pyelonephritis, bacteraemia, septicaemia and liver abscess. Treatment is challenging as most of the infecting isolates have shown multiple drug resistance.

Investigation into human intestinal carriage of ESBL-KP and clonal relatedness among ESBL-KP isolated from faecal samples in Iran was made by Aghamohammad et al. (2020). Rectal swabs (120) were collected from inpatients of intensive care unit (61) and from outpatients (59) and 22/120 (18.3%) ESBL-KP was isolated with 81% $bla_{\mathrm{CTXM\text{-}15}}$. The most prevalent virulence gene detected was *Ompk35* in 86.3% of the isolates.

30.8 Disease

Klebsiella pneumonia can infect blood, bladder and UTI, brain, eyes, liver, lungs and wounds. Brief symptoms:

Pneumonia—is common. It occurs in community setting such as mall and more so in hospital setting. Transmission is human to human. Persons at risk are old age, long course of antibiotics and corticosteroids; hospitalisation, wounds, users of breathing machine, catheter or intravenous, surgery, solid organ transplant. Symptoms: chest pain, shortness of breath, cough, yellow or bloody mucus, fever, chills. The sputum produced by those with *S. pneumonia* was 'blood-tinged' or 'rust-coloured'; however, the sputum produced by persons infected with *K. pneumoniae* was 'currant jelly' because *K. pneumoniae* causes significant inflammation and necrosis of the surrounding tissue.

Bacteremia, endophthalmitis, sepsis—complications associated with pneumonia include bacteremia, extension of infection from lungs to other organs/systems and sepsis. About half of bacteraemia occurs after pneumonia and has a potential to progress into sepsis if not treated immediately. Bacteraemia patients show high fever, chills and shaking. Endophthalmitis cases have blurred vision, photophobia, pain in the eye, redness; white or yellow discharge.

UTI—*K. pneumoniae* infects urinary tract commonly of old women and through catheter used in hospital. Infection ranges from asymptomatic to severe. Patient reports fever, chill, nausea, vomiting and pain in the upper back and pelvic region. Specific signs and symptoms are cloudy/bloody and strong-smelling urine, discomfort in lower abdomen, frequent urge for and burning sensation during urination.

Pyogenic liver abscess—may occur in diabetic and those on prolonged antibiotic therapy. Patient complains of pain in the right upper abdomen, nausea, vomiting and diarrhoea. There may be fever.

Skin or soft tissue infection—is characterised by fever and flu-like symptoms with pain, redness, swelling, necrotising fasciitis, cellulitis and myositis.

Meningitis—it occurs in hospital setting. Membrane around brain and spinal cord is infected and inflamed. Cases report high fever, nausea, vomiting, stiff neck, headache, photophobia and confusion.

30.9 Diagnosis

Aghamohammad et al. (2020) used the following method for screening and isolating ESBL-*K. pneumoniae:* for isolation cefotaxime supplemented MacConkey agar was used. PCR was performed to detect ESBL, carbapenemase and virulence factor genes. Experiments for conjugation and replicon typing based on PCR were performed. Clonal relatedness was studied using multilocus sequence typing (MLST) and multiple locus variable number tandem repeat analysis (MLVA).

30.10 *K. oxytoca*

E. coli and *Klebsiella* are the opportunistic pathogens and leading cause of severe diseases. Majority of *Klebsiella* are *K. pneumoniae. K. oxytoca* makes small case reports and studies. *K. oxytoca* is commonly isolated from clinical samples of blood and respiratory secretions of patients in hospital. It has clinical significance in patients admitted to intensive critical care units (ICCU), neonatal care units (NCU) and weak, immunocompromised patients. The prevalence of *K. oxytoca* varies from 2% to 24%. The multidrug-resistant strains could be fatal to immunocompromised and those with comorbidities. It has been causally associated with a wide range of pathologies, diarrhoea, haemolytic colitis, infective endocarditis, respiratory and urinary tract infections. Chronic pneumonia confounded with pulmonary tuberculosis in a 50-year-old male smoker was diagnosed on sputum and bronchial aspirate culture (Gera et al. 2015). *K. oxytoca* isolation from blood and urine diagnosed infection and medical investigation revealed pathology in more than one organ in a 73-year-old man (Memon et al. 2018). He had nephrolithiasis, 21 mm left side ureteral stone and hydronephrosis; underwent emergent nephrostomy tube replacement, symptoms of cardiac fibrillation and arrest due to tricuspid valve endocarditis.

K. oxytoca produces cytotoxins, tilivalline and tilimycin responsible for pathologies (Neog et al. 2021). Pathogenic mechanism: Studies suggest that *K. oxytoca* impairs intestinal barrier. Impairment is possibly caused by two ways: (a) the cytotoxin (tilivalline/tilimycin) dependent mechanism works by increasing cellular apoptosis; (b) independent of cytotoxin, the paracellular pathway is weakened through the tight junction proteins claudin-5 and 8 (Hering et al. 2019; Neog et al. 2021).

In a military hospital study, 654/17,335 samples tested positive for *Klebsilella*. Most (96.48%) were *K. pneumonia* and (3.52% or 23 patients) *K. pneumoniae* isolates from neonatal care unit at a tertiary centre were ESBL producing (*drug resistant*). *K. oxytoca* isolates were sensitive to colistin and tigecycline but resistant to many other drugs. These KPC-producing bacteria are less sensitive to aminoglycosides and quinolones. Of *K. oxytoca* isolates, 58% were KPC producers. It easily develops resistance to drugs and is capable of producing extended-spectrum ß-lactamases (ESBLs), AmpC lactamases, *Klebsiella pneumonia* carbapenemase (KPC) and aminoglycosides-modifying enzymes (Singh et al. 2016). Most *K. oxytoca* infection is asymptomatic. It is being recognised as an important pathogen for nosocomial infections in cohorts of hospitalised patients.

30.11 Epidemiology and Clinical Importance of *K. pneumoniae* Carbapenemases (KPC)

E. coli and *Klebsiella* of the family *Enterobacteriaceae* are opportunistic pathogens and important causes of nosocomial infections. They have acquired genes for antimicrobial resistance and virulence factors through horizontal transfer of genetic material. Carbapenemases in *Enterobacteriaceae* make them resistant to carbapenems, drugs of choice for treatment. The three molecular classes of beta-lactamase: A, B, and D represent carbapenemases in *Enterobacteriaceae. Klebsiella pneumonia* carbapenemase (KPC) is a class A beta-lactamase and is transferable to other gram-negative bacteria. KPCs have a great potential to spread due to their localisation on mobile genetic elements. Therefore, rapid detection of KPC-carrying bacteria with phenotypic and confirmatory molecular tests is essential.

These markers can be used to trace the pathogen, track the route of spread and finally establish the causal association with infection/outbreak.

KPC-producing *Klebsiella pneumonia* isolates have caused outbreaks in Israel, Greece, South America and China and have spread rapidly to the USA, Europe, Asia and Australia. Hoenigl et al. (2012) made a retrospective observational study on an outbreak of KPC-producing *Klebsiellaoxytoca* (October 2010-February 2011) in Austria. Five patients (P1-5) with serious morbidities (e.g., ischaemic heart, CAD, etc.) occupied the same ICU room. The P1 suffering with ischaemic heart hospitalised for 31 days in other ICUs introduced the first isolate of KPC-producing *K. oxytoca*. It caused UTI and ventilator associated pneumonia (VAP). Infection spread horizontally to the other four patients. Isolations made periodically, the last made in February 2011 from bronchoalveolar lavage fluid from P5 belonged to the same clonal group. All the detected KPC-producing *K. oxytoca* strains were multi-drug resistant. Therapeutic options were limited. The strains exhibited susceptibility to colistin, fosfomycin, tigecycline and amikacin only. Systemic anti-infective treatment for KPC- producing *K. oxytoca* infection was successful. Labrador and Araque (2014) reported the first case of KPC-2-producing *K. oxytoca* isolated in a paediatric patient admitted to ICU with nosocomial pneumonia in Venezuela. This strain also coproduced other β-lactamases as CTX-M-8 and TEM-15.

30.12 Prevention

Epidemiological studies of ESKAPE pathogens, particularly *K. pneumoniae* are desired to elucidate the development of drug resistance and virulence, and transmission pathways between humans, animal hosts, foods and the environment.

Generate/compile data on:

- The general distribution and antibiotic resistance in *K. pneumoniae* in domestic animals, wildlife, environment and food
- Transmission of bacteria with antibiotic-resistance or their corresponding resistance determinants between animal and man and country to country
- Increased awareness of public health and veterinary health is required
- Monitoring of MDR pathogens in animal, food and environment
- Further investigation of MDR pathogens in animals and the food chain is required to elucidate transmission of AMR genes

References

Aghamohammad S, Badmasti F, Solgi H, Aminzadeh Z, Khodabandelo Z, Shahcheraghi F (2020) First report of extended-spectrum betalactamase-producing *Klebsiella pneumoniae* among fecal carriage in Iran: high diversity of clonal relatedness and virulence factor profiles. Microb Drug Resist 26(3):261–269

Davis GS, Waits K, Lora Nordstrom L, Weaver B, Aziz M, Gauld L et al (2015) Intermingled *Klebsiella pneumoniae* populations between retail meats and human urinary tract infections. Clin Infect Dis 61(6):892–899

Dorman MJ, Feltwell T, Goulding DA, Parkhill J, Short FL (2018) The capsule regulatory network of *Klebsiella pneumoniae* defined by density-TraDISort. mBio 9(6):e01863-18

Gera K, Rosha R, Varma-Basil M, Shah A (2015) Chronic pneumonia due to *Klebsiella oxytoca* mimicking pulmonary tuberculosis. Pneumonol Alergol Pol 83(5):383–386

Harada K, Shimizu T, Mukai Y, Kuwajima K, Sato T et al (2016) Phenotypic and molecular characterization of antimicrobial resistance in *Klebsiella* spp. isolates from companion animals in Japan: clonal dissemination of multidrug-resistant extended-spectrum β-lactamase-producing *Klebsiella pneumoniae*. Front Microbiol 7:1021

Hering NA, Fromm A, Bucker R, Gorkiewicz G et al (2019) Tilivalline- and tilimycin-independent effects of *Klebsiella oxytoca* on tight junction-mediated intestinal barrier impairment. Int J Mol Sci 20(22):5595

Hoenigl M, Valentin T, Zarfel G et al (2012) Nosocomial outbreak of *Klebsiella pneumonia* carbapenemase-producing *Klebsiella oxytoca* in Austria. Antimicrob Agents Chemother 56(4):2158–2161

Labrador I, Araque M (2014) *Case report* first description of KPC-2-producing *Klebsiella oxytoca* isolated from a pediatric patient with nosocomial pneumonia in Venezuela. Case Rep Infect Dis 2014:434987

Memon W, Miller M, Shabbir Z (2018) *Klebsiella oxytoca* tricuspid valve endocarditis in an elderly patient without known predisposing factors. BMJ Case Rep 2018:bcr2018225352

Neog N, Phukan U, Puzari M, Sharma M, Chetia P (2021) *Klebsiellaoxytoca* and emerging nosocomial infections. Curr Microbiol 78(4):1115–1123

Singh L, Cariappa MP, Kaur M (2016) *Klebsiellao xytoca*: an emerging pathogen? Med J Armed Forces India 2016(72):s59–s61

Wareth G, Neubauer H (2021) The animal-foods-environment interface of *Klebsiella pneumonia* in Germany: an observational study on pathogenicity, resistance development and the current situation. Vet Res 52:16

31 Aeromonas hydrophila

Aeromonads are important pathogens for fish leading to economic loss to aquaculture/industry and simultaneously for humans causing water and foodborne gastroenteritis, travellers' diarrhoea and a number of serious infections such as septicaemia, sepsis, necrotising fasciitis and complications. *Aeromonas hydrophila* is found in all forms of water, fresh, sea, estuarine and brackish. It is able to survive cold temperatures, aerobic and anaerobic conditions. It can use organic matter in water for growth.

The genus *Aeromonas,* family *Aeromonadaceae* comprises of mesophilic and psychrophilic species that are pathogenic to warm and cold-blooded animals. The mesophilic species—*A. hydrophila, A. caviae, A. sobria, A. veronii* and *A. schubertii* and the non-motile, psychrophilic *A. salmonicida* (a fish pathogen) have been associated with a wide range of infections in human—diarrhoea, sepsis, wound infections, eye, urinary-, respiratory- and hepatobiliary tract infections and necrotising fasciitis. The mesophilic *Aeromonas* are emergent agents of foodborne illness.

A. hydrophila are gram-negative, oxidase-positive, facultative anaerobic, glucose fermenting, non-sporing motile rods of 1–3 μm, tolerate sodium chloride 0.3–0.5%. Identification requires a combination of tests, biochemical, matrix-assisted laser desorption/ionisation time of flight mass spectrophotometry (MALD-TOFMS) and 16S ribosomal nucleic acid (rRNA) sequencing. Multilocus phylogenetic analysis (MLPI) needs five or more housekeeping genes. There are 32 species.

31.1 Virulence Factors

Gonçalves Pessoa et al. (2019) described the virulence factors and the respective genes. Virulence factors are cellular and extracellular. *A. hydrophila* invade Hepa 2 cells through adhesins and pili. Biofilm production confers resistance to bactericidal agent; promotes adhesion to abiotic solid surface and host cells, the first step to

K. G. Narayan et al., *Veterinary Public Health & Epidemiology*,
https://doi.org/10.1007/978-981-19-7800-5_31

infection process. Glycerophospholipid: cholesterol acyltransferase or GCAT (gene '*gcat*') is one of the virulence factors in *A. salmonicida* complex. It is a haemolytic enterotoxin. It becomes more toxic with LPS than alone. A number of cell-surface proteases enhance virulence. A number of extracellular toxins and enzymes have also been described. These are extracellular proteins such as aerolysin, lipase, chitinase, amylase, gelatinase, haemolysins and enterotoxins.

31.1.1 Enterotoxins

Cytotoxic and two types of cytotonic enterotoxins are well known. Cytotoxic enterotoxin promotes degeneration and contributes to gastroenteritis. Cytotoxic enterotoxin (gene '*act*') has cytotoxic, haemolytic and enterotoxic activities, effects degeneration of villi and mucus producing cells in human bloody diarrhoea and generates inflammatory response leading to systemic involvement.

Cytotonic enterotoxins are related with non-bloody diarrhoea. The heat labile cytotonic enterotoxin (gene '*alt*') is degraded at 56 °C in 10 min and the heat stable (gene '*ast*') at 100 °C in 30 min. These cause cytotoxic effect on hamster ovarian cells, fluid secretion in rat ileum and secretion of cyclic AMP and prostaglandins in intestinal cells. Seven isolates of *Aeromonas* from raw meat and human diarrhoea were studied for virulence genes. Most had at least one enterotoxin-coding gene.

Plasmid-encoded cytotoxin similar to Shiga-like toxin1 from *A. hydrophila* and *A. caviae* production is variable. Shiga-like toxins (Stx1 and Stx2) have been identified in animal isolates. One part of the toxin binds to the surface of hosts' cells and the other part having enzymatic property inhibits protein synthesis of the host's cells.

Haemolysins (aerolysin) from many strains of *A. hydrophila* and *A. sorbia* are heat labile beta-haemolysin with phospholipase A and C activity and cause cytoplasmic leakage by forming pores in the cell membrane, ultimately apoptosis of host's cells.

31.1.2 Specialized Protein Secretion Machinery (TTSS)

After entry in host, *Aeromonas* spreads through blood stream to the first available organ. It has been proposed that specialised protein secretion machinery (TTSS) is triggered. Of the six secretion systems of gram-negative bacteria, four types, II–VI, are reported in the genus *Aeromonas.* The extracellular release of virulence factors protease, amylase, DNases and aerolysin is TTSS type II mediated. The type III is widespread in relation to virulence and responsible for injecting harmful proteins directly into the hosts' cell cytoplasm. ADP-ribosylation toxin of *A. hydrophila* (human diarrhoeal isolate) and *A. salmonicida* (fish pathogen) and *A. jandaei* GV17 (fish and human pathogen) is translocated through TTSS and delivered into the hosts' cell cytoplasm causing interruption of NF-kB pathway, cytoskeletal damage and apoptosis.

Virulence factors are detected by genome sequencing and annotation. Detection of genes such as '*aer*' and '*ast*' in samples of water—tap, bottled and well, raises a serious concern.

31.2 Public Health Problem

Aeromonas is an emerging public health problem, associated with septicaemic conditions and gastrointestinal in a variety of aquatic organisms and a number of extra-intestinal pathologies in immunocompetent and immunocompromised human. They infect gastrointestinal system, and if not treated properly have the potential to cause systemic infection and septicaemia. The pathogens may infect the hepatobiliary and respiratory systems, eyes, skin, bone and joints. *Aeromonas* have been associated with rare systemic cellulitis, inflammation of connective tissues necrotising fasciitis; myonecrosis, necrosis with/without gas gangrene; erythema with necrotic centre; osteomyelitis; septicaemia, chill, fever, hypotension with high mortality; pneumonia, peritonitis; cholecystitis acute gallbladder infection; conjunctivitis, corneal ulcer, endophthalmitis.

31.3 Epidemiology

A number of factors such as age (children more susceptible), compromised defence system (leukaemia, carcinoma, HIV, transplant) and underlying illness (e.g., cirrhosis of liver) appear predisposing. Genetic plasticity and diverse virulence factors and a number of bacteria determine infection and pathology.

The increase in environmental temperature during summer increases bacterial load in vehicles of infection such as drinking water by mesophilic species. Extra-intestinal infections, such as bacteraemia and septicaemia also increase. Rains lower salinity in water, favour the bacteria, thus increase the prevalence of related diseases.

Infection with aeromonads reportedly appear to be prevalent in developing countries such as India, Bangladesh, China, Vietnam, Iran, Libya, Egypt, Nigeria, Brazil and Venezuela (Bhowmick and Bhattacharjee 2018).

31.4 Sources

Aeromonas have adaptation capacities that enable them to colonise diverse aquatic and terrestrial environments, especially low temperature and their inhabitants. Natural sources of *Aeromonas* are soil, plants, fruits, vegetables, birds, meat, reptiles, fish, crustacea and amphibians.

Aeromonads are autochthonous to fresh and marine water and are readily isolated from nutrient-poor and rich environments and from drinking water supply system. Pathogenic *Aeromonas,* which have been isolated from both unchlorinated and chlorinated water, are able to grow at 4 °C and hence can be detected in water throughout the year and in many geographical areas. Mesophilic aeromonads can utilise a variety of organic compounds available in water.

Leeches, seafoods, fish, shellfish, and marketed meats from lamb, beef, pork and poultry, vegetables, sprouts constitute sources for human infection.

In Turkey, 126 new isolates of *Aeromonas* from red meat, raw chicken, minced meat and fish samples were studied and *A. hydrophila, A. caviae* and *A. sorbia* were identified (Erdem et al. 2011). *A. caviae, A. hydrophila* and *A. sobria* have been isolated from meat, milk and dairy products; and plants, lettuce (except *A. sobria*). Meat products harboured greater number of *A. caviae* and *A. hydrophila* than vegetables. According to Bhowmick and Bhattacharjee (2018), 13.4% of animal-origin food samples, the highest being fish were contaminated with *Aeromonas.* Drinking water may be contaminated with non-culturable *Aeromonas.* Genetic sequencing of 16S rRNA led to detection.

Some of the species may be introduced into foods from sources such as soil, animal faeces, and water for irrigation and during agricultural practices.

Mode of infection includes ingestion of contaminated food and water (scuba divers) causing gastroenteritis and direct contact (of lacerated injury/fracture) with aquatic environments leading to systemic infection.

Aeromonas have been frequently isolated from dairy, pork or beef products, fish, seafood and vegetables. *A hydrophila* and *A. veronii* have been isolated from intestine of *Musca domestica* (Gonçalves Pessoa et al. 2019); contamination of finished ready-to-eat food is possible.

Animal farming and aqua culture activities such as ranching, crustacean breeding and aviculture present risk of direct transmission as *Aeromonas* colonise in the settings. Elevated environmental temperature is prevalent during summer, which favours infection.

31.4.1 Pathogenic Species

Common human pathogenic species are *A. hydrophila*, *A. caviae* and *A. veronii* bv. Sobria. *A. jandaei*, *A. veronii* bv. *veronii*, *A. schubertii*, *A. popoffi* are also known to infect human, the last one causes urinary tract infection. *A. salmonicida* is a pathogen for cold-blooded animals. It has been isolated from blood of a human patient.

31.4.1.1 Gastri-intestinal

Aeromonas spp. are potential pathogens of gastroenteritis, and malignancy, liver cirrhosis, post liver transplantation in immunocompromised patients. Gastrointestinal pathogenic *Aeromonas* spp. escape gastric acidity, reach intestine, attach to epithelium, produce biofilm, colonise and elaborate virulence factors to cause gastroenteritis. *A. hydrophila* was more prevalent in samples of extra-intestinal infections and has the potential to cause serious disease. According to Gonçalves Pessoa et al. (2019), the frequency of species of *Aeromonas* associated with 96% of gastroenteritis cases was *A. hydrophila* (14.5%), *A. caviae* (37.6%), *A. veronii bv. Sobria* (27.2%) and *A. dhakensis* (16.5%). Zhou et al. (2019) reported prevalence of *A. caviae* (43.9%), *A. veronii* (35.7%), and *A. dhakensis* (12.2%) in the intestinal tract of adult patients of diarrhoea.

Gonçalves Pessoa et al. (2019) described an outbreak of acute gastroenteritis in a village of Bhutan caused by *A. hydrophila*. Thirty-three of 55 people who consumed contaminated mutton developed the disease. Three forms of gastroenteritis may be caused: (a) secretory watery diarrhoea—cholera like rice-water stool, vomiting more common; (b) dysenteric acute diarrhoea with blood and mucus (considered most severe); and (c) common chronic diarrhoea lasting >10 days. Most cases are self-limiting.

Aeromonas colitis may affect any segment but most common are ascending and transverse segments, causing ischaemic colitis or Crohn's disease. Ileal ulceration, intestinal haemorrhages and bowel obstruction may occur.

Treatment Rehydration and third generation cephalosporins, fluoroquinolones and aminoglycosides for gastroenteritis.

31.4.1.2 Extra-intestinal

Common isolates from extra-intestinal infections were *A. hydrophila* (29.4%), *A. caviae* (29.4%) and *A. dhakensis* (23.5%). *A. hydrophila* appear to be more frequently associated with extra-intestinal infection (29.4%) than with intestinal (1%) infections. *Aeromonas* were associated with malignancy and liver-transplant related cholecystitis. Most isolates (82.3%) were MDR compared to 30.6% isolates from intestine. The number and type of virulence genes varied and with no significant relation with invasion.

Skin and soft tissues infection Infecting *Aeromonas* settle down on wounds with the help of adhesins, produce proteases to damage hosts' tissues and enter; deeper *Aeromonas* infection causes mild pustules to serious morbid conditions such as cellulitis, necrotising fasciitis, myonecrosis, septic arthritis and septic shock. Infection during medicinal procedures, e.g. such as leech therapy, and surgeries, e.g. appendectomies, cause soft tissue infection. Post burn immersion in contaminated water led to infection with *A. hydrophila* and *A. caviae* (Bhowmick and Bhattacharjee 2018).

Blood infection LPS make most *Aeromonas* resistant to host's complement pathway. Most septicaemia causing species belong to serogroups O:11, O:16, O:18 and O:34 suggesting the virulence role of LPS. Septicaemia and sepsis are commonly caused by *A. hydrophila sensustricto*, *A. caviae* and *A. veronii* bv. Sobria and less commonly *A. jandaei*, *A. veronii* bv. *Veronii* and *A. schubertii* in immunocompromised, malignancy and comorbid cases. *A. hydrophila* caused meningitis in a premature born baby (Kali et al. 2016). Invasive procedures such as catheters, endoscopy and surgical interventions introduce *Aeromonas*.

Health of Other Terrestrial and Aquatic Animals

Aeromonas have been associated with pathological conditions in warm-blooded and aquatic animals, e.g. isolated from purulent exudate of bronchopneumonia in wild boar, from septicaemia in crocodile and red leg disease in frogs with internal haemorrhages and sometimes fatal (Gonçalves Pessoa et al. 2019). Every year, fishes die in mass due to *Aeromonas*-associated diseases resulting to huge economic loss. Pathologies include haemorrhagic septicaemia (lesions—scale shedding, haemorrhages in gills and anal areas, ulcers, abdominal swelling, exophthalmia), fin rot, tail rot, ulcers. *A. salmonicida sensustricto* caused furunculosis in salmonids characterised by haemorrhages. *A. hydrophila* and *A. veronii* caused septicaemia in a variety of fishes, viz. carp, tilapia, salmon, freshwater prawn, etc.

Treatment Antibiotics are useful; chloramphenicol, tetracycline, nitrofuran derivatives, etc. Terramycin in fish hatchery; fluoroquinolone administered as prophylactic during medicinal leech attachment.

31.5 Diagnosis

Isolate growing as yellow colonies on isolation agar, gram negative, motile, rod, positive for indole, catalase, oxidase, VP, citrate, TSI; utilising lactose, glucose, trehalose, starch; hydrolyse gelatine but MR and urease negative was most likely *A. aeromonas*. Sarkar et al. (2012) observed that direct sequencing of the 16S rRNA gene identified *A. hydrophila* as the most prevalent species in the waterways, food samples such as raw milk and meat in West Bengal, India.

31.6 Prevention and Control

Hygienic practices and correct food processing techniques are major contributors to avoid contamination by *Aeromonas* as well as other types of microorganisms.

Control of *Aeromonas* in water supply: An increasing number of *Aeromonas* in water is indicative of general deterioration of quality of water. Managing filter beds prevents regrowth. Temperature <14 °C, free chlorine residue >0.1 to 0.2 mg/L and reduced organic matter and are important for control. Use 1% sodium hypochlorite solution or 2% calcium hypochlorite solution.

References

Bhowmick UD, Bhattacharjee S (2018) Bacteriological, clinical and virulence aspects of Aeromonas-associated diseases in humans. Pol J Microbiol 67(2):137–149

Erdem B, Kariptas E, Cil E, Isik K (2011) Biochemical identification and numerical taxonomy of *Aeromonas* spp. isolated from food samples in Turkey. Turk J Biol 2011(35):463–472

Gonçalves Pessoa RB, de Oliveira WF, Marques DSC, Dos Santos Correia MT et al (2019) The genus *Aeromonas*: a general approach. Microb Pathog 130:81–94

Kali A, Kalaivani R, Charles PMV, Seetha KS (2016) *Aeromonas hydrophila* meningitis and fulminant sepsis in preterm newborn: a case report and review of literature. Indian J Med Microbiol 34:544–547

Sarkar A, Saha M, Roy P (2012) Identification and typing of *Aeromonas hydrophila* through 16S rDNA-PCR fingerprinting. J Aquacult Res Dev 3:146

Zhou Y, Yu L, Nan Z, Zhang P, Kan B, Yan D, Su J (2019) Taxonomy, virulence genes and antimicrobial resistance of *Aeromonas* isolated from extra-intestinal and intestinal infections. BMC Infect Dis 19:158

Staphylococcus aureus 32

Staphylococcus aureus is an important zoonotic pathogen. It can cause a wide range of illnesses, commonly mastitis (bovine, ovine, caprine), bacteraemia and foodborne intoxication in human. Bacterial toxins are considered as the third most common cause of foodborne outbreaks worldwide (Grispoldi et al. 2021). Staphylococcal enterotoxins accounted for about half of all the foodborne outbreaks linked to bacterial toxins in 2015 in the European Union (EFSA 2016). *S. aureus* food poisoning is one of the most common foodborne diseases worldwide, causing an estimated 241,000 illnesses per year in the United States; actual episodes/cases could be more as many sporadic ones are not reported (Kadariya et al. 2014).

32.1 *Staphylococcus aureus*

Staphylococci are ubiquitous, can be found in air, dust, sewage, water, environmental surfaces, humans and animals. According to Hennekinne et al. (2012), there are over 50 species and subspecies of Staphylococci with potential to produce coagulase. Coagulase negative staphylococci play a role in fermentation of milk and meat products. Association of *Staphylococcus* enterotoxin and Methicillin resistant *S. aureus* (MRSA) with coagulase- negative are emerging (Salamandane et al. 2022). Only coagulase positive strains have been evidenced in food poisoning. *S. aureus* is coagulase positive and a common coloniser of skin and nasal mucosa of human and animals. It was first identified as a cause of bacteraemia with high mortality. It was largely controlled with the advent of penicillin. Strains of *S. aureus* acquire multiple drug resistance to beta-lactam antibiotics through natural selection or by horizontal gene transfer. Strains resistant to methicillin, oxacillin and cephalosporins are designated methicillin resistant *S. aureus* (MRSA). Methicillin sensitive *S. aureus* (MSSA) are susceptible to these antibiotics. MRSA strains are important drug resistant pathogens, able to thrive in the presence of antibiotics and difficult to treat. The *mecA* gene in MRSA stops beta-lactam antibiotics from

K. G. Narayan et al., *Veterinary Public Health & Epidemiology*,
https://doi.org/10.1007/978-981-19-7800-5_32

inactivating bacterial transpeptidases and cell wall synthesis continues. This gene is used as biomarker. A number of different genetic lineages of MRSA with varying virulence may arise from MSSA strains.

MRSA strains were detected in the beginning as hospital-acquired infection and later as community-acquired and livestock-acquired in hospital, community and intensive farm settings, respectively.

32.2 Common Characters of *S. aureus*

S. aureus is a gram-positive, cocci appearing in grape like cluster. It is oxidase negative, catalase and coagulase positive. It is facultative anaerobic and able to grow in a wide range of temperature and survive in dry and stressful environment.

S. aureus is a common coloniser of mucosa of nostrils and are found on skin and hair of warm-blooded animals including food animals and human, epidemiologically important niche easily contaminating foods and entering the food processing chain.

Hennekinne et al. (2012) have summarised the conditions of growth and enterotoxin production (Table 32.1).

32.3 Virulence Factors

(a) capsules, slime and biofilm formation; (b) binding proteins for collagen, fibrinogen, elastin, penicillin, beta-lactamase, alpha protein, teichoic acid; (c) enzymes such as coagulase, staphylokinase, DNase, phosphatase, lipase, phospholipase, hyaluronidase and (d) exotoxins (SEs), toxic shock syndrome toxin 1, leucocidin, haemolysins and exfoliatin.

S. aureus is thus able to colonise mammalian skin, evade hosts' defence and causes disease in animals and human beings. The principal *S. aureus* exotoxins

Table 32.1 Conditions for growth and enterotoxin production

	Growth		Enterotoxin production	
Conditions	Optimum	Range	Optimum	Range
Temperature	37 °C	7–48 °C	37–45 °C	10–45 °C
pH	6–7	4–10	7–8	4–9.6
aW (water activity)	0.98	0.83–0.99 (aerobic); 0.90–0.99 (anaerobic)	0.98	0.85–0.99 (aerobic); 0.92–0.99 (anaerobic)
NaCl %	0	0–20	0	0–10
Redox potential (Eh)	> +200 mV	<−200 to > +200 mV	+200 mV	<−100 to > +200 mV
Atmosphere	Aerobic	Anaerobic-aerobic	Aerobic (5–10% dissolved O_2)	Anaerobic-aerobic

involved in food poisoning (in bold face), and the responsible '*gene*' listed by Abril et al. (2020) are as follows:

1. The toxic shock syndrome exotoxin 1—**(TSST-1)** is governed by the gene '*tst*'.
2. SE exotoxins and those commonly involved in food poisoning are **SEA, SEB, SEC1, SEC2, SEC3, to SEE, SEG to SER** and **SEU**. The responsible genes are '*sea to see, seg* to *ser,* and *seu*'.
3. SE-like toxins are **SEG, SEH, SEI, SER, SES, SEIY,** and **SET** and the respective genes are '*seg, seh, sei, ser, ses, seiy* and *set*'. These do not induce emesis or have not been tested for it.
   The above three exotoxins act as super antigen.
4. Leucocidins—**Panton-Valentine leucocidin (PVL), LukPQ, LukMF, LukAB,** and **LukED.** The genes are '*lukPV, lukPQ, lukM, lukA and lukB genes, and lukED*'.
5. Haemolysin—**α haemolysin (Hla)** and **β haemolysin (Hlb),** the genes are '*hla* and *hlb*'.
   Leucocidins and haemolysins are pore forming toxins.
6. Exfoliative Toxins—**(ETs) ETA** to **ETE** and the Genes Are '*eta* to *ete*'

These act as serine proteases that specifically cleave desmoglein 1 (Dsg1).

There is a wide variety of toxigenic *S. aureus* genomic types that cause clinical diseases. Strains from bovine mastitis frequently produce enterotoxins (SE) G to Q, involved in mammary gland inflammation. Environmental conditions influence the mechanisms that regulate the expression of SEs, hence the concentration of SEs is different when the bacterium is grown in laboratory.

The community associated MRSA isolates contained pathogenicity islands encompassing new exotoxin genes. The mobile genetic elements such as plasmids, staphylococcal cassette chromosome can also contain SEs gene clusters. Some exotoxin genes are placed in clusters within the pathogenicity islands as revealed by gene sequencing. Genetic diversity is high among the naturally occurring strains of *S. aureus.* Isolates from intra-mammary infection in bovine, caprine and ovine show close relationship but existence of specific clonal types for each animal group and probably with distinct virulence mechanisms. Small colony variants develop for better adaptation and survival in mammalian cells. Such phenotypic mutations are unstable, and reversion occurs.

32.4 Pathogenesis

Haemolysins—α, β and δ toxins attack cell membranes. Hla (α haemolysin) enables adhesion to epithelial cells and disrupts osmosis irreversibly causing cell death of a variety of cells including blood cells and endothelial cells. Beta haemolysin (Hlb) is sphingomyelinase, haemolyse sheep red blood cells. Hlb of *S. aureus* helps adhesion and bacterial multiplication. Hla increases the damaging effects by facilitating cell lysis. These exotoxins damage mammary epithelial cells causing mastitis.

Exfoliative toxins (ETs) damage keratinocytes in human and animal skin. The exfoliation of skin in different hosts is caused by A, B and D exfoliative toxins.

Leucocidins have seven different types. These kill bovine neutrophils, macrophages and monocytes and affect the immune system. *S. aureus* pore-forming toxins (PFTs), α-toxin and leukocidins are specific and have binding sites for mammalian species.

TSST-1 causes hypertension, rash, fever, constitutional symptoms, and multi-organ failure, finally resulting in death.

Staphylococcal super-antigens interact with the major components of histocompatibility complex class II (MHC-II) and T cells are activated to cause cytotoxin flush. These are pyrogenic toxins.

32.5 Food Poisoning

The causative linkage of staphylococci to food poisoning has interesting history described by Hennekinne et al. (2012). Vaughan and Sternberg linked micrococcus, or some other microorganisms present in the cheese to food poisoning in 1884. A decade after this in 1894, Denys considered meat from a cow that died of pyogenic staphylococci caused poisoning. Owen recovered staphylococci from dried beef that caused poisoning. Direct proof was brought out by Barber in 1914 by demonstrating staphylococci in unrefrigerated milk from a cow suffering with staphylococcal mastitis. In the spring of 1918, staphylococci contaminated sausage caused poisoning involving 2000 soldiers. Experimental proof of intoxication was brought by Dack et al. (1930). Haemolytic *Staphylococcus* was isolated from a sponge cake that caused intoxication in 11 individuals. Three human volunteers took culture filtrate orally and experimental rabbit was injected intravenously. They developed nausea, vomiting, chilliness and diarrhoea 3 h after, and the rabbit suffered with diarrhoea and died.

Hennekinne et al. (2012) described some subsequent outbreaks and listed selected ones that occurred between 1968 and 2009.

Staphylococcal food poisoning caused illness in one or two persons to a large number of victims especially among school children. The 1968 outbreak among school children in Texas that had 1300 cases was caused by contaminated chicken salad. In a school in Kentucky, contaminated 2% chocolate milk caused an outbreak with >1000 cases in 1985. Four thousand persons suffered in Brazil after eating contaminated chicken, roasted beef, rice and beans in 1998. In Osaka, Japan low-fat milk ingestion led to 13,420 cases.

Various types of freshly made ice cream were served in a party with 31 participants. Food poisoning led to 13 cases; 7 had to be hospitalised. Ice cream carried large number of coagulase positive *S. aureus* and SE. Investigation identified spa-type t127 sea + in ice cream and five victims. Either a contaminated ingredient or equipment was used (Fetsch et al. 2014).

According to Abril et al. (2020), there are 23 antigenically different SEs of which A–D are well characterised and account for 95% of SFP with SEA and SED being most common. SEA and SED are stable under a wide range of acidity and water activities. There are 220–240 amino acids with molecular weight ranging from 25 to 30 kDa. They are resistant to low pH, freezing and drying. The bacterium is killed by heat treatment, but the SEs and TSST-1 survive.

The isoforms of SEA are stable and survive proteolytic enzymes such as pepsin, trypsin, chymotrypsin, renin and papain. SEB is most likely to be inactivated by pepsin digestion at pH 2.0. TSST-1 is stable to heat, pepsin and trypsin digestion.

SE-like toxins identified are SEG, SEH, SEI, SER, SES, SEIY, and SET. These do not induce emesis.

S. aureus food poisoning (SFP) outbreaks occur by eating or drinking staphylococcal enterotoxins (SEs) along with the contaminated foodstuffs or drink. The infective dose of SE is small, 100 ng for children and few micrograms for adult.

32.6 Source of *S. aureus*

S. aureus adopts one of several paths to contaminate dairy food destined for human consumption. Humans and livestocks are the primary source. Cross-contamination is the most common way of introduction into foods. Other source could be dairy animals, soiled udder, milking equipment, workers and environment of dairy food industry. Kadariya et al. (2014) cited prevalence of methicillin susceptible and methicillin resistant *S. aureus* in bulk tank milk and herd prevalence in Minnesota as 84% and 4%, respectively. The estimated prevalence of *S. aureus* in bulk milk tank was 31% in Pennsylvania and 35% in cow milk samples in Louisiana. Enterotoxin genes and production of SEs from *S. aureus* of bovine origin have been documented. Bovine mastitis as the source of poisoning among consumers of unpasteurised milk was reported in Brazil. Milk from ovine and caprine mastitis was equally potential source of poisoning. Poor hygienic handling of cooked foodstuffs, abuse of storage temperature result into growth and exotoxin production. MRSA from an asymptomatic food handler caused gastroenteritis via contaminated coleslaw.

Food rich in starch and protein generally promote growth and production of *exotoxins* by *S. aureus*.

Foods such as milk and dairy products, eggs, poultry and cooked meat products (enterotoxins are heat stable) such as ham or corned beef; cream-filled baked goods, especially those not cooked after handling, e.g. puddings, pastries, sandwiches, sliced meat, meat salads are associated with *Staphylococcus* food poisoning. The amino acids and low molecular weight peptides support the growth of *S. aureus*. Spray drying of milk may not eliminate staphylococci present. Contaminated foods are not altered, has no bad smell or spoiled appearance. SEs are heat stable and can withstand heat at 121 °C for 10 min. Pasteurisation at 72 °C/15 s does not destroy SEs completely. Crude SEA in broth and in mushrooms remains active after treatment of heat 100 °C/2 h and 121 °C/28 min, respectively (Hennekinne et al. 2012).

Bacteria in general and *S. aureus* in particular quickly adapt to stress factors (new conditions) by regulating expression of genes associated with physiological features including production of enterotoxins. Foods present a highly complex matrix consisting of factors impacting growth, duration of lag phase, expression of genes controlling virulence factors and enterotoxin include temperature, pH, sugar or salt concentration, water activity (aW), presence of competitive microorganisms, etc. According to Grispoldi et al. (2021), ESB and SEC appear more sensitive to aW. The lower limit of 0.85 is shown in Table 32.1. SEA production is increased in a condition of mild stress posed by 2% NaCl as it leads to phage induction. Nitrites used as preservative and colour fixative in cured meat have little or no effect on growth and enterotoxin production in the concentration used. SEs are optimally produced under aerobic condition. However, the addition of 10% dissolved O_2 in vacuum-packed ham and sausages may increase the production of SEB ten times. Starter cultures, *Lactobacillus* spp., *Lactococcus* spp. and *Enterococcus faecalis* are potentially inhibitory to growth and enterotoxin production.

32.7 Symptoms

The onset is rapid. The incubation period is short. Victims report sudden start of vomiting, diarrhoea, nausea and abdominal cramps appearing as early as 30 min and commonly 2–6 h after consuming contaminated food or drink. Duration of illness is short, may be 1 day. The attack rate may be up to 85% and case fatality is low.

Enterotoxin molecules settle in the intestine to cause inflammation. Enteritis involves jejunum and ileum, mucosa of which is severely damaged. SEs and TSST-1 act as super-antigens (SAgs), trigger MHC class II response resulting in a massive cytokine secretion, inflammation and toxic shock syndrome (TSS). TSST-1 is a potent toxin reported in 0.006 cases per 100,000 people (Abril et al. 2020).

32.8 Diagnosis

Symptoms, rapid resolution, history of eating suspected foodstuffs are strong indications. Detection of Staphylococci ($\geq 10^5$/g) in suspected foodstuffs, stool and vomit is confirmatory. *S. aureus* may not be detected by culture in the events when food is contaminated, and toxin is formed prior to cooking.

Isolates may be evaluated for ability to produce toxins.

Enterotoxin may be assayed by using bioassays, molecular biology and/or immunological techniques.

32.9 Treatment

- Plenty of fluid supplement orally or if needed i/v and anti-emetic medicine.
- Use of antibiotic is not indicated as toxin is not affected by it.

32.10 Prevention

Proper hygiene and sanitation during food preparation, after preparation and before eating should be maintained. The bacterium is inactivated by heating: 57.2 °C/80 min, 60.0 °C/24 min, 62.8 °C/6.8 min, 65.6 °C/1.9 min and 71.7 °C/0.14 min (Hennekinne et al. 2012). Thorough cooking of food assures safety.

Foods stored between 4.4 °C (40 °F) to 60 °C (140 °F) permit rapid growth. Ready-to-eat foods or leftovers for eating later should never be left for >2 h or 1 h if the atmospheric temperature is >32.2 °C (90 °F). Conditions of storage: refrigerate in wide shallow container as soon as possible (https://www.cdc.gov/foodsafety/diseases/staphylococcal.html).

Sanitation steps:

- Clean, separate, cook and chill are steps for safety of foods.
- Hand wash with soap for 20 s—before eating, during and after preparing food; post-use of toilets, changing baby's diaper, touching pets and animals.
- Health of food handlers: not suffering with diarrhoea and vomiting; without cut or wounds on hands and wrists (use gloves while preparing foods).

General recommendation include: (a) hygiene and sanitation cover from 'farm to fork', (b) rapid detection of contamination with and *S. aureus* including MRSA and ETs for surveillance and outbreak investigation (Kadariya et al. 2014). Bacteriophage and biotyping were used for surveillance.

32.11 MRSA or Methicillin-Resistant *Staphylococcus aureus*

MRSA cause infections of skin, lungs and other tissues in community settings. Infections may turn severe, sepsis if neglected. In hospital settings, post-surgery surgical site infection, pneumonia and bacteraemia occur.

An estimated 2.0 billion are carriers of *S. aureus* and about 2.7% carry MRSA (https://en.wikipedia.org/wiki/Methicillin-resistant_Staphylococcus_aureus). A similar estimate from US CDC report 33% carriers of *S. aureus* in their nose and MRSA carriers 2%. Anybody can get infected. Injection of drugs (drug addicts; opioid epidemics) is 16 times risky. Carriers of MRSA (about 5% patients in the US hospitals), a member of a crowd and activities where skin to skin contact cannot be avoided, abraded skin, sharing common facilities or equipment such as medical devices are associated with risk of infection. MRSA infection spreads in community by contact with infected people and wounds, contaminated objects such as razors and towel.

32.11.1 Symptoms

MRSA infection of skin causes painful small red warm bumps that resemble pimples, spider bites, or boils filled with pus and fever. The bumps progress to large eventually open and look like deep boils filled with pus. Most of the community associated MRSA infections are localised affecting skin and soft tissues and treatable.

32.11.2 Diagnosis

MRSA is confirmed by laboratory diagnosis and reference laboratories. Specimens may be pus, sputum, blood and urine.

PCR offers quick diagnosis and is important for appropriate treatment.

32.11.3 Prevention

Pus contains MRSA. The wound has therefore to be kept covered with clean and dry bandage. Those in close contact should wash hands with soap and water and rub hands with alcohol-based sanitiser after contact with wound, bandage and clothing. Personal items of the patient should not be shared.

References

Abril AG, Villa TG, Barros-Velazquez J, Canas B et al (2020) Review *Staphylococcus aureus* exotoxins and their detection in the dairy industry and mastitis. Toxins 12:537

Dack GM, Cary WE, Woolpert O, Wiggers H (1930) An outbreak of food poisoning proved to be due to a yellow hemolytic *Staphylococcus*. J Prev Med 4:167–175

EFSA (2016) The European Union summary report on trends and sources of zoonoses, zoonotic agents and food-borne outbreaks in 2015. EFSA J 14(12):4634

Fetsch A, Contzen M, Hartelt K, Kleiser A, Maassen S et al (2014) *Staphylococcus aureus* food-poisoning outbreak associated with the consumption of ice-cream. Int J Food Microbiol 187:1–6

Grispoldi L, Karama M, Armani A, Hadjicharalambous C, Cenci-Goga BT (2021) *Staphylococcus aureus* enterotoxin in food of animal origin and staphylococcal food poisoning risk assessment from farm to table. Ital J Anim Sci 20(1):677–690

Hennekinne JA, De Buyser ML, Dragacci S (2012) *Staphylococcus aureus* and its food poisoning toxins: characterization and outbreak investigation. FEMS Microbiol Rev 36(4):815–836

Kadariya J, Smith Tara C, Thapaliyal D (2014) *Staphylococcus aureus* and staphylococcal food-borne disease: an ongoing challenge in public health. BioMed Res Int 2014:827965

Salamandane A, Oliveira J, Coelho M, Ramos B et al (2022) Enterotoxin- and antibiotic-resistance-encoding genes are present in both coagulase-positive and coagulase-negative foodborne *Staphylococcus* strains. Appl Microbiol 2(2):367–380

Streptococcus suis

33

Streptococcus suis is an emerging human pathogen originating naturally from pigs. Almost all pigs carry this bacterium asymptomatically. The disease is characterised by meningitis, sepsis, loss of hearing, endocarditis, arthritis and haemorrhagic skin lesions and is life threatening with mortality of 3–18%. It was first reported in 1954 in pigs and 1968 in human in Denmark. The prevalence is coincident with high density of pigs reported mostly in Southeast Asia. The pork industry is expanding geometrically so also the number of potentially exposed human to *S. suis* infection.

33.1 Aetiology

S. suis belongs to the family *Streptococcaceae*, genus *Streptococcus.* It is gram-positive, capsular, spherical peanut shaped bacterium seen as single, pair or short chain under a microscope. It is aerobic but growth is enhanced in micro aerophilic condition. It is alpha-haemolytic on bovine and sheep blood agar. *S. suis* produces biofilm that protects from unfavourable external conditions such as desiccation, oxidative stress and UV exposure allowing long persistence.

For serotyping, 1–35 antisera against capsular polysaccharide (CPS) antigens were used. The serotype SS2 is recognised as the most virulent. Multilocus sequence typing (MLST) genotypes *S. suis* into many different sequence types (STs). Serological and sequence typing together provide more precise evidence of zoonotic linkage between pig and human strains.

33.2 Epidemiology

The number of reported human cases increased dramatically post epidemics of 1998 and 2005 in China. More than 30 countries/regions reported sporadic to outbreaks occurrence. According to Goyette-Desjardins et al. (2014), 1642 human cases were

K. G. Narayan et al., *Veterinary Public Health & Epidemiology*,
https://doi.org/10.1007/978-981-19-7800-5_33

reported till 31 December 2013. Ninety per cent were from Asia. Vietnam, Thailand and China accounted for 83% of total worldwide cases. Europe accounted for 8.5% of cases, mostly (71.4% cases) from the Netherlands, the United Kingdom, France and Spain. These countries have developed pig industry. Endemicity in East and Southeast Asia may be due to high density of pigs, relatively large number of backyard farms and slaughtering practices without proper preventive measures; wet markets and consumption of ill pigs and/or of uncooked or undercooked pork products. Most of the published reports from the world over on the isolates of *S. suis* are from the US and Canada, of which 97% are from Canada. This does not reflect high number of cases. The rate of isolation of *S. suis* serotype 2 from pigs and cases of pig diseases were lower than in Europe and Asia. Possibly, the strains prevalent in the US and Canada were less virulent. Sporadic cases were also reported from elsewhere in the world.

33.2.1 Distribution of Serotypes

The distribution of serotypes of *S. suis* of 4500 serologically identified strains reported between 1 January 2002 to 31 December 2013 worldwide was reviewed by Goyette-Desjardins et al. (2014). Accordingly, serotypes 2 and 3 are prevalent throughout the world, and SS2 is the most common. Other serotypes in North America and Canada were 1/2, 8 and 7 in clinical cases in pigs. Brazil recorded SS2 from a mean of 57% cases in pigs, followed by serotypes 1/2, 14, 7 and 9 in decreasing order. In Europe, serotypes 9 followed by 2, 7, and 8. Serotype 3 prevailed in Spain and 9, 2, 7, 1 and 4 in the Netherlands. Asia reported vast majority of clinical cases in pigs, China and South Korea accounting for 14% and the prevailing serotypes in decreasing order were 2, 3, 4, 7 and 8.

33.2.1.1 Infection in Animals

It seems *Streptococcus suis* is widely distributed in nature and maintained by circulation in various species of mammals and birds. Nearly 80% of pigs are healthy carriers of *S. suis*. Nasal cavities, tonsils, and upper respiratory, genital, and alimentary tracts are colonised by multiple serotypes (serotypes 1–9 and 14). It mainly affects piglets up to 10 weeks of age, peaks during weaning about 6 weeks of age. Susceptibility generally wanes post-weaning. *S. suis* can invade multiple organs, cause severe inflammation and breach blood-brain barrier. The first sign of disease is pyrexia, death without any premonitory signs. Common manifestations are meningitis and septicaemia besides endocarditis, pneumonia and arthritis. Overall morbidity is around 5%, ranging from <1% to >50%. There is huge economic loss.

Transmission Pig-to-pig transmission is both vertical and horizontal. Piglets born of sows with vaginal or uterine infection may get infected before birth, at birth or soon after birth by ingesting secretion and excretion from uterus and vagina (Dutkiewicz et al. 2017). Horizontally, infection is transmitted through respiratory (oro-nasal) route, commonly through a 'nose-to-nose' contact between infected and uninfected pigs, especially when the animals show clinical signs of infection. SS2 is the most pathogenic for pigs and man and account for 97% of all human cases. Aerosol transmission from infected to a swine free from this pathogen may occur. Serotypes causing sporadic and epidemics 1, 2, 4, 5, 9, 14, 16, 21, 24 and 31 have been reported from many countries.

Predisposing factors include comorbidity (pseudorabies, influenza), stress, overcrowding, poor housing and ventilation, and immunosuppression.

Other animals infected are ruminants, cats, dogs, deer, horses and wild boars. Most human cases occurred among hunters and handlers of wild boar carcass in France, the UK, the Netherlands and Denmark and were due to serotype 2. Serotypes 4 and 14 from wild boar caused meningitis and septicaemia.

33.2.1.2 Infection in Human

S. suis infection in human affects multiple organs causing severe pathology such as endocarditis, cellulitis, arthritis, pneumonia, peritonitis, spondylodiscitis, uveitis and endophthalmitis. Serious manifestations are meningitis, septicaemia and streptococcal toxic shock-like syndrome.

Serotype 2 has the zoonotic potential. It accounted for 84.6% of isolates from nasal cavities of healthy persons occupationally exposed to pig and pig meat related activities for long period as compared to those not occupationally exposed. Butchers, abattoir workers and meat-processing employees carried it. Studies in the Netherlands revealed 6% veterinarians and 1% pig farmers were seropositive to serotype 2.

Transmission *S. suis* is transmitted directly through contact during handling infected carcass or meat. The bacterium enters through abrasion or cuts in hands and skin.

Risk factors *S. suis* infection may cause an insignificant transitory colonisation of respiratory mucosa or subclinical to serious disease. According to Ho et al. (2012), SS2 human meningitis in Vietnam was associated with three important factors: (a) eating 'high risk' dishes popular in Southeast Asia, (b) occupational exposure to pigs and pork related products and (c) preparation of pork in presence of skin lesions. Odd ratios were 11.9 and 3.0 for those slaughtering and cutting carcass/processing sick/dead pigs, respectively. Other risk activities were sharing accommodation with pigs and consuming pork; housewives exposed while handling contaminate pork in kitchen.

Over 98% households consume pork in Vietnam, mostly purchased fresh. Eleven percent of samples of internal organs were contaminated with serotype 2 in Vietnam. Wet market in Hong Kong had 6.1% pork positive.

In Vietnam, the local delicacies are pig blood, tonsils, uterus and intestine. *Tiet canh* is commonly consumed during family celebrations in Vietnam. It is made with chopped cooked pork mixed with blood in any form, fresh, uncooked and coagulated. Adults and not children commonly consumed *Tiet canh*—probable reason for more meningitis among adults. '*Tiet canh has health benefits'*—prevailing belief (Huong et al. 2014).

People ignore the 'ban on selling it'. Based on a case-control study in Vietnam, Ho et al. (2012) identified risk factors of *S. suis* meningitis were high risk dishes including undercooked pig blood and pig intestine, occupation related to pigs and exposure to pigs or pork in presence of skin injury.

Goyette-Desjardins et al. (2014) reviewed the risk factors associated with *S. suis* human disease. As compared to non-exposed, slaughterhouse workers were 1500 times at risk of getting *S. suis* infection in the Netherlands. The estimated annual risk of getting *S. suis* meningitis were 3.5 for slaughterhouse workers, 1.2 for butchers and 2.7 for pig breeders per 100,000. The annual incidence for the occupational groups was 350 times higher than the general population in Hong Kong. The amount of contact between people and pork carcasses in Asia may explain the differences observed in the Netherlands and Hong Kong (1500 vs. 350). Comorbidities such as splenectomy, diabetes mellitus, alcoholism, malignancy and structural heart diseases increased the chance of infection.

33.2.2 Sequence Types and Distribution

S. suis strains have been genotyped into many different sequence types (STs) by multilocus sequence typing (MLST). Sequence typing of serotype 2 *S. suis* (SS2) strengthens evidence of zoonotic association as isolates from pigs and human. The distribution of SS2 across the world is further refined with sequence types. It tends to explain virulence. SS2 ST data from a few countries for a little over a decade are available.

Kerdsin et al. (2020) evaluated whether these STs were potentially zoonotic. They characterised pulsotypes of isolates from healthy slaughterhouse pigs and compared that with Thai human isolates present in the database and in previous reports. There are 11 sequence types found in *S. suis* serotypes 2 and 14. Seven, ST1, ST25, ST28, ST103, ST104, ST105 and ST237 caused human infections in Thailand. *SS 2* and *14* with STs and pulsotypes identical to human isolates were common in healthy slaughterhouse pigs suggesting zoonotic transmission.

The serotype 2 of *S. suis* is predominant in Asia and represented 90% of cases of diseased pigs in the mainland China. The predominant STs were ST1, ST7 and ST28 and were mostly associated with cases of pneumonia. In Japan, ST1 and ST28 were isolated from endocarditis cases on pigs and accounted for 8% and 76% of isolates of SS2. In the US, 75% strains were ST28, followed by ST25 (10%) and ST1 (15%). The proportion of ST25 and ST28 were 54% and 46%, respectively.

ST1 has global distribution while ST7 is reported from mainland China and Hong Kong and caused the 1998 and 2005 epidemics. ST1 is associated with the disease in both pigs and humans in Europe, Asia (Cambodia, mainland China, Hong Kong, Japan, Thailand and Vietnam) and Argentina. The sequence types ST101–104 are endemic to Thailand only and cause meningitis and non-meningitis cases. Sequence typing tends to explain virulence. Strains isolated from clinical cases carried one or the other of the virulence factors.

33.3 Virulence Factors

So far, almost 60 bacterial components have been identified to be involved in the infection and/or pathogenicity of *S. suis* (Feng et al. 2014).

According to Guillaume Goyette-Desjardins et al. (2014), the most popular virulence markers used in association of serotypes are SLY (sly), MRP (mrp) and EF (epf) and are mainly associated with SS2 strains. ST1 strains from both pigs and human cases carried these virulence markers (SLY1 MRP1EF1).

Serotype 2 ST1 is associated with septicaemia and meningitis in both pigs and humans in different parts of the world. ST1 and ST7 predominated among the isolates from Chinese patients since the last outbreak in 2005. A study of complete genomes (Zhou et al. 2017) showed 'pathogenicity island 89 K PAI' (a novel DNA segment of 89 kb in length named as 89 K Pathogenicity Island) in strains linked to 'epidemics' and not in strains linked to 'sporadic' infections. The isolates from the two successfully treated cases of meningitis were identified as SS2 ST7 without pathogenicity island 89 K PAI, logically coincident with the absence of STSS in patients (Jiang et al. 2020). The 'pathogenicity island 73K PAI' carries elements linked to streptococcal toxic shock syndrome (STSS).

33.4 Pathogenesis

Dutkiewicz et al. (2018) described four stages of pathogenesis. First, the bacteria adhere and colonise the mucosal and/or epithelial cells surfaces of hosts, pigs and human. This is followed by the invasion of deeper tissues and entry to blood stream freely or mounted on monocytes. Fatal septicaemia may result. In the third stage, *S. suis* enters into organs, crosses blood-brain barrier or blood-cerebrospinal fluid barrier to invade the central nervous system causing meningitis. Inflammatory response is the fourth stage causing systemic and CNS infection. There is an excess production of pro-inflammatory cytokines causing septic shock and/or acute inflammation of CNS. A fulminant inflammation of brain may occur causing intracranial complications such as oedema, increased intracranial pressure, cerebrovascular insults, cochlear sepsis leading to deafness.

33.5 Disease

S. suis may temporarily colonise the mucosa of nasal cavity, tonsils, pharynx and oral cavity. The infection may result into subclinical infections, sero-conversion, followed by serious disease. The serotypes causing serious illness were SS2 and SS14, responsible for 74% and 2%, respectively. Serious illness manifests as meningitis, sepsis (bacteraemia, septicaemia) and streptococcal toxic shock syndrome. The serotype SS2 accounted for 68.1% of meningitis and 26.9% of septic shock, while serotype 14 accounted for 50% of meningitis and 21.4% of septic shock. The serotype SS2 was associated with a number of serious inflammatory conditions such as pneumonia, pulmonary oedema, myocarditis, endocarditis, septic arthritis, etc.

Mai et al. (2008) studied 450 adult patients of bacterial meningitis in Vietnam. *S. suis* was the most common (33.6%) pathogen. Most strains (91/92) were SS2. Exposure to pigs or pork was reported by one third of the patients. Mild to severe loss of hearing was most common (66.4%) and mortality (2.6%). Severe deafness was related to age, odd ratio of 3.65. Quantitative real-time polymerase chain reaction detected the bacterial DNA in 63% of CSF specimens collected 6–10 days after antimicrobial therapy.

Rajahram et al. (2017) reported two cases aged 41 and 44 years of age from Malaysia. One was a pig farmer and the other a butcher. Both patients presented a 2-day history of fever. One presented meningitis associated bacteraemia, hearing loss and vestibular symptoms; suffered with headache, vomiting, neck pain and behavioural changes. Examination revealed disorientation, confused state, Glasgow Coma Scale (GCS) 7/15. The other case had fever with chills, headache and vomiting.

Outbreaks have occurred in rainy season (June–September) in China and Thailand and warmer months (April–October) in Vietnam.

33.6 Symptoms

S. *suis* caused meningitis, septicaemia and arthritis. Incubation period ranged between 3 h and 4 days (average 2.2).

Meningitis is an inflammation of the lining that covers the brain and spinal cord (the meninges) presents with a brief influenza-like prodroma ending in loss of hearing.

Mai et al. (2008) studied meningitis cases among adults in Vietnam. The common symptoms were headache, stiff neck, vomiting, body ache, temperature (38 °C), skin haemorrhage, pneumonia, diarrhoea, focal neurological signs, monoplegia, hemiplegia and cranial nerve palsy and coma. The median duration of illness was 4 days (range of 1–21 days). The haemorrhage on skin may present as extensive petechiae, purpura, and ecchymoses may be haemorrhagic bullae.

A 67-year-old man was admitted to the Affiliated Hospital of Xuzhou Medical University. He had a 2-day history of headache and fever, and 1 day disturbance of consciousness, stiff neck, difficult speech and temperature of 38.7 °C. Blood and CSF proved positive for *S. suis*. The case was diagnosed as purulent meningitis and sepsis. The second reported cases also showed impaired consciousness and nucha rigidity. CT scan showed cerebral inflammation (Jiang et al. 2020).

Feng et al. (2014) summarised the septicaemia and toxic shock syndrome caused by SS2.

Septicaemia is life threatening. It is in fact bacteraemia with sepsis causing multiorgan failure. Generally, SS2 infection occurring as local infection due to cut injury in skin leads to septicaemia. The patient reports fever with chills, increased rates of heart/respiration, falling blood pressure, looks pale and may fall unconscious. Leaking blood vessels under skin cause petechiae and rashes. Meningitis and septicaemia may occur in the same patient.

Streptococcal toxic shock syndrome (TSS), arthritis and subacute endocarditis are other forms of disease.

Tang et al. (2006) described the outbreak (June to August 2005) that occurred in China. There were 204 cases and 38 deaths. Cases included farmers, butchers and a veterinarian. They got infected through the cuts and skin injuries on hands and legs, manifesting as acute illness, diarrhoea, distal part of the extremities had erythematous blanching rash including blood spots and petechia. Severe cases had coma. There was autolysis of liver and spleen. Histopathology revealed degeneration of hepatic cells surrounding the central vein. One death was due to meningitis and had fever, chills, headache, vomiting and meningism.

TSS refers to highly invasive infection of deep tissues and bacterial super antigens, staphylococcal and streptococcal exotoxins are involved. There is sudden onset of high fever, hypotension, diarrhoea, petechiae, disseminated intravascular coagulation and acute renal failure. In an outbreak of SS2 infection in Sichuan, China, Yang et al. (2006) recorded 38% TSS cases with 58% fatality and septicaemia or meningitis cases.

33.7 Diagnosis

It is based on clinical observation followed by mandatory laboratory confirmation. Specimens used are body fluids, CSF. Laboratory tests are as follows:

- Selective media-based microbiological cultivation and identification tests: isolation of alpha haemolytic streptococci, optochin-resistance, Voges-Proskauer, salicin, trehalose, and 6.5% sodium chloride followed by agglutination test with a panel of 35 antisera.
- Serological tests such as agglutination test, ELISA (whole-cell antigen-based indirect ELISA and purified capsular polysaccharide antigen-based indirect ELISA), fluorescent antibody tests.
- Molecular techniques—PCR-based detection techniques targeting 16S rRNA gene or serotype specific *cps* genes increased the sensitivity and specificity of *S. suis* detection in clinical specimens.

Treatment: Penicillin, Amoxicillin.

33.8 Prevention

- Good farm management, biosecurity.
- Increased awareness.
- *S. suis* caused disease should be considered 'industrial disease'. Appropriate legislation and regulations are expected to reduce human infection and suffering.
- Enhanced detection of *S. suis* through improved diagnostic service, training at the National institute of Hygiene and Epidemiology, updating surveillance and control of epidemic to include *S. suis* were adopted by Ministry of Health, Government of Vietnam in 2007 (Horby et al. 2010). The authors observed 'Research collaborations can efficiently inform and influence national responses if they are well positioned to reach policy maker'.

References

Dutkiewicz J, Sroka J, Zając V et al (2017) Streptococcus suis: a re-emerging pathogen associated with occupational exposure to pigs or pork products. Part I – Epidemiology. Ann Agric Environ Med 24(4):683–695. https://doi.org/10.26444/aaem/79813

Dutkiewicz J, Zając V, Sroka J, Wasiński B, Cisak E et al (2018) *Streptococcus suis*: a re-emerging pathogen associated with occupational exposure to pigs or pork products. Part II—pathogenesis. Ann Agric Environ Med 25(1):186–203

Feng Y, Zhang H, Wu Z, Wang S, Cao M, Hu D, Wang C (2014) *Streptococcus suis* infection: an emerging/re-emerging challenge of bacterial infectious diseases? Virulence 5(4):477–497

Goyette-Desjardins G, Auger JP, Xu J, Segura M, Gottschalk M (2014) *Streptococcus suis*, an important pig pathogen and emerging zoonotic agent-an update on the worldwide distribution based on serotyping and sequence typing. Emerg Microbes Infect 3(6):e45

Ho DTN, Le TPT, Wolbers M, Cao QT, Nguyen VMH et al (2012) Correction: risk factors of *Streptococcus suis* infection in Vietnam. A case-control study. PLoS One 7(5). https://doi.org/10.1371/annotation/25743e50-5a58-4fb6-b466-9a345311d4a8

Horby P, Wertheim H, Ha NH, Trung NV, Trinh DT et al (2010) Stimulating the development of national *Streptococcus suis* guidelines in Viet Nam through a strategic research partnership. Bull World Health Organ 88(6):458–461

Huong VT, Hoa NT, Horby P, Bryant JE et al (2014) Raw pig blood consumption and potential risk for *Streptococcus suis* infection, Vietnam. Emerg Infect Dis 20(11):1895–1898

Jiang F, Guo J, Cheng C, Gu B (2020) Human infection caused by *Streptococcus suis* serotype 2 in China: report of two cases and epidemic distribution based on sequence type. BMC Infect Dis 20:223

Kerdsin A, Takeuchi D, Nuangmek A, Akeda Y, Gottschalk M, Oishi K (2020) Genotypic comparison between *Streptococcus suis* isolated from pigs and humans in Thailand. Pathogens 9(1):50

Mai NT, Hoa NT, Nga TV, Linh LD, Chau TT et al (2008) *Streptococcus suis* meningitis in adults in Vietnam. Clin Infect Dis 46(5):659–667

Rajahram GS, Hameed AA, Menon J, William T, Tambyah PA, Yeo TW (2017) Case report: two human *Streptococcus suis* infections in Borneo, Sabah, Malaysia. BMC Infect Dis 17(1):188

Tang J, Wang C, Feng Y, Yang W, Song H et al (2006) Streptococcal toxic shock syndrome caused by *Streptococcus suis* serotype 2. PLoS Med 3(5):e151

Yang WZ, Yu HJ, Jing HQ, Xu JG, Chen ZH et al (2006) An outbreak of human *Streptococcus suis* serotype 2 infections presenting with toxic shock syndrome in Sichuan, China. Zhonghua Liu Xing Bing Xue Za Zhi 27(3):185–191

Zhou Y, Dong XX, Li ZW, Zou G, Lin L, Wang XH et al (2017) Predominance of *Streptococcus suis* ST1and ST7 in human cases in China, and detection of a novel sequence type, ST658. Virulence 8(6):1031–1035

Clostridium perfringens

34

Clostridium perfringens are a gram-positive spore forming rod shaped anaerobic bacteria. These are found commonly in intestines of man and animals and are ubiquitously distributed in soil and sewage. They are associated with intestinal and histotoxic infections in man and animals.

The generation time <10 min increases *C. perfringens* burden in foods, intestine and wounds in a short time. They produce some 20 exotoxins, i.e. virulence factors targeting a number of tissues causing a variety of pathologies upon invading a host. Gahari et al. (2021) have listed these, respective functions, targets, genes, etc.

Classification of *C. perfringens* is based on the production of four typing toxins (alpha, beta, epsilon and iota) and Types A–E are classified based on the production of these. Gas gangrene in human is caused by type A. Type C causes enteritis necroticans in human. Type F produces *C. perfringens* enterotoxin (CPE) and not beta, epsilon and iota toxins; causes food poisoning and antibiotic associated diarrhoea (AAD). Type G produces NetB toxin and causes necrotising enteritis in chicken (Table 34.1).

C. perfringens is the second most common cause of food poisoning in the US (CDC 2019).

The available epidemiological data reveal that *C. perfringens* ranks after *Salmonella* spp., *Campylobacter* spp. and *Staphylococcus aureus* as bacterial agent of foodborne illness in developing countries.

C. perfringens type A accounts for >95% of global isolates and diseases associated with CPE usually represent it. *Acute food poisoning* occurs when the heat resistant spores of contaminating *C. perfringens* survive cooking process, dormant spores are stimulated by heat to germinate and propagate in food. Large number of bacterial cells survive stomach acid and begin sporulating in the intestine during which CPE is produced. A contaminated food held or served at 10–54 °C allows growth of *C. perfringens*. Large number of vegetative cells is ingested. These sporulate and release CPE into the intestinal lumen. CPE is 35 kDa polypeptide and (intestinal) enzyme resistant (Ghoneim and Hamza 2017).

K. G. Narayan et al., *Veterinary Public Health & Epidemiology*,
https://doi.org/10.1007/978-981-19-7800-5_34

Table 34.1 Toxinotypes of *C. perfringens* and diseases

Type	Alpha	Beta	Epsilon	Iota	CPE	NetB	Disease
A	+	–	–	–	–/+	–	Human—gas gangrene
							In several animals; haemorrhagic gastroenteritis in dogs and horses; possibly, enterotoxaemia and GI disease of ruminants, horses, pigs
B	+	+	+	–	–	–	Lamb dysentery
C	+	+	–	–	+	–	Human—enteritis necroticans (pig-bel, Darmbrand)
							Haemorrhagic and necrotising enteritis of several neonatal animals; struck
D	+		+	–	–	–	Enterotoxaemia in sheep, goat, cattle; enterocolitis in goats
E	+	–	–	+	–	–	Possibly gastroenteritis in cattle, rabbit
F	+	–	–	–	+	–	Human food poisoning, AAD and sporadic diarrhoea
G	+	–	–	–	–	+	Necrotic enteritis in poultry

The *cpe* is located on chromosome of some strains and on plasmid on others; usually the strains that cause acute food poisoning carry *cpe* on chromosome and those causing non-foodborne diarrhoea carry *cpe* on plasmid.

Ghoneim and Hamza (2017) studied prevalence of *C. perfringens* in retail foods, faecal carriage among food handlers and also examined diarrhoeic stool in part of Egypt. All isolates were PCR characterised as *C. perfringens* type A. At the level of slaughterhouse, percent of meat from cattle and buffalo positive were 52.9% and 43.5%, respectively. *C. perfringens* was added from the environment of butchers to raise these to 69.2% and 88.2% respectively. The isolation rate from meat products was 30% in beef burgers, 10% in sausage, 40% in beef luncheon meat, 10% in frozen kofta, 5% in canned beef and 20% in tuna; 55% of food handlers were carriers; faecal sample was positive. Three of 90 diarrhoeic faeces had CPE, detected by ELISA.

The gene *cpe*—isolates represented one each from meat of cattle and buffalo from meat shop, food handlers' stool and two from tuna. *C. perfringens* count in tuna was low.

The criteria for assigning *C. perfringens* to a foodborne disease are (a) clinical presentation, (b) a load of viable cells 10^5/g of suspected food and (c) faecal count of spores 10^6/g. Detection of *cpe* gene is NOT included in the criteria.

C. perfringens type F causes food poisoning. *C. perfringens* CPE producing strains carry the gene *cpe* and such strains are <5% globally. The gene *cpe* may be located on chromosome or large plasmids. It is located on chromosome of most *~70% type F food poisoning strains* which are widely distributed in retail raw meats and fish and form heat resistant spores. The resistance phenotype of *chromosomal-cpe* isolates includes resistance of both vegetative cells and spores which manifest enhanced resistance to heat, osmotic stress from sodium chloride and nitrites employing multiple mechanisms.

C. perfringens is associated with 5–15% of non-foodborne gastrointestinal conditions in human, sporadic diarrhoea and antibiotic associated diarrhoea (AAD). Almost all strains carry plasmid *cpe* gene. The AAD occurs when *C. perfringens* type F from nosocomial environment colonises the gastrointestinal tract. The duration of disease is long (several weeks) and severe in elderly.

34.1 Common Vehicles/Sources

Beef, poultry, turkey and other meat products contaminated commonly with faecal matter. There is a possibility of endogenous contamination with *C. perfringens*, spread from natural intestinal habitat of stressful meat food animal before slaughter. Other sources of contamination may be water, animals and human under low level of sanitation.

C. perfringens type F is resistant to cooking, refrigerator/freezer temperature and food preservatives (nitrite, osmotic stress and pH extremes). Storage at 4 or −20 °C for 3–6 months leads to average log reduction of spores by 0.3–0.6 (Gahari et al. 2021). *C. perfringens* type C, the Darmbrand strains also form heat resistant spores and is associated with foodborne diseases in human. The spores of type F chromosomal *cpe* strains and type C Darmbrand strain are reduced by one log in ≥30 to 120 min of heating at 100 °C (D_{100} value). It produces four Small Soluble Proteins that provide special protection to spore DNA against heat, chemical and UV radiation. Spore size, coat thickness, mineral concentration, dipicolinic acid, metal ions and protoplast-sporoplast ratio also contribute to spore heat resistance (Orsburn et al. 2008).

C. perfringens enterotoxin (CPE) is produced during sporulation. CPE constitutes >15% of proteins inside sporulating cells. Sigma K, Sigma E and Sigma F are sporulation-associated sigma factors in many *Bacillus* spp. and *Clostridium* spp. seem to play an important role in regulating production of sporulation and CPE.

The gene *cpe* is often present on conjugative plasmids facilitating transfer of this gene to another strain of *C. perfringens* and if this transfer happens during infection, it will potentiate pathogenesis. The *cpe* gene may be mobilised by the associated insertion sequence.

It happens in food establishment. Large chunk of meat is cooked and improperly held. Highly resistant spores survive in improperly held or cooked meat. The vegetative form multiplies actively during gradual cooling and produce exotoxin. Doubling time is short. The burden of *C. perfringens* type A reach 10^6 to 10^7per gram. Consumers ingest large number of bacteria, infected and suffer. Large meats (roasts or turkeys) are commonly incriminated. Therefore, number exposed/eating contaminated meat is large. Generally, institutions need to cook large meats to prepare for large number of people. *C. perfringens* food poisoning outbreak involves large number of people. Sporadic infections go undiagnosed.

The culinary process, especially heating large pieces of beef/pork for preparation of stock should be followed by immediate sharp cooling.

34.2 Pathogenesis

CPE is 319 amino acids polypeptide. CPE belongs to the family of aerolysin pore-forming toxin. The C terminal mediates binding to receptor molecule, claudin. The N-terminal is used for oligomerisation of the bound toxin into a pre-pore forming a β-barrel that inserts into the host cell membrane to create an active pore. There is efflux of ions such as potassium, influx of extracellular ions including calcium. It triggers a toxin dose-dependent cell death. Low CPE dose (~1 μg/mL) causes modest pore formation, a limited calcium influx and a mild activation of calpain that triggers caspase-3 dependent apoptosis. High CPE doses (~10 μg/mL) form large numbers of pores, allowing a massive calcium influx, strong calpain activation to cause a necrotic death. Dead cells release a cytotoxic factor that kills CPE-insensitive cells contribute to the disease.

Human infection occurs by ingestion of food prepared from contaminated meat or fish.

CPE is produced only by sporulating *C. perfringens*, released along with endospores in the intestines, which causes shortening of villus, desquamation of intestinal epithelium, mainly small intestine and ileum in particular. Colon is also focally affected.

Incubation period is usually 8–16 h. Diarrhoea and abdominal cramps commonly reported. Duration of illness is generally 12–24 h. Old and debilitated patients may die. Around 26 deaths are reported in the US annually as reported by Shrestha et al. (2018) who cited two outbreaks of unusual severe food poisoning resulting into deaths of healthy and young ones. The victims were special, recipient of psychoactive medications in psychiatric institutions. The medication caused severe constipation leading to increasing the CPE-intestine contact time, increased uptake, enterotoxaemia. CPE reached and damaged internal organs such as liver and kidney resulting in hyper-potassaemia causing cardiac arrest.

34.3 *C. perfringens* Type C

Isolates of *C. perfringens* producing alpha and beta toxins, causing necrotic enteritis in Germany produced heat resistant spores, were designated type F, later realised it was a variant of type C.

C. perfringens type C producing beta-toxin caused enteritis necroticans (EN), syn. Darmbrand among malnourished in post-World War II Germany. The disease is necrohaemorrhgaic and enterotoxemic. The gene, *cpb* is located on plasmid. Some strains produce low amounts of both CPB and CPE, and the two toxins can act synergistically. CPB is synthesised in intestine.

Predisposing factor or comorbidity is associated with enteritis necroticans.

Known as Pig-bel in Papua New Guinea, it caused deaths among children during 1960s and 1970s. They barbecued pig in pit dug in ground. *C. perfringens* type C in soil or pigs contaminated the food. Beta toxin was produced in intestine of those who consumed contaminated barbecued pig. The people were poor and malnourished (protein in particular) and had low level of intestinal trypsin. They ate sweet potato which contains trypsin inhibitor. CPB is rapidly inactivated by trypsin, but they were naturally susceptible.

Outbreaks of enteritis necroticans occur sporadically in malnourished population of developing countries and occasionally among individuals with pancreatic pathology such as diabetes (Shrestha et al. 2018).

Enteritis necroticans is a serious disease. The affected portion of intestine requires surgical removal.

34.3.1 *Cpe* Negative *C. perfringens* Type A

Epidemiological characters of outbreaks and clinical symptoms of food poisoning resembling those caused by *C. perfringens* occurred in 1997 in Tokyo, Osaka and Tochigi. The isolates were non-CPE producers and did not harbour the gene *cpe*.

Irikura et al. (2015) studied the strain W5052 from the Tokyo outbreak. The culture supernatant evoked the death of the L929 and Vero cells, swelling and fluid accumulation of the ileal loops of rabbits, suggesting the presence of enterotoxin. L929 cells do not have receptor for CPE. Antiserum CPE did not neutralise the enterotoxic activity suggesting new toxin. This new toxin was iota-like enterotoxin, CPILE (*C. perfringens* iota like enterotoxin) having two components CPILEa and CPILEb.

Yonogi et al. (2014) studied the toxin and the responsible genes. It is a novel toxin, Binary Enterotoxin of *C. perfringens* (BEC), BECa and BECb similar to other members of Binary toxin family, such as *C. perfringens* iota toxin and caused acute gastroenteritis. The BEC produced fluid accumulation in rabbit ileal loop and suckling mouse assay. Binary toxin family toxins are composed of two components, one enzyme and the other binding, e.g., *C. perfringens* iota, *C. spiroforme* iota-like, *C. difficle* Cdt and *C. botulinum* C2. The binding components bind to the receptor cell and the enzymic component is translocated into the cytosol. The BECa has the ADP-ribosylating activity, possibly destroys filamentous actin.

The *becAB* genes were located on 54.5-kb pCP13-like plasmids.

Distribution of *becAB* gene was studied in 26 CPE positive and negative *C. perfringens* isolates from diarrhoeal and healthy human faeces, only one isolate from heathy faeces was found positive, apparently rare distribution. BEC-positive *C. perfringens* was isolated from roasted beef served at the dinner in the Tochigi outbreak and was suspected in the Osaka outbreak in the epidemiological investigation.

34.4 Diagnosis

Epidemiological investigation of *C. perfringens*, particularly involved in food poisoning led to development of serotyping using 91 sera. This failed to type many isolates. Toxinotyping and currently genotyping are preferred.

Genes encoding beta, epsilon and iota toxins are encoded on plasmids. Toxinotyping is fundamentally genotyping. PCR is done. Determination of *cpe* gene and production of CPE protein in isolates from affected patients and suspected food establishes food poisoning and its cause. CPE kills Vero cells.

PCR and the reversed-passive latex agglutination test are available for the detection of the *cpe* gene and CPE protein.

Treatment—Symptomatic, mepacrine may be effective.

Prevention—thorough cooking, hold food at either <4 or >65 °C.

34.5 Histotoxic Infections

Gas gangrene or myonecrosis is necrotising skeletal muscle and subcutaneous tissue infection caused by *C. perfringens* type A. Wound infection with vegetative cells or spore occurs. Multiplication and toxin production induce severe and extensive necrosis rapidly. Local oedema is seen. If disease progresses, bacteraemia, sepsis, shock and death may occur. Clinically, patient reports pain, local oedema and fever.

This was most common cause of amputation and often deaths among soldiers during World War II. Incidence is low presently. Lethality continues to be high 5–30% in treated cases and 100% if untreated. Treatment include surgery, antibiotic and hyperbaric oxygen.

References

Centres for Disease Control and Prevention (CDC) (2019) Surveillance for foodborne disease outbreaks United States, 2017: annual report. U.S. Department of Health and Human Services, Atlanta

Gahari IM, Navarro MA, Li J, Shrestha A, Uzal F, McClane BA (2021) Pathogenicity and virulence of *Clostridium perfringens*. Virulence 12(1):723–753

Ghoneim NH, Hamza DA (2017) Epidemiological studies on *Clostridium perfringens* food poisoning in retail foods. Rev Sci Tech 36:1025–1032

Irikura D, Monma C, Suzuki Y, Nakama A et al (2015) Identification and characterization of a new enterotoxin produced by *Clostridium perfringens* isolated from food poisoning outbreaks. PLoS One 10:e0138183

Orsburn B, Melville SB, Popham DL (2008) Factors contributing to heat resistance of *Clostridium perfringens* endospores. Appl Environ Microbiol 74(11):3328–3335

Shrestha A, Uzal FA, McClane BA (2018) Enterotoxic Clostridia: *Clostridium perfringens* enteric diseases. Microbiol Spectr 6(5). https://doi.org/10.1128/microbiolspec.GPP3-0003-2017

Yonogi S, Matsuda S, Kawai T, Yoda T, Harada T et al (2014) BEC, a novel enterotoxin of *Clostridium perfringens* found in human clinical isolates from acute gastroenteritis outbreaks. Infect Immun 82:2390–2409

35 Botulism

Botulism is a serious foodborne life-threatening intoxication caused by ingestion of foods containing botulinum exotoxin which is a neurotoxin. It is a public health problem. Outbreaks of botulism are serious. Respiratory distress and paralysis in botulism do not allow time. Treatment has to be initiated before laboratory diagnosis to save life.

35.1 Aetiology

Botulism is a neurological disease of man and animals. It is characterised by flaccid paralysis, especially of respiratory muscles causing respiratory distress and even death. There is inhibition of secretions from glands such as salivary, lachrymal, and sweat controlled by cholinergic nerves. The toxin blocks the release of neurotransmitter, acetylcholine at the neuromuscular junction and other cholinergic neurones. The disease is caused by botulinum neurotoxins (BoNTs) which cause proteolytic cleavage of SNARE (soluble N-ethylmaleimide-sensitive-factor attachment protein receptor) proteins involved in the exocytosis of neurotransmitters.

35.2 Botulinum Neurotoxins (BoNTs)

There are nine toxin serotypes (A, B, C, D, E, F, G, H, or H/A, or F/A, X). Types A, B, E, F and H cause human disease. Type C causes limber neck in poultry and type D botulism in other mammals. Barash and Arnon (2014) described *C. botulinum* type H, the new toxin in the last 40 years from an 'infant botulism'. This was supported with gene analysis (Dover et al. 2014). Type H produces most lethal toxin, 2 ng by injection and 13 ng by inhalation is lethal. Type G does not cause any disease. Some strains produce small amount of other than the main toxins and are designated as Ab, Af, and Bf (capital letters for main toxin). The neurotoxin

K. G. Narayan et al., *Veterinary Public Health & Epidemiology*,
https://doi.org/10.1007/978-981-19-7800-5_35

degrades rapidly at 100 °C. It is resistant to digestive enzymes and hence causes botulism after ingestion.

Sequencing of BoNT gene and study of BoNT amino acid sequences revealed 41 BoNT subtypes and multiple variants of a toxin serotype. A strain may possess one, two or three neurotoxin genes. The one having three forms up to three toxins, e.g. A, B, and/or F. A variation of >2.6% amino acids led to a subtype. A strain may be referred to by their type and/or subtype of neurotoxin gene, e.g. strain type A B5F2 is a *C. botulinum* type A having genes encoding for botulinum neurotoxin subtype B5 and F2.

Botulinum neurotoxins are zinc metalloproteases acting on SNARE (soluble N-ethylmaleimide-sensitive factor attachment protein receptors) proteins. Cleavage of SNARE proteins prevents the release of acetylcholine at the neuromuscular junction, resulting in flaccid paralysis. All BoNTs have the same structure, functions and cause same toxic effects. Most have similar mechanism of action. BoNTs consist of light and heavy chains connected by a disulfide bond. Of the two domains of the heavy chain, the C-terminal mediates binding to receptor and the N terminal translocation of the light chain across endosomal membrane. LC acts as protease in neurones to cleave a set of proteins. The interaction with distinct receptors and cleavage sites differs (Rasetti-Escargueil et al. 2020).

35.2.1 C. botulinum

BoNTs (A-H) are produced commonly by a heat resistant spore forming bacillus, *Clostridium botulinum.* Tryptose sulphite cycloserine agar is used to isolate. It can be grown between pH 4.8 to 7.0; is a lipase positive (iridescent colonies on egg yolk agar) and fails to use lactose as primary C-source.

Some strains of *C. butyricum* and *C. baratii* have been implicated as agents of infant botulism (Suen et al. 1988a, b). These produce types E and F toxin. *C. botulinum* is able to transfer neurotoxin gene to any other clostridia naturally. *C. botulinum* is known to have four distinct groups, I-IV, based on ability to digest complex proteins and also molecular properties. Group I include proteolytic *C. botulinum* types A, B and F. Nontoxigenic strains are referred to as *C. Sporogenes* (Anonym 1999). Group II includes saccharolytic *C. botulinum* E, F and certain strains of type B. Group III has weak proteolytic *C. botulinum* C, D. *C. botulinum* type G belongs to group IV, is neither proteolytic nor saccharolytic and renamed as new species—*C. argentinense* (Suen et al. 1988).

Summary of characters of *C. botulinum* Group I and II is presented in Table 35.1.

Genetic diversity and spread of Group I (proteolytic *C. botulinum* types A, B and F and non-toxigenic strains are referred to as *C. sporogenes)* were studied by Brunt et al. (2020). These bacteria make two major lineages based on core genome single-nucleotide polymorphism: (a) *C. botulinum* Group I and (b) C. *sporogenes.*

Most strains of Group I possessed neurotoxin genes of types A, B, and F.

Some strains of *C. sporogenes* possessed type B neurotoxin gene caused five foodborne outbreaks in France, the UK, and Australia wherein ham, meat, and fish

Table 35.1 Characters of *Clostridium botulinum* Groups I and II (Carter and Peck 2015)

Characters	*C. botulinum* Group I (proteolytic *C. botulinum*)	*C. botulinum* Group II (non-proteolytic *C. botulinum*)
Neurotoxins formed	A, B, F, H[a]	B, E, F
Ferment glucose	+	+
Ferment maltose	V	+
Ferment fructose	V	+
Ferment sucrose	–	+
Ferment mannose	–	+
Proteolysis[b]	+	–
Liquefaction of gelatin[b]	+	+
Lipase production	+	+
Lecithinase	–	–
Degradation of chitin	+	+
Minimum growth temperature	12 °C	3 °C
Optimum growth temperature	37 °C	30 °C
Minimum pH for growth	4.6	5.0
NaCl concentration preventing growth	10%	5%
Minimum water activity for growth with NaCl	0.94	0.97
Minimum water activity for growth with glycerol	0.93	0.94
Spore heat resistance[c]	$D_{121^\circ C} = 0.21$ min	$D_{82.2^\circ C} = 2.4/231$ min[d]
Non-neurotoxigenic equivalent clostridia	*C. sporogenes*[e]	No species name given

V Some trains positive, others negative

[a]More than one type of toxin may be formed; type H neurotoxin, yet to be verified

[b]Proteolytic—degrades native proteins, e.g. coagulated egg white, cooked meat particles, casein. Derive protein and gelatine degraded by both *C. botulinum* Groups I and II

[c]Decimal reduction time (D-value; time to a ten-fold reduction in viable spores) at specified temperature determined in phosphate buffer pH 7.0

[d]D-value without/with lysozyme during recovery

[e]*C. sporogenes*, strain PA 3679 is a non-toxigenic putrefactive strain spores of which have higher thermal resistance than spores of *C. botulinum* Group I is widely used for validation of thermal processing in food industry (121 °C/3 min)

were incriminated foods and B2, B1, and B6 were the neurotoxins, respectively. Two outbreaks of infant botulism caused by B6 and B1 toxins were reported from Australia and the USA, respectively. One outbreak of wound botulism caused by B2 was reported in Italy.

A new cluster of five strains of *C. sporogenes* possessed *C. botulinum* type B1 neurotoxin gene. The toxin genes were primarily carried on plasmid and the strains were likely to lose.

35.2.1.1 Botulinum Toxin Producing Clostridia

Clostridium including *Clostridium botulinum* (groups I to III), *C. argentinense, C. baratii* type F neurotoxin– Le^+/Li. *C. butyricum* type E has been associated with foodborne botulism in China, Italy, Japan, and India. The toxigenic isolates are anaerobic, subterminal spore forming, lipase, lecithinase and gelatine, nitrate-reduction negative, produce type E toxin. Nontoxigenic Li^-/Le^-isolates are aerobic, nitrate reducer and form terminal spore (Dykes et al. 2015).

35.2.1.2 Non-Clostridia (Rasetti-Escargueil et al. 2020)

BoNT related sequences have been detected in non-clostridial strains. These are:

bont/Wo or bont/I from *Weissella oryzae*, a bacterium of fermented rice, bont/J (ebont/F or bont/En) from *Enterococcus faecalis* strain from cow faeces, and Cp1 from *Chryseobacterium piperi* from sediment. A BoNT-like neurotoxin (PMP1) specific of invertebrate (Anopheles mosquito) has been characterised from a *Paraclostridium bifermentans* strain.

No active human or animal botulism has been reported in the non-clostridial strains.

C. botulinum are anaerobic and found in soil, bottom sediments of streams, lakes, river, or sea/coastal waters in form of spores that remain dormant for years. The spores require warm temperatures, a protein source, an anaerobic environment, and moisture to become active and produce toxin. Decomposing vegetation and insects provide such condition in nature. Spores are not killed by boiling. Heating expels dissolved oxygen from heat treated foods and creates anaerobic condition. Protein of food, low-salt, low-acid (pH 4–6), low-sugar, and ambient temperatures during cooling enable the growth of *C. botulinum* and toxin production.

35.3 Epidemiology

In 1735, food poisoning associated with eating German sausage was recorded. 'Botulus' is a Latin word for sausage, hence named botulism in 1870. The causative bacterium was isolated in 1895. It produced neurotoxin. It is the most toxic substance (lethal dose 1.3–2.1 ng/kg in human beings) and considered Category A bioweapon. One kg would be enough to kill the entire population.

Therapeutic and cosmetic use of botulinum toxin has grown tremendously during past decades.

Pharmaceutical use lies in the treatment of strabismus (deviation of eye), blepharospasm, hemifacial spasm, oesophageal stricture, spasmodic dysphasia, congenital pelvic tilt and failure of cervix and Wilson's disease.

Cosmetic use of BOTOX (BoNT-A is botulinum toxin A) has the approval of the FDA for treatment of wrinkles, underarm sweating and muscular pain. Other preparations are Dysport, Xeomin, and Neurobloc.

35.3.1 Source

Improperly cooked/processed foods are implicated in food poisoning. Commercial canning employs 'botulinum cook' to ensure destruction of spores. Therefore, most of the poisoning is reportedly caused by 'home canned, home bottled' or inadequately cooked, lightly preserved, or fermented foods that have been left for some time during which the bacterial spores germinate and produce toxins. A variety of foods have been implicated in botulism: low acid preserved spinach, mushrooms, beans, beets, carrot juice, garlic or herbs, baked potatoes wrapped in aluminium foils; canned fermented, salted and smoked fish, tuna; meat products such as sausage, ham, ready-to-eat foods in low oxygen-packaging.

Waterborne botulism is a theoretical possibility, but water sanitation is effective to detoxify botulinum toxin. Growth and toxigenesis can be prevented by a combination of low temperature, acid and salt.

35.3.2 Modes of Infection (Forms of Botulism)

'Food poisoning form' is the commonest and ingestion of toxin containing food is the route. *'Intestinal form or floppy baby syndrome'* is caused by infection of intestines followed by establishment and toxin production in situ. Infant botulism occurs like this and is more common in <6 months age group. Honey is the most common source. It is rare in infants >6 months and adults as natural defences protect.

'Wound form of botulism' is infection of wounds with bacterial spores followed by germination growth and toxin production. Drug addicts may inadvertently inject spores of *C. botulinum* with contaminated product or needle. It may take 2 weeks for symptoms to appear.

'Iatrogenic or botulism of undetermined origin' may be observed in adults *'adult intestinal botulism'*, usually not linked with ingestion of food. *C. botulinum* spores may be ingested by adults (including >6 months age) without causing any symptoms.

The source of spores is generally undetermined. Possible sources determined in some cases include refrigerated cream of coconut, blackberries, tuna and/or spaghetti with meat sauce, vacuum-packaged hashed beef, and peanut butter.

The adult intestinal tract has a healthy microbiome which generally does not support spore germination and toxin production. Predisposing factors are: those altering normal gut floras—such as antibiotic therapy, surgery, inflammatory bowel disease, Meckel's diverticulum. The spores of BoNTs producing clostridia transit to intestine upon ingestion germinate, multiply, and colonise (focal or entire lumen) the large intestine and produce toxin. *C. botulinum, C. baratii* type F and *C. butyricum* type E have caused adult intestinal botulinum toxaemia (Harris et al. 2020).

Overdose of BOTOX may also be dangerous. It should be administered under medical setting in doses tailored for customer.

'Botulism from biological warfare' – Botulinum toxin has been weaponised by many countries. Weaponisation with botulinum toxin H is a matter of concern as there is no antitoxin. Botulinum toxin is inactivated in water, faster in chlorinated water. Aerosolisation would be most appropriate. The median lethal dose for humans has been estimated at two nanograms of botulinum toxin per kilogram of bodyweight. Symptoms appear in one to three days or longer depending upon the amount of toxin inhaled. Symptoms and the manner these appear are same as in case of foodborne botulism.

The patient's clothing may cause additional exposure to the patients and others. Immediate shower given to patient, clothing be washed with soap and water (Botu lism who.int.10 January 2018).

Person to person transfer of botulism does not occur. All forms of botulism are neuroparalytic; call for medical emergency because it often ends fatally.

35.3.3 Public Health Reports

Fleck-Derderian (2017) reviewed the data on botulism. During 1920 to 2014 there were 197 outbreaks, most (55%) occurred in the US. Outbreaks were point source, 70% of large and 77% of small ($\leq$ 11 cases) significantly associated with commercial foods. Almost half of the outbreaks were caused by type A botulinum toxin and cases required mechanical ventilation.

The frequency of toxin types A, B, E and F causing outbreaks was 34%, 17%, 16% and 1%, respectively. The number of cases per outbreak ranged between 2–97 with a median of 3. The mean incubation period was one day. An average of 34% cases required mechanical ventilation.

International Network of Food Safety Authorities (INFOSAN) is managed jointly by FAO and WHO. National surveillance system, such as the US CDC is linked with it. *Cl. botulinum* types A, B, E, and F caused 34%, 16%, 17%, and 1% foodborne outbreaks globally from 1920–2014. *C. baratii* caused type F outbreak. In the US, there were 153 to 205 confirmed and 16 probable cases between 2012–2016. Most of these (71% to 88% each year were 'infant botulism', remaining shared between foodborne and wound botulism (https://www.healio.com/news/infectious-dis ease/20200319/botulism-a-rare-lifethreatening-illness. March 23, 2020).

A single case of botulism is treated as public health emergency as it can signal an outbreak. On April 21, 2015, the Fairfield Medical Centre (FMC) and Fairfield Department of Health contacted the Ohio Department of Health (ODH) about a suspected botulism patient. Within 2 hours of notification four more patients reported and later in the afternoon one died of respiratory failure. Investigation revealed it was the largest outbreak in the past four decades in the US involving 77 persons. All affected persons had eaten at the same widely attended church potluck meal on April 19. The risk ratio for potato salad was 13.9. Serum and stool samples from 19 cases investigated were positive for *C. botulinum* type A (Carolyn et al. 2015).

Botulism does not allow time to save life. The implicated food and also the species of *Clostridium* could be unconventional and unsuspected.

C. butyricum E outbreak involving 34 children of a rural school was reported by Chaudhry et al. (1998). Two died on way to hospital and the third even before initiating treatment. They reported abdominal pain, nausea, chest pain and difficult breathing. Eight were discharged after 24 hours; rest had to be taken to Ahmedabad, India for emergency treatment for ptosis, pupillary mydriasis, extraocular palsies, and impaired consciousness. Two continued with respiratory distress, required ventilation, and took about a month to recover after the administration of antitoxin (ABE). All had eaten *ladoo* (a local sweet), curd, buttermilk, *sevu* (crisp made of gram flour), and pickle. No toxin was detected in these and serum from eight cases (sampling delayed by a week). Leftover food items were cultured. *Sevu* yielded pure culture of *C. butyricum* Li $^-$ and gelatine $^-$. Toxin in broth culture was type E botulinum toxin. Tox -gene was also detected. The outbreak was caused by contaminated *sevu.*

C. baratii F botulism in France has been investigated (Mazuet et al. 2017). About 40–50 cases of botulism occur every year in France. Ham and its preparation made in home or small-scale enterprises generally are implicated. The first episode consisted of two cases in a family. The second episode of *C. baratii* F botulism in France consisted of a cluster three cases. The incubation period was short (mean 32 hours). The cases were more likely foodborne than intestinal colonisation. The cases developed quadriplegia and respiratory failure. All cases required prolonged respiratory assistance. One of them had high level of toxin in serum and remained paralysed for two weeks. *C. baratii* F was isolated from ground meat used for preparation of Bolognese sauce consumed by the three victims and their stool. BoNT was detected at 40 and 2000 MLD (mouse lethal doses)/g in the stools of two patients, respectively and BoNT/F gene was identified. Genetic studies showed distant relationship with the earlier strains from the US and China suggesting distinct origin.

In 2012, 160 lab-confirmed cases were reported to CDC (http://www.cdc.gov/ncezid/dfwed/PDFs/bot-overview_508c.pdf). Foodborne-, infant- and wound-botulism accounted for 16%, 72%, and 5%, respectively. Type A botulism was most common (76%), followed by 12% each of types B and E. Cases ranged between 15 to 77 years of age, median was 33 years. Most (88%) were males. There were four outbreaks (events with two or more cases) and one death. Implicated eatables were an illicit alcoholic beverage 'pruno' brewed (from potato) by prisoners, beets and pasta in meat sauce, both home canned.

Twenty eight states reported 122 infant botulisms in 1–53 weeks infants; median 19 weeks; 60% were male. Type B toxin accounted for the most (54%), additional one case each due to Ba and Bf toxins. Types A and F accounted for 42% and 3% respectively. There was no death.

Eight cases of 'wound botulism' without any death were reported from three states. Botulinum toxin type A accounted for 88% and type B for the remaining. All but 2 were drug users. Males (75%) predominated with 47 years as the median age.

Five cases could not be associated with any specific aetiology. Type A botulinum toxin was the commonest (3 or 60%), followed by types B and E or F each causing botulism in most (4 or 80%) males of 50 years as median age.

'Wound botulism' is important as is often incorrectly diagnosed as drug-related complication and the course is severe. Diagnosis in injecting drug users (IDU) is further complicated because of multiple health problems due to malnutrition, poor hygiene and underlying co-infections. Schroeter et al. (2009) investigated outbreak of wound botulism in IDU. Between October and December 2005, 16 cases of wound botulism in IDU were notified to the health authorities of North Rhine-Westphalia, Germany. All patients used contaminated injection drugs. *C. botulinum* was cultivated from clinical samples of six patients and molecular typing revealed that these were identical.

35.4 Symptoms

The preformed toxin in food is produced as a progenitor BoNT in association with haemagglutinin (HA) and non-toxic non-haemagglutinin (NTNH) as 'complex BoNT'. These protect BoNT from degradation by stomach acidity and intestinal protease. HAs facilitates paracellular passage of this complex. Free BoNT is able to pass through intestinal cells by transcytosis. BoNT crosses stomach acid barrier, enters intestine, passes to lymphatic and blood circulation and then disseminates to peripheral nervous system. Botulinum toxin blocks nerve function leads to paralysis.

Incubation period, period between eating food containing botulinum toxin and appearance of symptoms is usually 12 to 36 hours, (minimum four hours to maximum 8 days). There is no fever. The onset usually involves cranial nerves. Feeling of weakness, fatigue and vertigo is followed by diplopia, blurred vision, drooping eyelid, dry mouth, thick feeling tongue, difficulty in swallowing and speaking, slurred speech, vomiting, constipation. There is progressive weakness of muscles of neck, arms, chest (respiratory) and lower body say knee shows reduced or absent deep tendon reactions.

Signs include extra-ocular palsy, pupils' reaction sluggish, ptosis, facial paralysis, impaired gag reflex, objective evidence of declining respiratory function.

Sometimes respiratory symptoms may precede observable paralysis of more skeletal muscles. There is compromise of upper airway and not paralysis of diaphragm. Paralysis of respiratory muscles leads to difficult breathing, respiratory failure, coma and even death in about 5–10%. Consciousness is not lost.

35.4.1 Infant Botulism

Symptoms in 'infant botulism' include hoarse, altered cry, moan, whimper, loss of appetite, difficulty in suckling, weak suck, constipation, loss of head control. Blood and stool samples are tested for toxin. Most botulism is caused by *C. botulinum* types A and B. *C. butyricum* type E caused infant botulism was first reported in 1987 and has since been reported from Italy, Japan, the Republic of Ireland, England, and the US (Dykes et al. 2015).

35.5 Diagnosis

Neurological examinations should uncover the cranial nerve palsies, symmetric, bilateral and descending. Sometimes, neurological examination is pushed back to attend to the rapidly progressing or advanced respiratory symptoms that need immediate support.

Classical triad—bulbar palsy and descending paralysis, absence of fever, clear senses and mental status strongly suggest botulism. Add to this history. However, confounding syndromes and conditions such as Guillain-Barré syndrome, stroke, acute flaccid myelitis, tick paralysis, and myasthenia gravis need to be ruled out by brain scan, spinal fluid examination, nerve conduction test (electromyography, or EMG), and a tensilon test for myasthenia gravis.

Confirmatory diagnosis requires laboratory tests for botulinum toxin and/or *C. botulinum.* Detection of BoNT in suspected food samples, stool, stomach content, and blood/serum (in per-acute cases) is attempted.

According to Rasetti-Escargueil et al. (2020), detection of toxin in serum should be attempted in all cases of toxaemia, such as foodborne and wound botulism. Toxin remains more stable in blood. Sampling between 1–4 days after ingestion has maximum chances of detection. A very prolonged period of toxaemia may be ≥120 days.

Nearly 70% (56–82%) patients of foodborne botulism had detectable toxin in their serum. Serum of few asymptomatic persons sharing the contaminated food also proves BoNT positive. Intestinal botulism in adults including >1 year old – Serum samples collected between 5 and 22 days, maximum 47 days after ingestion tested positive because there is a progressive growth of *C. botulinum,* toxin production and toxaemia.

Amount of toxin ingested and time of sampling after ingestion affect the detection in serum, likely due to intestinal absorption and/or clearance and elimination in individuals. In infant botulism, likelihood of toxaemia is less because toxin is partly excreted with stool and remaining is trapped by the enteric nervous system resulting into loss of intestinal motility and secretions. No toxin is left to enter blood circulation. Only 28% samples were positive.

Infants' stool would be the ideal sample for detection of BoNT (87%),

Excretion of the causative bacteria and toxin may continue for several months in infant and adult botulism. Symptoms persist and recur in the latter.

Diagnostic tests:

- Mouse inoculation test, the gold test, is done for demonstration of toxin and toxin type. It takes 24–96 hours for the result to be available.
- ELISA and electrochemiluminescent may also be done.

- Quantitative PCR identifies A, B, E, F genes (Peck et al. 2011).
- Multiplex PCR assay is rapid and inexpensive (Williamson et al. 2017).

Molecular studies demonstrated genomic diversity within BoNTs producing species. The multiplex marker can differentiate quickly BoNTs producing isolates within *C. botulinum* group I, *C. sporogenes* and two major subgroups of *C. botulinum* group II. These bacteria could be identified in mixed cultures, potentially environmental and clinical samples.

The in vitro methods do not detect the full biological activity of BoNTs. However, their sensitivity is high and can better differentiate botulism from autoimmune neuropathies and myasthenia. In vitro test based on endopeptidase activity are promising (Rasetti-Escargueil et al. 2020).

35.6 Treatment

Outbreaks of botulism are rare. Yet it is a Public Health emergency. Rapid identification and locating source, differentiating between 'natural', 'accidental', and 'potential deliberate', preventing additional cases and treatment are essential.

Equine anti-BoNT is available as heptavalent (all types), trivalent (ABE) for adults and adults including children aged >1 year. Human anti BoNT/A and anti BoNT/B immunoglobulin is available for infant botulism. The antibodies neutralise the toxins before binding to neuronal cells. Ideal is to administer the antibodies early, < 24 hours of the onset of symptoms.

Therefore, early diagnosis and initiation of management is important.

Severe cases require intensive medical care, breathing machine and effective nursing for long until respiratory function spontaneously recovers. Complete recovery is time taking. Recovery is not complete in most of the cases. Regeneration of neuromuscular tissues takes months. Long term effects are dry mouth, fatigue, weakness, difficulty in performing strenuous works, shortness of breath, dizziness. There may be psychological effect—a feeling of less peaceful.

In case of 'inhalation botulism', all efforts are made to prevent exposure of others. Patients need to be showered to remove all traces of toxin. His clothing is removed, sealed in plastic bags and washed thoroughly with water and soap.

Wound botulism requires surgical removal to remove the bacteria, followed by flush of antibiotic to destroy the left over.

35.7 Prevention

Acidic foods (pH < 4.6) do not favour growth of *C. botulinum* but fail to degrade any pre-formed toxin. Spores in pickles may not pose a problem. Storage below 3 ° C, very low levels of moisture, high level of oxygen or high ratio of dissolved sugar are unfavourable. Boiling at 100 °C (internal temp. >85 °C) for 5 to 10 minutes destroys toxin and should be followed for ready-to-eat foods; else follow the instructions on the packages of such foods.

Regulatory authorities to check if producers of canned foods follow the standard 'botulinum cook'—121 °C for three minutes and also do 'sample check' from food stores. Public need to be educated on (a) to discard 'cans showing bulge'; (b) 'home canning'—destruction of *C. botulinum* spores by using pressure canners/cookers, hygiene, refrigeration for storage; preferring acid fruits/vegetables only or acidifying items such as tomatoes, garlic, herbs; (c) baked in aluminium foils items like potatoes to be kept hot till consuming or storing in refrigerator.

Un-eviscerated fish, fish products—smoked, dried, salt-cured—are considered unsafe. Seeking medical care for infected wounds and not using 'injectable addictive drugs' will take care of 'wound botulism'. Honey or corn syrup being highly concentrated sugar solution is safe for persons one year and above and not for infants as the sugar is diluted in their low oxygen, low acid digestive system. Cleanliness in house prevents accumulation of dust under carpet, on floor and dining table or kitchen tabletops.

35.7.1 Public Health Agency

Public should be educated and made aware about botulism, safe foods and safe canning. Public Health agency should have ready panel of knowledgeable physicians, health departments and laboratories for diagnosis and investigation and centres where antitoxin is available and can be quickly delivered. BOTULINUM HELP LINE should be notified and easily accessible.

Molecular epidemiological investigation into botulism outbreaks and cases should be carried out. The genome sequences enable enhanced isolate discrimination and spread, determination of botulinum neurotoxin sub-type variant, association with foodborne, infant and wound botulism, epidemiology, and geographic origin. This helps risk assessments and prevention and/or minimising outbreaks.

References

Anonym (1999) Rejection of *Clostridium putrificum* and conservation of *Clostridium botulinum* and *Clostridium sporogenes* opinion 69. Judicial Commission of the International Committee on Systematic Bacteriology. Int J Syst Bacteriol 49 Pt 1:339

Barash JR, Arnon SS (2014) A novel strain of *Clostridium botulinum* that produces type B and type H Botulinum toxins. J Infect Dis 209(2):183–191

Brunt J, van Vliet AHM, Carter AT, Stringer SC et al (2020) Diversity of the genomes and neurotoxins of strains of *Clostridium botulinum* group I and *Clostridium sporogenes* associated with foodborne, infant and wound botulism. Toxins 12:586

Carter AT, Peck MW (2015) Genomes, neurotoxins and biology of *Clostridium botulinum* group I and group II. Res Microbiol 166(4):303–317

Chaudhry R, Dhawan B, Kumar D, Bhatia R et al (1998) Outbreak of suspected *Clostridium butyricum* botulism in India. Emerg Infect Dis 4:506–507

Dover N, Barash JR, Hill KK, Xie G, Arnon SS (2014) Molecular characterization of a novel Botulinum neurotoxin type H gene. J Infect Dis 209(2):192–202

Dykes JK, Lúquez C, Raphael BH, McCroskey L, Maslanka SE (2015) Laboratory investigation of the first case of botulism caused by *Clostridium butyricum* type E toxin in the United States. J Clin Microbiol 53:3363–3365

Fleck-Derderian S, Shankar M, Rao AK, Chatham-Stephens K et al (2017) The epidemiology of foodborne botulism outbreaks: a systematic review. Clin Infect Dis 66(suppl_1):S73–S81

Harris RA, Anniballi F, Austin JW (2020) Adult Intestinal Toxemia Botulism. Toxins (Basel) 12(2):81

Mazuet C, Legeay C, Sautereau J et al (2017) Characterization of *clostridium baratii* type F strains responsible for an outbreak of botulism linked to beef meat consumption in France. PLoS Curr 9:ecurrents.outbreaks.6ed2fe754b58a5c42d0c33d586ffc606

McCarty CL, Angelo K, Beer KD, Cibulskas-White K, Quinn K, de Fijter S, Bokanyi R, St. Germain E, Baransi K, Barlow K, Shafer G, Hanna L, Spindler K, Walz E, DiOrio M, Jackson BR, Luquez C, Mahon BE, Basler C, Curran K, Matanock A, Walsh K, Slifka KJ, Rao AK (2015) Large outbreak of botulism associated with a Church Potluck Meal — Ohio. MMWR 64 (29):802–803

Peck MW, Stringer SC, Carter AT (2011) *Clostridium botulinum* in the post-genomic era. Food Microbiol 28(2):183–191

Rasetti-Escargueil C, Lemichez E, Popo MR (2020) Toxaemia in human naturally acquired botulism. Toxins (Basel) 12(11):716

Schroeter M, Alpers K, van Treeck U, Frank C, Rosenkoetter N, Schaumann R (2009) Outbreak of wound botulism in injecting drug users. Epidemiol Infect 137:1602–1608

Suen JC, Hatheway CL, Steigerwalt AG, Brenner DJ (1988) *Clostridium argentinense sp.* nov.: a genetically homogeneous group composed of all strains of *Clostridium botulinum* type G and some nontoxigenic strains previously identified as *Clostridium subterminale* or *Clostridium hastiforme*. Int J Sys Bacteriol 38:375–381

Suen JC, Hatheway CL, Steigerwalt AG, Brenner DJ (1988a) Genetic confirmation of identities of neurotoxigenix *Clostridium baratii* and *Clostridium butyricum* implicated as agents of infant botulism. J Clin Microbiol 26:2191–2192

Williamson CHD, Vazquez AJ, Hill K, Smith TJ, Nottingham R, Stone NE et al (2017) Differentiating Botulinum neurotoxin-producing clostridia with a simple multiplex PCR assay. Appl Environ Microbiol 83(18):e00806–e00817

Campylobacteriosis 36

Campylobacteriosis is a bacterial zoonosis characterised by enteritis often requiring hospitalisation. It is the most common zoonosis transmissible mainly through poultry meat in the EU (EFSA 2010).

36.1 Aetiology

The causative agent belongs to the family *Campylobacteraceae*, genus *Campylobacter.* These are gram-negative, non-sporing, helical shape, motile oxidase positive bacteria. Generally, growth temperature is 37 °C, not <32 °C; optimum for *C. jejuni* and *C. coli* is 42 °C which are most common pathogenic species. *C. lari, C. fetus,* and *C. upsaliensi* also cause illness.

Campylobacteria are most unlikely to grow at chilling temperature maintained while processing, handling of carcass, and in refrigerated storage. These may persist at these temperatures, e.g. for weeks at 4 °C during storage of meat. Freezing is inimical, the bacterial count reduces by 2-log by freezing broiler meat. Freezing at −15 °C for 3 days inactivates, but it fails to eliminate from contaminated frozen foods. Heating destroys Campylobacteria. D_{55} in heart infusion broth for *C. coli* is 6.6. ± 0.5 and D_{57} in ground chicken breast, for *C. jejuni i*s 0.79 (Silva et al. 2011).

36.2 Burden

Campylobacteriosis is the most common reported foodborne zoonoses in the EU and the US. Most campylobacteriosis are sporadic, pass unidentified and unreported unless part of a reported outbreak.

The global burden of foodborne diseases is high causing sickness in 1/10 people and loss of 33.0 million healthy life years. Most foodborne diseases cause diarrhoea. *Campylobacter* is one of the four key global causes of diarrhoeal diseases.

K. G. Narayan et al., *Veterinary Public Health & Epidemiology*,
https://doi.org/10.1007/978-981-19-7800-5_36

Campylobacteriosis is the most common reported foodborne zoonoses in the EU and the US.

According to EFSA (2021), broiler meat and milk were most commonly associated with foodborne campylobacteriosis in the EU. Campylobacteriosis was the most common cause of gastroenteritis since 2005. The occurrence maintained a stable trend during 2015–2019. The EU recorded incidence of 59.7/100,000 (220,682 cases) in the year 2019 with 319 outbreaks involving 1254 cases of illness and 125 hospitalisations without any deaths. As compared to the incidence in 2018, there was reduction by 6.9%.

According to the European Union One Health (2020) Zoonoses report, Campylobacteriosis is the most frequently reported foodborne illness in the EU with over 246,000 cases/year. The actual number is believed to be nearly nine million per year responsible for an estimated annual loss of 2,4 billion euros. Human got infected commonly by eating uncooked chicken, ready-to-eat foods and contact with raw chicken. Chicken and chicken meat alone accounted for 20–30% of cases.

Scallan et al. (2011) analysed the US data (mostly 2000–08) and found that 55,961 of 228,744 hospitalisations were caused by eating contaminated foods. Bacteria were responsible for 64% of these. In the US, FoodNet diagnosed 20 cases/100,000/year while CDC 1.5 million infections/year.

According to Huang et al. (2015) campylobacteriosis is a notifiable disease and is leading cause of human enteric infections in Canada. On an average 34.9 cases/100,000 are reported. The peak period lies between June to September (summer) with lowest number of cases reported in February–March. *C. jejuni* is frequently the cause.

36.3 Epidemiology

36.3.1 Source

Campylobacter are relatively fragile, cannot survive desiccation and oxidative stress but can form biofilm and remain viable in it. Antimicrobial resistant variants may survive better in food chain. These survive in water. Survival is long (10 months) in compost. Survival in stockpile of farmyard manure is dependent upon temperature, 2–5 days at 50 °C and 32 days at approximate 15–20 °C.

C. jejuni is commonly isolated from poultry but also from cattle, sheep, goats, dogs and cats. *C. coli* is common in pigs but also in poultry, cattle and sheep. The birds including wild birds and animals do not manifest any symptom. Chicken carry 10^8CFU/g in intestinal content. Human cases continue shedding *Campylobacter* in faeces after clinical recovery. In-contact symptomless shedders occur.

Whiley et al. (2013) reviewed the literature on the environmental sources of *Campylobacter* spp. Water from rivers, lakes, streams and coasts has been associated with waterborne infection. *Campylobacter* survive for long in subsurface aquifers of groundwater as favourable conditions are available—almost constant temperature, absence of UV, and desiccation. Large aquifers deliver water to big cities and are potential risks. Certain protozoa present in drinking water system for broiler internalise *Campylobacter* spp. The protozoan cyst provides protection against environmental conditions, may be disinfectant also. Thus protected, *Campylobacter* spp. may spread through water and air. Risk of *Campylobacter* infection is high during rainy season. Contamination levels increase through sewage overflow and agricultural runoff.

Recreational water may become a source. Also, playground is often contaminated with droppings of wild birds, stray dogs, cats and reptiles and constitutes source of infection among children. Whiley et al. (2013) cites nine cases of *C. fetus* sub spp. *tsetudinum* subsp. nov of reptile origin.

Campylobacter contaminated poultry meat, red meat, raw milk, dairy products and fish and fishery products, mussels and fresh vegetables and untreated water are often sources of infection. De Haan et al. (2013) studied multi location sequence (MLST) of the isolates of *C. jejuni* in opined that natural water and poultry are the important sources of human infection.

Contact borne infection in human occurs; sources can be infected poultry and pets.

36.3.2 Modes of Human Infection

Modes of human infections are (a) commonly ingestion of inadequately cooked foods, un-sanitised water, and (b) contact as may occur among pet owners, farmers, butchers and meat/poultry processing plant workers.

Human carriage and human to human transmission seems to be more frequent in developing countries. Humans are likely to get infection through direct contact with animals, chicken and their produce and contaminated water. In developed countries poultry and their products are most common sources.

Campylobacteriosis affects older children and young adults, can be severe requiring hospitalisation and treatment with antimicrobials. In developing countries, *C. jejuni* infection is common in children <5 years, especially <1 year. Infection is subclinical or milder in young adults.

In Europe smaller distinct outbreak peak is observed in winter also in addition to the common and sharp summer peaks since past 8 years including 2019. The winter peak is limited to the first 3 weeks of the year, suggesting coincidence with Christmas and New Year celebrations and increased travel during the holidays. Preparations like meat fondue or tabletop grilling are popular during the festive season and might be responsible for *Campylobacter* transmission.

Most (80%) foodborne campylobacteriosis may be traced to chicken reservoir (Whiley et al. 2013). In the US, a study of common source campylobacteriosis during 1997–2008 revealed that 86%, 9%, and 3% were linked to eating of foods, drinking water and animal contact, respectively (Taylor et al. 2013). The EFSA's Biological Hazards Panel confirmed that poultry meat was the major (if not the largest) source. The home (poultry farm) and transit of *Campylobacter* to broiler meat consumers follows.

36.3.3 *Campylobacter* Infection in Birds

Campylobacter can appear in broiler chicken as early as 14 days age at the rearing centre. The infective dose for broilers was 20–90 CFU of *Campylobacter* and within 6 h of infection colonisation occurred. Caeca is the most favoured site (10×) compared to oesophagus and small intestines and the bacterial count reached 11 $\log_{10}$ CFU in 2 days. *C. jejuni* maintained motility in the mucus layer of the crypts of intestinal epithelium and utilised nutrients.

The source of infection seems to be environment of a broiler house because poultry feed generally tested negative and feed environment is unfavourable.

Lapses in maintaining high biosecurity and farm hygiene, farm visitors including managers and auditors from other contaminated farms are the likely sources of infection because infected flocks shed huge number of *Campylobacter*, 6–9 logs CFU/g of caecal contents or fresh faeces. The spread of infection is rapid (estimated at 2.37 birds/day). The prevalence of Campylobacteriosis in flocks reaches 100% within days or 1 week of introduction of infection. The spread is rapid in summer. Infection is very likely to persist to normal broiler slaughter age.

Preventing spread between flocks of a broiler farm is very difficult. *Campylobacter* and *Salmonella* infection in birds are common. However, there are epidemiological differences between Salmonellosis and Campylobacteriosis. *Camylobacter* but not *Salmonella* is more likely to be introduced into broiler flocks at any stage of their life. Vertical transmission is uncommon in Campylobacteriosis. Culling and vaccination to control salmonellosis is not applicable to campylobacteriosis. Poultry feed is generally free from *Salmonella*. Broiler house environment can be maintained *Salmonella*-free. It is possible to control *Salmonella* with basic precaution such as disinfectant boot dips or boot changes.

Prevalence of *Campylobacter* in the Member States of the European Union was revealed that proportion of samples positive for *Campylobacter* was much higher in population of pigs and cattle than the respective fresh meats examined at the levels of processing and retail. This was not so with broiler and broiler meat (EFSA 2012). Handling, preparation and consumption of broiler meat directly accounted for 20–30% human cases of campylobacteriosis and 50–80% might be attributed to chicken broiler reservoir.

36.3.4 *Campylobacter* Contamination of Broiler Meat

Carriage of *Campylobacter* from farm to finished poultry meat studied (Franz et al. 2012) by examining specimens at three levels viz., prevalence at the farm—arrival at the slaughterhouse—exit of chilled dressed broiler from slaughterhouse. Prevalence of *Campylobacter* in the chilled dressed broiler was significantly ($p = <0.001$ and

<0.005) associated with the prevalence at the two preceding levels. Thirty three per cent of packed chicken products were *Campylobacter* positive and 51% originated from infected flocks.

A logistic slaughter can be planned (Sasaki et al. 2013). When *Campylobacter* – negative flocks were slaughtered prior to positive flocks, no chicken product was positive. Tang et al. (2020) used label tracking method combined with Hazard Analysis Critical Point determination to determine contamination from rearing to slaughtering. The contamination was highest at the level of evisceration. It decreased sharply at cooling (one *C. jejuni* and one *C. coli*) and partition stages (one *C. coli*). The distribution of *Campylobacter* during broiler chicken production was dynamic—*C. jejuni* 66.3% during rearing and *C. coli* 60.4% of *Campylobacter* isolates during slaughtering. On sequence typing, *C. jejuni* found to has 4 sequence types (STs) and 6 STs of *C. coli*. Core genome of isolates from tag-labelled samples at different stages elucidated transmission routes. Two antimicrobial drug resistance genes were observed.

Verhoeff-Bakkenes et al. (2011) observed higher contamination rate in raw fruits and vegetables than in packaged ones.

Prevalence of *Campylobacter* in broilers was 13% in 2019. Forty one per cent of broiler carcasses (neck skin samples) were positive, with 15% showing more than the limit of 1000 CFU/g. The proportion of *Campylobacter*-positive samples within the categories 'ready-to-eat' and 'non-ready-to-eat' food was 0.2% and 20.6%, respectively.

Kottawatta et al. (2017) reported *Campylobacter*-contamination of broiler meat in Sri Lanka. *Campylobacter* colonised broiler flocks were 67%; 59% of meat were contaminated at retail. The level of contamination after semi-automated processing was 27.4% compared to 48% after wet market processing. The contamination occurred even when *Campylobacter*-free broilers were processed, 15% with semi-automated processing vs 25% after wet market processing. Most isolates were characterised as *C. coli* than *C. jejuni*.

The prevalence of *Campylobacter* spp. in broiler in in organised and unorganised units of poultry in has been reported. Organised units observed better hygienic practices as reflected in lower prevalence (Sharma et al. 2007; Rajkumar et al. 2010).

36.4 Symptoms

36.4.1 Campylobacteriosis in Human

Campylobacteriosis is often considered sporadic as most infections pass as part of small family outbreaks and self-limiting. Investigated-identified outbreaks are relatively uncommon. All age groups are affected, maximum <1 year and 15–29 years, more males than females suffer.

The incubation period is usually 2–5 days. *Campylobacter* is highly invasive. The infective dose is small, 500–800 bacteria. The invasive antigen *(Cia)* facilitates motility and the spiral shape enable penetration of gastrointestinal mucus. Flagella are important for motility, formation of biofilm, host-cell interaction, adherence, cell invasion and colonisation. Enterotoxins and cytotoxins induce gastroenteritis, diarrhoea. As a response to infection immunoglobulins rise. IgA cross the gut wall to offer local protection. Inflammatory fever and diarrhoea are caused. Leucocytes and blood appear in stool.

Campylobacteriosis manifests as foul-smelling watery diarrhoea, fever, abdominal pain, nausea. Vomiting is not common, but diarrhoea may be severe and bloody. Pain is acute, periumbilical and confounded with appendicitis. There is inflammation of ileum, jejunum, colon and sometimes rectum. Illness lasts for several days to over a week with variable severity. Immunocompromised and young children may suffer with severe and life -threatening form of illness. There is bacteraemia and lesions may be seen in distant organs also. Campylobacteriosis is primarily gastroenteritis, but complications occur.

Guillain-Barre Syndrome (GBS) occurs in one in thousand cases of *C. jejuni* infection. GBS is an acute neuromuscular paralysis beginning several weeks after the onset of diarrhoea. Neuropathy is of wide range of types and severity. Maximum disability appears in less than a week and many cases are tetraplegic. The disability is prolonged, observed in 20%. Hyper-acute cases develop tetraplegia in 48 h, recover slowly and the residual disability is significant. Fatality may be 5%.

Reiter's syndrome is a reactive arthritis affects multiple joints and causes incapacitation. Approximately 1% of campylobacteriosis cases suffer with this. A variety of complications and syndromes such as 'irritable bowel', 'haemolytic uraemic', 'Chinese paralytic', abortion, meningitis, and hepatitis add to social and economic burden.

Direct spread of infection may lead to peritonitis, cholecystitis, pancreatitis and massive gastrointestinal haemorrhage. The infection may extend beyond intestine to cause a variety of complications like neonatal sepsis, septic arthritis, osteomyelitis, meningitis, and endocarditis.

36.4.2 Foodborne Outbreaks

Chicken

In Australia, *Campylobacter* was the leading cause of gastroenteritis among the notified enteric pathogens and accounted for 104.8–117.3/100,000 cases annually during 2007–11. Parry et al. (2012) reported an outbreak wherein *Campylobacter* survived the cooking and preparation of chicken liver pâté. Chicken liver can be contaminated both internally and externally. Cooking for 2–3 min after the core temperature reached 70–80 °C could reduce the presence of *Campylobacter* but the restaurant did sautéing before making the pâté. The relative risk for the 'chicken liver pate' was 16.7. Of 57 guests interviewed, 15 met the case definition of gastroenteritis of a median duration of 8 days. Two cases were <18 years, rest between 40–49 years; 51% were female.

The Vermont Department of Health (http://www.cdc.gov/mmwr/preview/mmwrhtml/mm6244a2.htm) reported a multistate outbreak in 2012. Chicken liver had been consumed. Of the six patients two were hospitalised. *C. jejuni* was isolated from chicken livers and identified by Pulsed-field gel electrophoresis. Chicken livers were not cooked thoroughly.

Chicken liver paste caused another outbreak in England at a wedding party. The preparation had violated the Foods Standards Agency's guidelines (Edwards et al. 2014).

Milk

Lahti et al. (2017) reported milk borne campylobacteriosis among children. A meal including unpasteurised milk was served in a dairy farm in Southwestern part of Sweden during a visit in April–May 2014. Of the 11 cases identified, seven were children 2–7 years of age. A retrospective cohort study and laboratory investigation established Campylobacteriosis. The attack rates were 45% and 42% among those who drank unpasteurised milk usually and those who drank during the visit. *C. jejuni* was isolated from 8 of the victims. Genotyping with pulsed-field gel electrophoresis and whole genome sequencing confirmed that human and cattle isolates of *C. jejuni* belonged to one cluster. The farm cattle were considered the source of infection. Contaminated unpasteurised milk was the vehicle.

36.4.3 Contact Borne

Puppies and cats brought recently may infect infants and young children who have not yet developed sanitary habits. Aged care facilities in Canberra, Australia had zoonotic campylobacteriosis. Two separate gastroenteritis outbreaks between April and June 2012 in nursing homes were traced to puppies. *C. jejuni* was isolated from faecal samples of human and canines. The latter extensively shed *C. jejuni*. Low dose was infective for the aged (aged care settings) despite varying degree of contacts with puppies. Health officials decided to ban puppy as companion animals in the aged care facilities [*Puppy ban over aged care illness scare. March 19*, 2013.: http://www.canberratimes.com.au/act-news/puppy-ban-over-aged-care-illness-scare-20130318-2gbkb.html#ixzz2SJ9D5qIT].

A contact borne multi-state outbreak of MDR *C. jejuni* in the USA was reported by the CDC on 15 April 2021 (*https://www.cdc.gov/campylobacter/outbreaks/puppies-12-19/index.html)*. A total of 56 (seven aged <5 years) people spread over 17 states were infected between 9 January 2019 to 1 March 2021. The median age was 40 years, range 2 months to 84 years; 55% female; 20% of those reported had to be hospitalised. There was no death. Whole genome sequencing of Campylobacteria isolated from ill people suggested a common source of infection and a part of an outbreak. The isolates were found to be genetically related to the 2016–18 infections linked to pet store puppies. The outbreak strain was isolated from two puppies purchased from the pet store and in the homes of ill people. Many (93%) ill and interviewed had contact with puppies a week before they fell ill; 55% of them reported contact with a puppy from a pet store. Some ill were employed of the pet store.

36.5 Diagnosis

Laboratory confirmation of suspected cases is required. Direct microscopic examination of specimens and suspected bacterial colonies show a characteristic cork-screw darting motile bacteria. Bacteriological cultural and identification is the gold test.

Multilocus enzyme, Pulsed-Field Gel Electrophoresis, whole genome sequencing, PCR targeting 16S ribosomal RNA are commonly used in epidemiological investigations.

Ivanova et al. (2014) claim that *C. jejuni*-specific primer *'C. jejuni hippuricase gene'* as target developed by them was highly sensitive, able to detect as low as one genome copy per reaction, compared with other tests. It was simple, easy and inexpensive.

The Polymerase Spiral Reaction (PSR) is an updated test that employs the dye HNB (Milton et al. 2021). *It is simple, rapid and sensitive test for screening samples of chicken and chicken-based products and does not require sophisticated instrument and trained personnel.* The test took 1 h 30 min to detect 1600 CFU/g of specimen.

36.6 Control

Culling of poultry to control avian influenza in the Netherlands in year 2003 concurrently reduced campylobacteriosis (Friesema et al. 2012).

Campylobacteriosis in poultry can be checked by biosecurity, infection of the flock and blocking transmission between flocks. Campylobacterial colonisation of broiler intestine can be reduced by the use of probiotics.

A high standard of hygiene and food preparation in Australia has minimised the impact of foodborne illness considerably.

Hygiene in the poultry meat production chain, from poultry farms through arrival, slaughter and processing at the slaughterhouse and market is required.

Awareness and emphasis on appropriate handling and cooking of high-risk foods are necessary to prevent outbreaks (Parry et al. 2012).

Freezing for 24 h at −25 °C-thawing-freezing for 24 h at −25 °C reduced the number of *Campylobacter* by three logs (Harrison et al. 2013).

36.7 Treatment

Cases generally respond to antibiotics, except when resistant strains are involved.

Probiotic strains of *Lactobacillus rhamnosus* GG and *Propionibacterium freudenreichii* ssp. *shermanii* JS and a starter culture *Lactobacillus lactis* ssp. *lactis* adhered well to intestinal mucosa to reduce binding by *Campylobacter* (Ganan et al. 2013).

Rehydrate and maintain electrolyte balance.

References

De Haan CPA, Lampen K, Corander J, Hanninen ML (2013) Multilocus sequence types of environmental *Campylobacter jejuni* isolates and their similarities to those of human, poultry and bovine *C. jejuni* isolates. Zoonoses Public Health 60:125–133

Edwards DS, Milne LM, Morrow K, Sheridan P, Verlander NQ et al (2014) Campylobacteriosis outbreak associated with consumption of undercooked chicken liver pâté in the East of England, September 2011: identification of a dose–response risk. Epidemiol Infect 142(2):352–357

EFSA (2010) EFSA confirms chicken meat major source of human cases of campylobacteriosis. https://www.efsa.europa.eu/en/press/news/biohaz100128

EFSA (2012) EU summary report on trends and sources of zoonoses, zoonotic agents and foodborne outbreaks 2010. EFSA J 10(3):2597

EFSA (2021) EFSA Scientific Report: The European Union One Health 2020 Zoonoses Report. EFSA J 19(12):6971. https://doi.org/10.2903/j.efsa.2021.6971

Franz E, van der Fels-Klerx HJ, Thissen J, van Asselt ED (2012) Farm and slaughterhouse characteristics affecting the occurrence of *Salmonella* and *Campylobacter* in the broiler supply chain. Poult Sci 91:2376–2381

Friesema IHM, Havelaar AH, Westra PP, Wagenaar JA, van Pelt W (2012) Poultry culling and Campylobacteriosis reduction among humans, the Netherlands. Emerg Infect Dis 18(3): 466–468

Ganan M, Martinez-Rodriguez AJ, Carrascosa AV, Vesterlund S et al (2013) Interaction of *Campylobacter* spp. and human probiotics in chicken intestinal mucus. Zoonoses Public Health 60(2):141–148

Harrison D, Corr JEL, Tchórzewska MA, Morris VK, Hutchison ML (2013) Freezing as an intervention to reduce the numbers of Campylobacters isolated from chicken livers. Lett Appl Microbiol 57(3):206–213

Huang H, Brooks BW, Lowman R, Carrillo CD (2015) Campylobacter species in animal, food, and environmental sources, and relevant testing programs in Canada. Can J Microbiol 61(10): 701–721. https://doi.org/10.1139/cjm-2014-0770

Ivanova M, Singh R, Dharmasena M, Gong C, Krastanov A, Jiang X (2014) Rapid identification of *Campylobacter jejuni* from poultry carcasses and slaughtering environment samples by real-time PCR. Poult Sci 93(6):1587–1597

Kottawatta KSA, Van Bergen MAP, Abeynayake P, Wagenaar JA, Veldman KT, Kalupahana RS (2017) Campylobacter in broiler chicken and broiler meat in Sri Lanka: influence of semi-automated vs. wet market processing on Campylobacter contamination of broiler neck skin samples. Foods 6(12):105. https://doi.org/10.3390/foods6120105

Lahti E, Rehn M, Ockborn G, Hansson I, Ågren J, Engvall EO, Jernberg C (2017) Outbreak of Campylobacteriosis following a dairy farm visit: confirmation by genotyping. Foodborne Pathog Dis 14(6):326–332

Milton AAP, Momin K, Priya GB, Das S, Angappan M, Sen A, Sinha DK, Ghatak S (2021) Development of a novel visual detection technique for *Campylobacter jejuni* in chicken meat and caecum using polymerase spiral reaction (PSR) with pre-added dye. Food Control 2021(126):108064

Parry A, Feamley E, Denehy E (2012) 'Surprise': outbreak of *Campylobacter* infection associated with chicken liver pâté at a surprise birthday party, Adelaide, Australia, 2012. Western Pac Surveill Response J 3(4):16–19

Puppy ban over aged care illness scare (2013). http://www.canberratimes.com.au/act-news/puppy-ban-over-aged-care-illness-scare-20130318-2gbkb.html#ixzz2SJ9D5qIT

Rajkumar RS, Yadav AS, Rathore RS, Mohan HV, Singh RP (2010) Prevalence of *Campylobacter jejuni* and *Campylobacter coli* from unorganised and organised small scale poultry dressing units in Northern India. J Vet Publ Health 8(1):1–5

Sasaki Y, Maruyama N, Zou B, Haruna M, Kusukawa M, Murakami M et al (2013) *Campylobacter* cross-contamination of chicken products at an abattoir. Zoonoses Public Health 60(2):134–140

Scallan E, Hoekstra RM, Angulo FJ, Tauxe RV, Widdowson M-A, Roy SL et al (2011) Foodborne illness acquired in the United States—major pathogens. Emerg Infect Dis 17(1):7–15

Sharma VK, Mishra SK, Mishra RK, Tamilselvan P, Mamarugan S (2007) Occurrence of *Campylobacter jejuni* in broilers from retail outlets. J Vet Publ Health 5(1):35–36

Silva J, Leite D, Fernandes M, Mena C, Gibbs PA, Teixeira P (2011) Campylobacter spp. as a foodborne pathogen: a review. Front Microbiol 2:200. https://doi.org/10.3389/fmicb.2011.00200

Tang Y, Jiang Q, Tang H, Wang Z, Yin Y, Ren F, Kong L, Jiao X, Huang J (2020) Characterization and prevalence of campylobacter spp. from broiler chicken rearing period to the slaughtering process in eastern China. Front Vet Sci 7:227. https://doi.org/10.3389/fvets.2020.00227

Taylor EV, Herman KM, Ailes EC, Fitzgerald C et al (2013) Common source of *Campylobacter* infection in the USA, 1997-2008. Epidemiol Infect 141(5):987–996

Verhoeff-Bakkenes L, Jansen HAPM, in't Veld PH, Beumer RR, Zwietering MH, van Leusden FM (2011) Consumption of raw vegetables and fruits: a risk factor for *Campylobacter* infections. Int J Food Microbiol 144:406–412

Whiley H, van den Akker B, Giglio S, Bentham R (2013) *Review:* the role of environmental reservoirs in human Campylobacteriosis. Int J Environ Res Public Health 10(11):5886–5907

37 Listeriosis

Listeriosis is an invasive infectious disease of a variety of animals including human beings. It is one of the most serious and severe but relatively rare foodborne diseases affecting mainly elderly, immunocompromised, and pregnant women, causing sepsis, affecting the central nervous system leading to lifelong sequelae and death. It is regarded as one of the causes of spontaneous abortions and stillbirth.

In adult ruminants, listeriosis is a circling disease characterised by encephalitis, meningoencephalitis, abortion, stillbirths, septicaemia, occasional mastitis, spinal myelitis, and keratoconjunctivitis. In young ruminants and monogastric animals, it is manifested by septicaemia and focal hepatic necrosis. In fowls, septicaemia, myocardial degeneration, and focal hepatic necrosis are common.

Its global occurrence is relatively low (0.1–10 cases/10^6) but the associated fatality rate is high, and this makes it a significant public health concern (WHO 2018). The annual numbers of cases in the USA are estimated at 1600 and nearly 260 died (https://www.cdc.gov/listeria/index.html). The rate of increase of multi country (>2 countries) events were: 1996–97—nil; 1998–2004—0.07 and 2012–2018—0.19; an overall increase of 171% of *Listeria monocytogenes* events (outbreaks and sporadic) reported to ProMED in the past 20 years. The food vehicles involved in these were not previously implicated. The outbreak in South Africa involved a contaminated vehicle, *polony*, and had to be recalled from as many as 15 countries (Angel et al., 2019).

37.1 Aetiology

Listeria monocytogenes and *L. ivanovii* (previously classified as *L. monocytogenes* serotype 5) are the two pathogenic species. *L. monocytogenes* affects man and a number of species of animals while *L. ivanovii* affects mainly ruminants and only occasionally human beings.

K. G. Narayan et al., *Veterinary Public Health & Epidemiology*,
https://doi.org/10.1007/978-981-19-7800-5_37

Table 37.1 Isolates of *Listeria* grouped into four lineages

Lineages	Serotypes	Prevalence/associated with
I	1/2b, 3b, 4b, 4d and 4e; (4d and 4e are considered as sub cluster of serotype 4b)	1/2a, 1/2b, and 4b) cause most (95%) human illness associated with outbreaks. 4b farm animal pathogen
II	1/2a, 1/2c, 3a and 3c 1/2b and 4b	Commonly cause animal cases; more prevalent in environmental and food samples; less from human clinical cases
III	4a, 4c (strains 4b subdivided into IIIA, IIIB, IIIC)—highly bio-diverse	Very rare, significantly more common in animals (non-human primates and ruminants) than human isolates
IV	Strains of IIIB—highly bio-diverse	

L. monocytogenes is a small motile (tumbling) at and around 25 °C, gram-positive, diphtheroid, coccobacillus, non-spore forming, facultatively anaerobic, and grows between 3–50 °C (optimum 30–37 °C) and pH 4.5–9.6. It is beta haemolytic. It can survive for several years in faeces—three and 16 ½ months in faeces of sheep and cattle, respectively, 2 years in dry soil and faeces; 11 ½ months in damp soil and 207 days on dry straw. It forms biofilm, survives at −20 °C for 2 years and remains viable after repeated freezing and thawing. It can grow at refrigeration temperature, high salt and nitrite concentration, and can resist common disinfectants. *L. monocytogenes* present intra-cellularly may survive pasteurisation. The D value is 0.9 s at 71.1 °C. The legal requirement for pasteurisation is heating at 71.7 °C for 15 s.

It has 13 known serovars identified based on the somatic and flagellar antigens—1/2a, 1/2b, 1/2c, 3a, 3b, 3c, 4ab, 4a, 4b, 4c, 4d, 4e, and 7. Based on multiplex PCR, four major serogroups are IIa (serovars 1/2a, 1/2c, 3a, and 3c), IIb (1/2b, 3b, 4b,4d, and 4e), IIc (1/2c and 3c) and IVb (4b, 4d, and 4e), targeting four marker genes.

Isolates may be grouped into four lineages based on evolutionary histories and pathogenic potential (Table 37.1) as follows:

Strains of serotype 4b originated from different sources and geographically dispersed regions in India. 68.8% of isolates had identical pulsotypes (Barbuddhe et al. 2016). The association of *L. monocytogenes with* spontaneous abortion and meningitis appeared low (1.47% of 481 samples). The isolates belonged to serotypes 4b, 1/2b, and 4e (Kalekar et al. 2015). Most (91.67%) of isolates from human and animal clinical cases fell into three serogroups: 4b, 4d, 4e, followed by 1/2a, 3a (5.56%) and 1/2b, 3b (2.78%). PFGE analysis indicated that foods of animal origin could be a significant source and spread of infection to human populations (Negi et al. 2015).

37.2 Epidemiology

L. monocytogenes is ubiquitous, occurs in human, animals, and foods worldwide. Listeriosis is less common in tropical and subtropical than in temperate and cold climates. The prevalence is sporadic and seasonal—maximum in December and May in the northern hemisphere but not so in the southern. It occurs in North America, Europe, the UK, New Zealand, Australia, and also in India.

It has been isolated from some 42 species of animals, 22 species of birds, fish, crustaceans, and insects (Veterinary Merck Manual 2006). *L. monocytogenes* infects almost all species of domestic animals (cattle, buffaloes, sheep, goats, occasionally horses and pigs), many species of poultry (hens, ducks, etc.), and rodents such as guineapigs, mice; cats, dogs, and rabbits, wild animals and fish.

37.2.1 Infection in Animals

Clinical cases occur mostly in ruminants. Birds may suffer from sub-clinical infections, and pigs rarely develop illness. Most infections are sub-clinical, sporadic and *Listeria* is shed in excretion and secretions. It has been isolated from infected man and animals' faeces, sewage, sludge, farm slurry, soil, wall, floor, and farm drains; feed-common is silage, water, nasal secretions, foetal discharges, aborted foetuses, urine, and ewes' milk. The period of shedding by sheep and goats, faeces is infective for 2–28 days, nasal secretions from 2–3 to 11–14 days post infection, and vaginal secretion and milk for 2 days after abortion. Isolation has also been made from the respiratory tract of ducks.

Direct contact transmission to human may occur with these, during handling and assisting in lambing.

In India, sporadic and few outbreaks of listeriosis have been reported in sheep, goats, calves, buffalo-calves, buffaloes, rabbits, guinea pigs, and chicks with fatality.

Source: Stored fodder and feed contaminated with *L. monocytogenes* from soil and decaying vegetables, and the environment and silage are the main sources of animal infection. After oral ingestion, the bacteria enter into intestinal mucosa in case of septicaemia.

Factors influencing animal infection include animal husbandry practices—feed and fodder, nutrition, sudden change in environment and feed, extreme weather—cold and wet; season (coincident with lambing) and size of the flock of the sheep.

Modes of infection: Ingestion or inhalation tends to cause latent infection, septicaemia, and abortion. Ingestion of infected silage cause nearly total latent infection. Infection through conjunctiva, buccal mucosa, or inhalation generally causes encephalitis.

Symptoms: *Listeria* localise in intestinal wall, medulla, and placenta. Listeriae might hide in the lymphatic system and Kupffer cells of the liver. It causes septicaemia followed by endometritis and abortion in ewes, does, cows, and she-buffaloes.

The incubation period is 1–2 weeks. Time elapsed between ingestion of contaminated feed and occurrence of outbreaks of encephalitis, septicaemia, and abortion are 3 weeks, 2 days, and 6–13 days, respectively.

Generally, the symptoms are mild. There is fever, 38.6–39.2 °C on day 4–6 post infection in calves, persisting for 8–10 days post infection in buffalo-calves. There is a mild diarrhoea and staggering gait. The clinical presentation of animal listeriosis can be distinguished and described as (a) septicaemia, (b) abortion, (c) encephalitis, (d) spinal myelitis, and (e) mastitis.

Septicaemia is least common, but fatality rate is high; occurs commonly in lambs, young calves, and piglets and is generally not associated with nervous signs.

Abortion occurs during late gestation in cows, sheep, and goats. It is sporadic in cattle. The attack rates of abortion in sheep and goats in an outbreak was10–15%.

Encephalitis, spinal myelitis. This is more common in monogastric animals, and principal lesion is focal hepatic necrosis, poor tone of jaw muscles, dropped jaw, drooling saliva, food hanging from mouth, retro- or ventro-flexed head but poll-nose relationship remains undisturbed; even if the position of head is corrected, it returns to its previous position, ataxia, always falling/leaning against fence/examiner on one side, while recumbent the animal moves legs but is unable to rise. Other symptoms are keratitis, corneal ulcer, strabismus, nystagmus, panophthalmitis, and pus in anterior chamber of eye(s) in cattle.

In experimental infection through tooth pulp, the organism travels through trigeminal nerve centripetally to brain to cause acute inflammation of brainstem. There is meningoencephalitis in young lambs infected intravenously. The ascending infection of sheep may result into spinal myelitis in all age group, accounting for about 0.8–2.5% of occurrence.

37.2.2 Poultry

L. monocytogenes in the poultry meat and products is a multifaceted potential hazard. Jamshidi and Zeinali (2019) reviewed papers on isolations from chicken flock and poultry meat and products. Poultry flocks spread it in the environment and carcass, fresh, wing, frozen, minced ready-to-eat chicken product, and barbecued chicken meat.

Cufaoglu and Ayaz (2019) detected *L. monocytogenes* in 12.3% of the chicken samples. The dominant serotype was determined as 1/2a (92.5%). ERIC-PCR fingerprinting identified ten different DNA profiles. Isolates were MDR resistant to six different antibiotics.

Three of five lytic bacteriophages isolated from waste waters and treated with *ClaI* and *SacI* were able to reduce up to 3.3 log CFU/ml *L. monocytogenes* count in 3 h of incubation at 4 °C. Results suggested that they could be used at final wash or at cooling step in poultry slaughtering process, as well as in decontamination of chicken meat parts.

Three serovars: 1/2a (87%), 1/2c (8%), and 1/2b (5%) of *L. monocytogenes* were detected in the chicken slaughtering line pointing to associated potential risk.

Contamination during processing was considerably indicated by observation of *L. monocytogenes* after packaging, evisceration, and precooling, respectively 8.3%, 2.8%, and 0.9%. The comparison among the isolation rates of *L. monocytogenes* in the cuts (breast fillets, drumettes, drumstick, thigh) and carcasses samples presented a statistically significant difference ($p = 0.017$), and the odds ratios indicated that the chance of the chicken cuts being contaminated by *L. monocytogenes* was twice and half higher than that observed for carcasses (Oliveira et al. 2018).

37.3 Pathogenesis

L. monocytogenes is both a saprophyte and a pathogen depending upon the location, environment, or a host.

L. monocytogenes is able to escape barriers such as stomach acidity, digestive enzymes, non-specific inflammatory attacks, and bile salts with the help of stress-response genes (opuCA, lmo1421, and bsh) and the related proteins.

The major virulence factors are haemolysin, listeriolysin O, invasion associated protein, phosphatidylinositol-phospholipase C (PI-PLC), and delayed type hypersensitivity factor. The primary site of infection is intestinal epithelium. *L. monocytogenes* invades macrophages and intestinal cells. D-galactose residues on its surface attach to D-galactose receptors on the wall of M cells and Peyer's patches in the intestine of hosts for translocating past the intestinal membrane. Its 'internalin (InlA/InlB)' attaches cell membrane 'cadherin' to invade hosts cells. The adhesion molecules are found on the intestinal cell membrane, blood-brain barrier, and foetal-placental barrier. Internalin InlC and InlJ participate in the post-intestinal stages of infection. It survives and grows in macrophages and monocytes as (a) superoxide dismutase protects against the cidal activity and (b) listeriolysin O disrupts the lysosomal membrane. *Listeria* is released in the cell cytoplasm to continue pathogenesis. The actin assembly-inducing protein of the bacteria uses the host cell's machinery to polymerise the cytoskeleton enabling its movement within and cell to cell.

Once blood borne, it spreads to mesenteric lymph nodes, liver, and spleen, and can cause septicaemia, infect macrophages, epithelial cells, endothelial cells, hepatocytes, fibroblasts, and neurons.

37.4 Listeriosis in Human

Human listeriosis is commonly a foodborne illness; less so is contact borne occupationally acquired. Most cases appear sporadic and detected outbreaks are small involving small number of people. Linking most cases to a common source or specific food is difficult. It occurs in two forms, invasive and non-invasive. The latter is more common. In the invasive form, *Listeria* spread from intestine to blood stream and other organs.

There is fever, myalgia often preceded by diarrhoea or other gastrointestinal disorder, stiff neck, confusion, loss of balance, and convulsion. The symptoms are limited to diarrhoea and fever in case of non-invasive form. The incubation period is usually 3–21 days but can be as long as 67 days. Long incubation period makes specific diagnosis difficult.

Compared to other foodborne diseases, hospitalisation is more common. It is the third leading cause of death.

The invasive form is a serious illness. Maternal transmission is high (ca 79%). Perinatal infection including abortion, stillbirth, neonatal sepsis, and meningitis are common. In neonatal listeriosis, symptoms develop within 7 days or classically within 1–2 days. Listeriosis is characterised by fever, myalgia, severe sepsis, meningitis (acquired transvaginally), stillbirth, and death in 20–30% of cases. *L. monocytogenes* is considered the third most important cause of meningitis and invades the spinal cord, brain, brain stem, and meninges; blood stream. It can cause corneal ulcer and pneumonia. In pregnant women (second to third trimester), it causes intrauterine and cervical infection resulting in abortion, stillbirth, or neonates with fetomaternal listeriosis beginning as flu or persistent fever and manifesting in granulomatosis (pyogenic granuloma spread through the body), septicaemia, and physical retardedness.

Occupationally, those assisting parturition, handling new borne calves and infected materials, and slaughterhouse workers are likely to get infection, especially if highly susceptible, although ingestion is the primary route.

The non-invasive form is febrile gastroenteritis manifesting in myalgia, headache, diarrhoea, and headache. Myalgia generally appears shortly after consumption of contaminated foods. Endocarditis, aseptic arthritis, and osteomyelitis may occur but rarely. The incubation period is short, only few days.

37.4.1 Factors Associated with Listeriosis

Listeriosis is dose dependent. Eating >0.04 or 100 CFU/g/ml is infective (WHO/FAO 2004). The probability of illness increases with higher dose. The ability of the food to support growth and measures to limit growth would favour or reduce the risk of foodborne diseases.

Listeriae-specific characters favouring foodborne infection, especially ready-to-eat (RTE) foods are (a) ubiquitous distribution, (b) soil, plant material-forage and surface water as principal reservoirs, (c) ability to multiply at 2–4 °C, and (d) opportunistic pathogen.

It is predominantly associated with ready-to-eat (RTE) foods of large and heterogenous category such as soft cheese, ice cream; salads (including coleslaw and bean sprouts), fresh vegetables and fruits; frankfurters, meat spread (paté), smoked fish (salmon), and fermented raw meat sausages. RTE foods are frequently industrially processed, stored in refrigerators and often consumed without further cooking. Dependence on RTE is high in industrially developed and developing countries.

Other factors determining its occurrence are: food habits, availability, socioeconomic condition, food storage, diagnosis, and reporting.

The social and economic impact is highest among the foodborne diseases although its occurrence is relatively rare.

High risk group includes pregnant (mostly third trimester) women (20× than healthy adults), elderly, and those with weak and/or compromised immunity such as on steroid therapy, transplant cases, and with comorbidities such as HIV/AIDS (300× than healthy adults), leukaemia, and cancer (WHO 2018). Neonates, young and old age (≥65 years), malnourishment, and concurrent diseases such as congenital heart, digestive disorders, and reproductive disorders such as obstetrics and abortions are also at risk.

Pregnancy-associated cases constituted 16.9% of cases (US Listeria initiative during 2004–07). Pregnant women and infants ≤28 days were affected. Maternal infection resulted into neonatal deaths and foetal loss (20.3%), meningitis (32.9%), and sepsis (36.5%). Pregnancy, Hispanic ethnicity, and Mexican style cheese were identified as risk factors (Jackson et al. 2010).

37.5 Contamination of Foods and Outbreaks

The overall occurrence of *L. monocytogenes* reported in India was summed up by Malakar et al. (2019) as follows: cattle faeces (6.0%), raw milk (8.0%), lassi (12.0%), dahi (16.0%), and ice cream (12.0%); fish intestine (1.03%), gill (0.85%), and flesh (0.43%) of samples. The prevalence of *Listeria* spp. in chevon, mutton, and swab samples was reported to be at 1.82%, 3.21%, and 6.66%, respectively.

An analysis of foodborne outbreaks data for the period 2008–2018 EU/EEA for the whole population was made (EFSA 2018). Blanched frozen vegetable (bfv) caused 46 cases requiring hospitalisation, five of them died only in 1 year (2018), compared to dairy foods which caused five outbreaks and 47 cases; fish and seafood nine outbreaks and 63 cases, and meat and meat products 16 outbreaks and 190 cases. Ready-to-eat (RTE) foods constitute the main vehicle of human infections.

Angel et al. (2019) analysed *L. monocytogenes* reported in ProMed during 1996–2018. Human infections are sporadic (11%) and foodborne (65%). Rates increased from 0.06 (1998–2004) to 0.28 (2012–2018), an overall increase of 366% ($p < 0.02$). Foods that were traditionally linked included unpasteurised milk and dairy products, soft cheese varieties; cooked, ready-to-eat sausages and sliced meats (deli meats); refrigerated seafood, smoked seafood, Pâtés and meat spreads. Novel foods linked to listeriosis were RTE: frozen fruits, fresh whole, and pre-cut fruits such as cantaloupe melon, stone fruits (nectarines, peaches, plums, pluots); blueberries, cranberries, peaches, raspberries, strawberries; ice cream, profiteroles, caramel apples; vegetables such as broccoli, cauliflower, peas, onions, peppers, sweet potatoes, corn, sprouts, packaged salad mixes, sandwiches, and wraps. In 24% of events, contaminated foods (not associated with cases) were recalled as precautionary measure and some of these were sandwiches, burritos and bakery products, frozen French fries, ready-to-eat cheeseburgers, varieties of sprouts, and sliced apple.

The rate of contamination of RTE foods in Austria such as smoked fish, seafoods, sausage, soft cheese, and cooked meat from supermarkets was higher than in the household. Eating foods with <100 cfu/g led to shedder status (Wagner et al. 2007). Awaisheh (2010) reported *Listeria* in ready-to-eat meat products (beef and poultry) in Jordan. PCR was used for species identification. The level of contamination was <100 cfu in 97.5%. *L. monocytogenes* was isolated from 23 beef and 18 poultry samples. Syne et al. (2011) observed contamination of 18.3% of retail ready-to-eat-meat products with *Listeria* spp. in Trinidad.

The outbreak in Haalifax, Novoscotia in 1981 is considered as the first foodborne listeriosis. There were 41 cases and 18 deaths, mostly pregnant women and neonates. A cabbage treated with infected sheep manure was used as an ingredient in coleslaw that caused the outbreak (Schlech III et al. 1983). In the recent past, sprouts, celery, and cantaloupe have caused outbreaks. The cantaloupe-caused outbreak in 2011 is the deadliest foodborne in the past 90 years in the US. The Rocky Ford-brand cantaloupe from a single farm, Jensen farms, was contaminated. The epidemic occurred from 31 July to 27 October 2011. Ninety-four percent (131/146) of infected persons distributed over 28 states had consumed the cantaloupe about a month earlier. Ninety-nine percent had to be hospitalised. Jensen farms had to recall some 4800 packages of fresh cut cantaloupe and cut mixed fruit containing it. Although it affected 1–96 years (median 77 years), most ill were <60 years, 58% were female (https://www.cdc.gov/listeria/outbreaks/hispanic-soft-cheese-02-21/details.html).

An outbreak which spread over four states in the USA occurred from 20 October 2020 to 17 March 2021. It affected 13 people of age 1–75 (median 52 years), seven were female. Most (12) were Hispanic. Twelve had to be hospitalised, one died. Two of the four pregnant cases aborted; one gave birth prematurely and the fourth continued pregnancy after recovery. Eight of eleven interviewed reported eating the Hispanic-style fresh and soft cheeses. Seven (88%) reported eating queso fresco—four specifically reported brands made by El Abuelito Cheese Inc., including El Abuelito brand and Rio Grande brand.

The WGS of *Listeria* isolated from El Abuelito brand queso fresco were closely related to the *Listeria* bacteria from sick people. Public health investigators used PulseNet system to identify illnesses that were part of this outbreak. The outbreak is over as of 14 May 2021.

The invasive listeriosis increased over the period 2009–13 in the EU and the European economic area (EFSA 2018). The monthly notified incidence rate for the period 2008–15 showed an increasing trend in the age group >75 years and females 25–44 years (probably related to pregnancies). The increased population size of the elderly and of susceptible in the age group >45 in both genders possibly accounted for the trend.

Quantitative modelling suggested that >90% of invasive listeriosis is caused by ingestion of RTE containing >2000 CFU/g; 1/3 of cases due to growth in the consumer phase.

A multi country outbreak of foodborne listeriosis in the EU occurred during 2015–18 was investigated (EFSA 2020/40). Investigation linked it to blanched frozen vegetable (bfv) eliminating other ready-to-eat food categories. *L. monocytogenes* ST6 was the most relevant pathogen. Compared to per serving cooked bfv, the probability of uncooked bvf causing illness among 65–74 years population was 3600 times. The Quantitative Microbiological Risk Assessment (QMRA) model was used to estimate the risk.

The factors likely to affect bfv are the quality of raw material (pH, $a_{w,}$ natural microbe, antimicrobial compounds) and water, food processing environment, and time-temperature combination for storage and processing (e.g., blanching, cooking).

Specific prerequisite programme and activities such as cleaning and disinfection of the food processing environment (FPE), water control, t/T control, and product information and consumer awareness were suggested for control.

37.6 Diagnosis

Listeriosis is an important disease of animals and also of human beings. The initial diagnosis of listeriosis is made based on clinical symptoms and detection of the bacteria in a smear. Laboratory investigation follows.

Its control in animals is important. Continuous monitoring of animals and farms for *Listeria* infection is required to prevent the spread to human and food production and processing establishments.

37.6.1 Clinical Diagnosis

- Clinical findings and post-mortem lesions may only be suggestive. Laboratory diagnostic methods are thus essential.
- CSF is cloudy, has inflammatory cells, increased mononuclear cells and lymphocytes and protein.
- Post-mortem may reveal meningeal congestion in sheep, panophtalmitis in cattle, yellow necrotic foci in liver, yellow to orange coloured meconium and small erosion in abomasum of aborted lamb.

37.6.2 Laboratory Diagnosis

37.6.2.1 Cultural and Histopathological

The following specimens may be useful—urine, faeces, milk, aborted foetus, meconium, abomasal scraping, vaginal secretion, liver with necrotic foci, spleen, endocardium, myocardium, endometrium placenta in case of abortion and septicaemia;

CSF/brain; vomitus, food/feed. Selective enrichment is achieved by cold and microaerophilic storage of specimens from the brain/CSF but not placenta and foetus. Small haemolytic zone around colony grown on sheep blood agar is seen.

Smear made with foetal abomasal scrapings may demonstrate large number of listeriae.

37.6.2.2 Biological Test

- Intracerebral injection of mouse with brain specimen kills in 2–3 days.
- Severe keratoconjunctivitis in rabbit or guineapig occurs in 24 h after instillation of culture into conjunctival sac (Anton test; https://en.wikipedia.org/wiki/Listeria_monocytogenes).

37.6.2.3 Serological

Tests include FAT/IFAT, IPT, ELISA, Dot-ELISA, AGPT, and CIEP using polyclonal and monoclonal antibodies for specific identification of agent.

Serological survey in animals sets up titres greater than 1:50/1:80 and use of mercaptoethanol to eliminate non-specific IgM.

Heat-killed cells or listeriolysin O antigens may be used for agglutination, AGPT, CIEP, ELISA, and Dot- ELISA tests.

Using listeriolysin O antigen one may use the following assays: ELISA, delayed type hypersensitivity reaction, and IFN-γ assay.

37.6.2.4 Nucleic Acid-Based Tests

Strains are diverse. Subtyping of isolates is necessary for population genetics, tracking source, and epidemiologic investigation. Two methods are phenotyping and genotyping. Serotyping is generally used in investigation of outbreaks and has low discriminatory power. Nucleic acid-based tests are better. Jamshidi and Zeinali (2019) summed up the procedures as follow:

- Random Amplification of Polymorphic DNA-Polymerase Chain Reaction (RAPD-PCR), which is cost effective especially for low number of strains.
- Repetitive Extragenic Palindromes-PCR (REP-PCR).
- Enterobacterial Repetitive Intergenic Consensus-PCR (ERIC-PCR) is highly reliable, simple, economic, and discriminatory (discriminates isolates of the same serotype).
- Pulsed field gel electrophoresis (PFGE), which is time consuming and difficult to standardise.

Pulsed-field gel electrophoresis (PFGE) is rapid and often employed as an initial screening tool.

EU/EEA-wide surveillance system was enhanced for listeriosis. Supranational WGS-enhanced surveillance was initiated in 2018 (Van Walle et al. 2018). The WGS used in South Africa and in other recent outbreaks has allowed the improved identification of genetically related isolates.

37.7 Treatment

A wide range of antibiotics is effective such as ampicillin, amoxicillin, tetracyclines, chloramphenicol, B-lactum antibiotics, aminoglycosides, trimethoprim, and sulphamethaxazole.

Strains of listeriae present a variable resistance to a wide range of drugs. It would be wise to get antibiotic-sensitivity test done to select the drug of choice. Treatment should commence before conception or during early pregnancy.

Supportive therapy is required to correct dehydration, acid base imbalance, and electrolyte disturbance.

37.8 Control in Animals

1. Feed should be stored in dry (not damp/moist) condition. Silage requires special attention. It should be adequately fermented.
2. A live attenuated vaccine in Norway reportedly reduced incidence to 1.5% from 4.0%.
3. As infected animals excrete organisms in excretion and secretion, detection and separation of such animals should be done.
4. Human beings-animal attendants, veterinarians, and consumers of milk/products need to take precaution. Personal protection such as the use of masks and gloves during handling of abortion cases, foetuses, and cultures in laboratory.

37.9 Control and Prevention in Humans

The very first foodborne listeriosis outbreak (Schlech III et al. 1983) illustrated the spread from farm to fork necessitating coverage of the entire chain.

L. monocytogenes persist for years or decades in food processing plant due to (a) growth in niches such cracks and crevices of surface, seals and gaskets which are difficult to clean, (b) biofilm formation, and (c) tolerance to sanitation.

Food safety approach aims at producing safe foods, reducing foodborne illness, gaining consumers' trust, and also improving national and international trade.

Risk assessment, management, and communication are considered to develop structured model to control food control system. One such model for *L. monocytogenes* was developed by WHO/FAO (Y5393e00_*L. monocytogenes*_riskassessment pdf. WHO/FAO 2004).

The following should be useful to control and prevent listeriosis:

1. Surveillance targeting RTE and in industrial countries.
2. Targeted intervention (Silk et al. 2012).
3. Recommendations which include (a) good manufacturing, handling, and storage practices extended to retail and service establishments, (b) training of food

handlers, workers, and managers, (c) educating consumers—cooking RTE before eating, and (d) peoples' participation.

Berzins (2010) observed that post-package pasteurisation of high- and low-fat content cooked sausages at temperatures higher than 55 °C was found to be effective in reducing contamination.

References

Angel ND, Amylee A, Lawrence C, Madoff BL (2019) Changing epidemiology of *Listeria monocytogenes* outbreaks, sporadic cases, and recalls globally: a review of ProMED reports from 1996 to 2018. Int J Infect Dis 84:48–53

Awaisheh SS (2010) Incidence and contamination level of *Listeria monocytogenes* and other *Listeria* spp. in ready - to- eat meat products in Jordan. J Food Prot 73:535–540

Barbuddhe SB et al (2016) Presence of a widely disseminated *Listeria monocytogenes* serotype 4b clone in India. Emerging Microbes Infect 5(6):e55

Berzins A (2010) Molecular epidemiology and heat resistance of *Listeria monocytogenes* in meat products and meat-processing plants and listeriosis in Latvia. http://www.researchgate.net/researcher/53539634_Aivars_Berzins

Cufaoglu G, Ayaz ND (2019) *Listeria monocytogenes* risk associated with chicken at slaughter and biocontrol with three new bacteriophages. J Food Safety 39:e12621

EFSA (2018) *Listeria monocytogenes* contamination of ready to eat foods and risk for human health in the EU. EFSA J 16(1):e05134

EFSA (2020) Public health risk posed by *Listeria monocytogenes* in frozen fruit and vegetables including herbs, blanched during processing. EFSA J 18(4):e06092

FAO (2004) Microbiological Risk Assessment Series 4. Risk assessment of *Listeria monocytogenes* in ready-to-eat foods. Interpretive Summary Y5393e00-L.monocytogenes-risk assessment.pdf

Jackson K, Iwamoto M, Swerdlow D (2010) Pregnancy-associated listeriosis. Epidemiol Infect 138: 1503–1509

Jamshidi A, Zeinali T (2019) Significance and characteristics of *Listeria monocytogenes* in poultry products. Int J of Food Sci 2019:7835253, 7 pages

Kalekar S, Doijad S, Poharkar KV, Rodriguez S, Kalorey DR et al (2015) Characterization of *Listeria monocytogenes* isolated from human clinical cases. Int J Med Health Sci 4(2):206–212

Malakar D, Borah P, Das L, Kumar NS (2019) A comprehensive review on molecular characteristics and food-borne outbreaks of *Listeria monocytogenes*. Sci Technol J 7(2): 2321–3388

Negi M, Vergis J, Vijay D, Dhaka P, Malik SVS et al (2015) Genetic diversity, virulence potential and antimicrobial susceptibility of *listeria monocytogenes* recovered from different sources in India. Pathog Dis 73(9):ftv093

Oliveira TS, Varjão LM, Nunes da Silva LS et al (2018) *Listeria monocytogenes* at chicken slaughterhouse: occurrence, genetic relationship among isolates and evaluation of antimicrobial susceptibility. Food Control 88:131–138

Schlech WF III, Lavigne PM, Bortolussi RA, Allen AC et al (1983) Epidemic listeriosis—evidence for transmission by food. N Engl J Med 308:203–206

Silk B, Date K, Jackson K et al (2012) Invasive listeriosis in the foodborne diseases active surveillance network (FoodNet), 2004–2009: further targeted prevention needed for higher-risk groups. Clin Infect Dis 54(Suppl 5):S396–S404

Syne SM, Ramsubhag A, Adesiyun AA (2011) Occurrence and genetic relatedness of *Listeria* spp. in two brands of locally processed ready-to-eat meats in Trinidad. Epidemiol Infect 139(5): 718–727

Van Walle I, Björkman JT, Cormican M, Dallman T et al (2018) European *Listeria* WGS typing group. Retrospective validation of whole genome sequencing-enhanced surveillance of listeriosis in Europe, 2010 to 2015. Euro Surveill 23(33):1700798

Veterinary Merck Manual (2006) Publisher – Merck &Co. Inc. Whitehouse Station, NJ, USA in association with Merial Ltd. http://www.merckvetmanual.com/mvm/indexjsp

Wagner M, Auer B, Trittremmel C, Hein I, Schoder D (2007) Survey on the *Listeria* contamination of ready-to-eat food products and household environments in Vienna, Austria. Zoonoses Public Health 54:16–22

WHO (2018) Listeriosis. https://www.who.int/news-room/fact-sheets/detail/listeriosis

Bacillus cereus 38

Of foodborne illnesses, *B. cereus* accounted for 2–5%, causing severe nausea, vomiting, and diarrhoea.

38.1 Aetiology

B. cereus sensu *lato* is an opportunist pathogen associated with food poisoning and occasionally soft tissue infections in human. *B. cytotoxicus* is a thermotolerant pathogen occasionally associated food poisoning. *B. cereus* group or *B. cereus* sensu *lato* consists of eight species: *B. anthracis, B. cereus* sensu *lato, B. cytotoxicus, B. mycoides, B. pseudomycoides, B. thuringiensis, B. toyonenesis,* and *B. weihenstephanensis.*

They are gram-positive spore forming rod-shaped motile bacterium.

38.1.1 Spores

B. cereus spores are destroyed by moist heat of 121 °C applied for >5 min (boiling, simmering, stewing, and steaming). Dry heat (grill, broiling, baking, roasting) of 120 °C for 1 h destroys all spores on the exposed surface.

38.1.2 Pathogenesis

These produce haemolysin Bl (Hbl); non-haemolytic enterotoxin (Nhe), and cytotoxin K(CytK), controlled by chromosomal genes *(nhe/hbl/cytK)* in small intestine of the victim to cause diarrhoeal form. The Hbl, Nhe, and CytK are pore forming, insert into cell membrane creating pores and eventual death.

K. G. Narayan et al., *Veterinary Public Health & Epidemiology*,
https://doi.org/10.1007/978-981-19-7800-5_38

The *ces* gene is the most relevant marker for the emetic syndrome caused by cereulide toxin and is produced only by emetic strains. It is a cyclic polypeptide. It binds to the 5-hydroxytryptamine 3(5-HT3) serotonin receptors and activate them leading to the stimulation of afferent vagus nerve. It is resistant to heat, acidity, and proteolysis.

B. cereus group (*B. cereus* sensu *lato*) produce heat labile enterotoxins during growth in small intestine that is diarrhoeagenic. They also produce cereulide, a single heat stable peptide. CytK, Nhe, and HBL toxins are also diarrhoeagenic.

38.1.3 The Phylogenetic Groups

The phylogenetic groups, species, growth temperatures and the distribution of and genes responsible for food poisoning of 391 isolates are summed up in Table 38.1.

Soil, food, and marine sponges are the common source. *B. cereus* sensu *lato* is a common contaminant of foods and spoilage, even at refrigerated temperature due to the hydrolytic enzymes of psychrotolerant strains, ability to grow at a wide range of pH, water activities and temperatures. It is able to form biofilm and adhere on industrial surface increasing the risk of contamination in face of inadequate cleaning procedures. Its detection in food chain may be due to the use of contaminated raw materials. Heat processing of foods favours selection of *B. cereus* sensu *lato* because of heat resistant endospores.

Prevalence of *B. cereus*-like isolates (grown on MYP agar) in Tunisia was 27.8% (191/687) of food samples examined. Most samples (77.5%) had a load of 10^3 cfu/g or ml (allowable level according to Public Health, 2009); 6.8% samples had >10^4/g or ml and these were freshly cut vegetables, cooked foods, cereal, and pastry

Table 38.1 Phylogenetic strains and characteristics (Guinebretière et al. 2010)

			% of strains tested carrying genes				
Phylogenetic groups	Species and other designation	Growth temp. °C	*hbl*	*cyt K-2*	*Cyt K-1*	*nhe*	*ces*
I (I-1, 2)	*B. pseudomycoides*	10–43	41–86	0	0	100	0
II	*B. cereus* II *B thuringiensis* II	7–40	61	13	0	100	0
III (III-1 to 4)	*B. cereus* III *B. thuringiensis* III *B. anthracis* (found only in subgroup III-4)	15–45	12–67	31–73	0	100	0–31
IV (IV-1 to 3)	*B. cereus* IV *B. thuringiensis* IV	10–45	29–34	86–97	79–97	100	0
V	*B. cereus* V *B. thuringiensis* V	8–40	88	0	6	100	0
VI (VI-1, 2)	*B. weihenstephanensis*, *B. mycoides*, *B. thuringiensis* VI	5–37	0–83	0	0	100	0
VII	*B. cytotoxicus*	20–50	0	0	100	100	0

products. A level of $<10^3$/g or ml can also cause food poisoning. It is important to understand that foods can easily be contaminated during handling and processing. They can directly or as an ingredient in processed foods cause poisoning because slow cooling after processing and extended storage at room temperature allow the germination of spores and the growth of bacteria. The surfaces of storage tanks, pipelines, etc. may also be a source of contamination.

PCR test targeting spore structural protein gene (*ssE*) specific to *B. cereus* group identified 91% (174/191). PCR positive isolates were prevalent mostly in cereal products (67.7%) and lowest in (4.8%) in dairy products.

The bacterial endospores which survived the cooking (≤100 °C) can cross the stomach acid barrier to cause illness. When such undercooked food is improperly refrigerated the spores germinate, bacteria grow and produce enterotoxin. Generally, germination and growth occur between 10 °C and 50 °C. Some strains can grow at low temperature. The toxin is highly resistant to heat and withstands a wide range of acidity (pH 2–11). The chances of foodborne illness are enhanced.

38.2 Symptom

B. cereus foodborne illness manifests in two forms—emetic and diarrhoeal.

Diarrhoeal form—IP 8–16 h, gastrointestinal pain and diarrhoea, often confounded with *C. perfringens* foodborne illness; a wide range of food is associated with this form.

Emetic form—The incubation period ranges between 1 and 5 h. Symptoms such as severe nausea, vomiting, and diarrhoea are confounded with *Staphylococcus aureus* foodborne intoxication. Commonly, starchy foods, rice cooked at a temperature and for a time insufficient to kill spores, followed by improper refrigeration, are associated with food poisoning. The toxin 'cerulide' is produced. Heating at 121 °C for 90 min does not inactivate it.

B. cereus causes chronic skin infection and keratitis.

38.3 Prognosis

Most emetic cases recover within 6–24 h. The toxin can cause fulminant hepatic failure in some cases. Septicaemia has been reported in newborns in the UK. They were given total parenteral nutrition that was contaminated.

38.4 Diagnosis

Isolation of >100,000/g from epidemiologically suspected food.

There are two, ISO 7932 and ISO 21871, (International Organization for Standardization) methods for isolation and enumeration of *B. cereus* (Wikipedia 2021).

B. cereus produces lecithinase and is unable to ferment mannitol. Mannitol egg yolk agar with polymyxin is useful. The colonies of *B. cereus* have violet-red background surrounded by a zone of egg yolk precipitate. For identification, the isolate is tested for motility, haemolysis, and rhizoid growth. *B. cereus* ferments ammonium salt-based glucose and not mannitol, arabinose, and xylose.

Vero cells and Caco 2 cells are used to test the cytotoxicity of culture filtrate to evaluate enterotoxicity.

Molecular typing relies on DNA sequencing. Pulsed-gel electrophoresis is useful for epidemiological characterisation and identifying phylogenetic group. It provides a more accurate indication of the associated risk.

38.5 Prevention

Critical points that need attention: (a) general hygiene from harvest through processing and prevention of cross contamination in kitchen, and (b) management of temperature after processing till consumption. Cooked foods should be consumed immediately or rapidly cooled to a temperature of <10 °C and stored in a refrigerator or at >50 °C.

References

Guinebretière MH, Velge P, Couvert O, Carlin F, Debuyser ML, Nguyen-The C (2010) Ability of *Bacillus cereus* group to cause food poisoning varies according to phylogenetic affiliation (groups I to VII) rather than species affiliation. Environ Microbiol 10:851–865

Public Health England [PHE] (2009) Guidelines for assessing the microbiological safety of ready-to-eat foods placed on the market. www.gov.uk/government/publications/ready-to-eat-foods-microbiological-safetyassessment-guidelines

Wikipedia (2021). https://en.wikipedia.org/wiki/Bacillus_cereus

Foodborne Parasites 39

Foodborne parasites are defined as 'any organism that lives in or on another organism without benefiting the host organism; commonly refers to pathogens, most commonly in reference to protozoans and helminths'. The diseases caused are 'neglected group'. Parasite spores, cysts, oocysts, ova, larval, and encysted stages can infect human and may be acquired from the environment, animals (domestic and game), and intermediate hosts. Ingestion of fresh, raw, uncooked, undercooked, processed foods generally causes illness of varying severity. Parasites do not replicate outside live host. A contaminated food along with the parasite is amplified during processing in some cases and the risk of infecting more than few is amplified (sausage made from meat of different origin).

Foodborne diseases in general and those caused by parasites in particular pass unreported. The WHO Foodborne Disease Epidemiology Reference Group (FERG) collects data on global occurrence and estimates the burden. The global burden of foodborne trematodiasis estimated from the data for the year 2005 revealed the number of infected—56.2 million, number with severe sequelae—7.8 million, and dead—7158 (Fürst et al. 2012).

The FAO/WHO expert committee (2014) identified foodborne parasites (Table 39.1). Multicriteria were agreed upon to rank these to recommend risk-management.

Parasites are ranked according to risk (Fig. 39.1).

Multiple criteria were decided. The risk managers put greater weight on potential for increased illness, trade relevance, and impacts to economically vulnerable communities than did experts, but all participants tended to put greater weight on public health criteria. These included the number of outbreaks, global distribution, morbidity rate, severity of illness, mortality rate, acute illness, chronic illness, and burden—disability, economic-, food-pathway trade- relevance. The experts made a score card based on the average of all elicited weights for the criteria. The ranking of foodborne parasites considering quantity and severity of illness, global distribution, increased human burden, trade disruption, and economics is presented in the figure

K. G. Narayan et al., *Veterinary Public Health & Epidemiology*, https://doi.org/10.1007/978-981-19-7800-5_39

Table 39.1 Foodborne parasites

Anisakidae
Anisakis simplex
Anisakis spp.
Pseudoterranova decipiens
***Paragonimus* spp.**
Paragonimus heterotremus
Paragonimus spp.
Paragonimus westermani
Paragonimus kellicoti
***Cryptospridium* spp.**
Crypto sporidium hominis
Crypto sporidium Parvum
***Sarcocystis*spp.**
Sarcocystis hominis
Sarcocystis fayeri
Sarcocystis Suihominis
Diphyllobothriidae
Diphyllobothrium latum
Diphyllobothrium spp.
Diplogonoporus grandis
***Spirometra* spp.**
Spirometra erinacei
Spirometra mansoni
Spirometra mansonoides
Spirometra ranarum
Spirometra spp.
***Fasciola* spp.**
Fasciola gigantica
Fasciola hepatica
***Toxocara* spp.**
Toxocara canis
Heterophyidae
Metagonimus spp.
Centrocestus spp.
Heterophyes spp.
Haplorchis pumilo
Haplorchis spp.
Haplorchis taichui
***Trichinella* spp.**
Trichinella britovi
Trichinella pseudospiralis
Trichinella native
Trichinella murelli
Trichinella papuae

(continued)

Table 39.1 (continued)

Trichinella zimbabwensis
Opisthorchiidae
Opisthorchis felineus
Opisthorchis viverrini

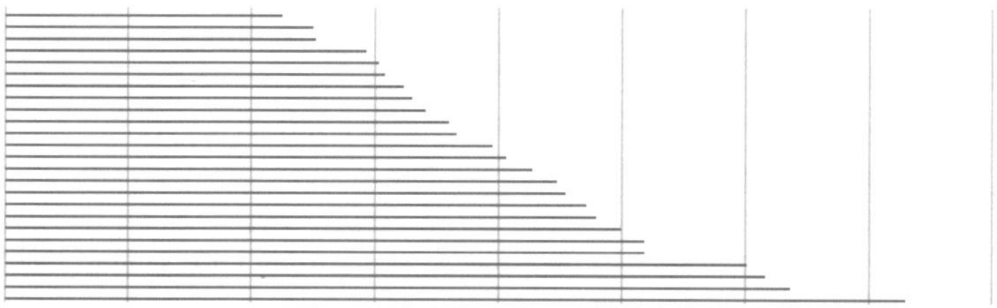

Fig. 39.1 FAO/WHO 2014: Global ranking of foodborne parasites using a multi-criteria ranking tool for scoring parasites, with weighting of scoring criteria based on criteria scores and weights (normalised overall score) elicited from expert meeting participants (Note: *Trichinella* spp.* includes *Trichinella* species except *T. spiralis*)

(normalised overall score). The top ranked parasites have already been identified by FERG and singled out as neglected tropical diseases by the WHO. Some of these are:

Taenia solium: Millions are infected and suffer with neurocysticercosis which is being increasingly reported; associated with traditional pig farming and pig farmers in the regions with poor sanitation and hygiene, and badly managed slaughterhouses; endemic areas are the Andean area of South America, Brazil, Central America, Mexico, China, India, Southeast Asia, and sub-Saharan.

Echinococcus granulosus (hydatid disease) and *E. multilocularis* (alveolar disease): Both represent a substantial burden on the human population; hydatid disease caused 1–3 million DALYs a year costing US$ 2.0 billion and alveolar disease nearly 650,000 DALYs/year; >1.0 million are affected at any one time with many showing severe clinical symptoms.

Toxoplasma gondii: The routes of infection are challenging, foodborne infection—via tissue cysts in various types of meat or organs, or via oocysts contaminating a wide range of food vehicles. Serious health consequences of infection affect all warm-blooded animals including human, 30% of global population infected; pregnant women and immunocompromised are at risk and may develop ocular problem later in life; foetal death, central nervous system abnormalities, or eye disease in child and lifelong suffering; behavioural changes, psychiatric disorder.

Trypanosoma cruzii: Chagas disease is severe and fatal but restricted to certain parts of Central and South America. FERG reported >11,000 deaths in 2004. Trypomastigotes survive in fruits, and juices may be disseminated globally.

Entamoeba histolytica (causing 20–70% fatality), although not a zoonosis, and *Cryptosporidium* spp. appear to be primarily transmitted through food handlers and contaminated water, which can enter the food chain causing illnesses attributed to fresh produce.

Entamoeba histolytica:

Amoebiasis is a common human enteric protozoan disease in tropics. Monkeys, chimpanzees, and apes are non-human hosts. Dogs and cats can be transiently infected but probably do not contribute to transmission. *Entamoeba histolytica* occurs in either trophozoites (fragile) form or cystic (resistant) form. The latter are infectious and commonly found in human stool of those suffering with mild form of disease or are asymptomatic. Survival period in cyst hosts' nails is 45 min, in water about 30 days and for 12 days in moist conditions. Cyst may contaminate the skin of hands and carried under nails and clothes of those who handle and work with non-human primate reservoirs. Infection is per-os, commonly called faecal-oral route and through contaminated water. Male homosexual relation can also be a means of transmission.

In asymptomatic form, the parasite lives upon bacteria and food particles in intestine and usually does not come in contact with the wall of intestines. Invasive amoebiasis is an incapacitating condition affecting male wage earners, requiring confinement or hospitalisation for 2–3 months. It has thus important social and economic consequences. It is potentially fatal. It affects 30–50 million, about 10–20% become clinically ill. The invasive form is seen in about 10%. It kills 55,000 every year. It is common in tropical areas and those who live in poor sanitary conditions, travellers, or are immunocompromised. Amoebiasis is common in China, Southeast and West Asia, and Latin America, especially Mexico. It is endemic throughout India affecting about 15% of Indian population.

Pathogenesis & Disease: *E. histolytica* or Histolytic = tissue destroyer; trophozoites invade the large intestinal wall, bore into walls resulting in colitis. *E. histolytica* secretes digestive enzymes for digestion of food and proteins it ingests. The same is used for digestion of cells of intestinal wall to create flask-shaped ulcersation (bore) and destroying phagocytes. Erythrocytophagocytosis is evidenced by presence of red cells inside amoeba seen during examination of stool.

They can enter the blood stream to invade organs like liver, sometimes spleen, lungs, and even brain. Amoebiasis can be dysentery (intestinal) or (extra-intestinal) liver abscess.

It takes about 2–4 weeks for symptoms to appear. Symptoms begin with constipation followed by water diarrhoea—foul smelling stool, gas, abdominal cramp, and tenderness. The disease may progress to acute form with fulminant mucoid and/or bloody dysentery and consequential anaemia with mild fever, chill, and myalgia. Unchecked or overlooked, there may be intestinal ulceration and perforation, peritonitis. The illness may be prolonged for months and years with remissions. The extension of infection to extra-intestinal organs causes amoebic abscess in liver (jaundice), lungs, pericardium, and the central nervous system. It causes ulceration, perforation, peritonitis, and anaemia.

Diagnosis is based on stool examination. Amoebiasis is preventable through personal hygiene and water sanitation. Chlorination (10 ppm) or heating water to 50 °C or freezing can eliminate cysts. Stool of non-human primates during quarantine should be examined, treated if positive. Metronidazole, paromomycin, iodoquinol, or other suitable drug may be used for treatment.

Cyclospora cayetanensis:

It is more likely anthroponotic. Dogs, ducks, and chickens are neither definitive nor intermediate hosts, although oocysts have at times been found in their faeces. Oocysts found in the faeces of non-human primates were not identical to those of *C. cayetanensis.* It is a coccidian parasite. Unsporulated oocysts in the stool of infected human form spores and become infectious in 7–15 days in the environment. Sexual and asexual multiplication occurs in the intestine of infected man and unsporulated oocysts form and released into the environment with faeces. The cycle of infection continues.

It is endemic in China, Cuba, Guatemala, Haiti, India, Mexico, Nepal, Peru, and Turkey. Infection in travellers suggest its prevalence in other tropical regions also such as Bali, Dominican Republic, Honduras, Indonesia, Papua New Guinea, and Thailand.

Faecal-contaminated drinking water, vegetables, herbs, fruits salads cause infection. The sporulated oocysts excyst in the gastro-intestinal tract, invade cells of small intestines, and cause gastroenteritis. Reportedly, the mean number of episodes of gastroenteritis caused by *Cyclospora* is 11_407 (CI: 137–37_673) with a 6.5% hospitalisation rate. Contaminated lettuce, chives, basil, snow peas, and berries (black berries and rasp berries) have caused infection.

Human infection is manifested as flatulence, watery diarrhoea, nausea, abdominal pain and anorexia, fatigue, and loss of weight. The duration of illness may be 7–15 days. Some cases may suffer with biliary disease, Guillain-Barrè Syndrome and Reiter's Syndrome. Children, old, and immunocompromised are at greater risk.

39.1 Risk Management

Surveillance and monitoring can trace back and locate 'high -risk' regions. Risk management could be applied at the levels of food production: (a) primary production, pre-harvest, (b) post-harvest, and (c) consumer level. Parasites could be prevented at the level of entry to soil, water, meat, and fish. Good farm practices, mass treatment of reservoir hosts, and control in aquaculture may be applied at the primary level of production. Further in the chain of production, the application of farm sanitation and hygiene can minimise faecal contamination of food items eaten uncooked such as lettuce, green vegetables, and salads. Faecal-oral route of transmission of parasites like *Cryptosporidium, Cyclospora, Echinococcus,* and *Giardia* can thus be interrupted. Post-harvest measures include the application of good agricultural practices (GAP) and hazard analysis critical control point (HACCP). Education of producers, processors, and consumers makes the application easy and sustainable. Freezing/cooking—time × temperature combinations, irradiation (for *Toxoplasma*, *Trichinella*) —are methods to destroy pathogens. Processors and consumers need to be made knowledgeable.

Summary of Practices

Pre-harvest control measures:

- Use of good quality water/water with permissible pesticides at prescribed dosage for irrigation and processing.
- Restricting access of livestock and other animals to crop lands and surface waters.
- Using only composted manure as fertilizer.
- Monitoring the health of farm workers and encouraging good hygiene.

Post-harvest level

- Use of good quality water for washing and processing produce.
- Monitoring and enforcing good personal hygiene in food handlers.
- Prevention of cross-contamination.
- Incorporation of HACCP plans.

Consumer level

- Good hygiene and avoidance of cross-contamination.
- Thorough washing of fresh produce.
- Storing produce at −20 °C for >24 h, or at −15 °C for at least a week.
- Cooking.

References

FAO/WHO (2014) Multi criteria - based ranking for risk management of food borne parasites. Microbiological Risk Assessment Series No. 23. Rome. 302pp

Fürst T, Keiser J, Utzinger J (2012) Global burden of human food-borne trematodiasis: a systematic review and meta-analysis. Lancet Infect Dis 12(3):210–221

One Health

40

Abstract

One of the greatest challenges to mankind has been the spread of infectious diseases that emerge or re-emerge at the interfaces of animals, humans, and the ecosystems in which they live. There are several contributing factors for this situation such as the exponential growth in human and livestock populations, rapid urbanisation, change in farming systems, close interaction between livestock and wildlife, encroachment in forest, ecosystems changes, and globalisation of trade in animals and animal product.

The exponential increase in the human population is not only putting pressure on land use, but also led to encroachment of natural forests and their rich and diverse fauna, thus, exposing mans and domestic animals to novel pathogens.

To minimise the global impact of zoonoses, especially those with pandemic potential, *One Health* concept evolved, which has been defined as 'the collaborative effort of multiple disciplines—working locally, nationally, and globally—to attain optimal health for people, animals and the environment'.

This will augment healthcare and public health efficiency; improve medical education and clinical care. Millions of lives will be protected. It is required that One Health stakeholders are connected, strategic networks /partnerships are created. Individuals and groups from around the world work together in the form of an organised team. The concept is accepted and implemented in one or the other forms in some advanced nations, others follow.

K. G. Narayan et al., *Veterinary Public Health & Epidemiology*,
https://doi.org/10.1007/978-981-19-7800-5_40

40.1 The Concept

Human beings have coexisted with animals, plants, and environment since ages. The 'interdependence of animal and human health' was first recognised by Rudolf Virchow in the nineteenth century and furthered probably by his disciple Osler (1849–1919) as 'one medicine' and revived by Dr. Calvin W Schwabe in 1960.

Driven by the current and potential movements of diseases between man, domestic animal, and wildlife, the Manhattan principle of One World One health (OWOH) was conceived on 29 September 2004. The essential feature was the recognition and need for interdisciplinary approach for combating the threatening diseases—West Nile virus, Ebola haemorrhagic fever, SARS, Monkey pox, mad cow disease, and avian influenza.

'"One World, One Health" is an interdisciplinary and cross-sectoral approach to promote and develop a better understanding of the drivers and causes resulting in emergence and spread of infectious diseases' (www.oneworldhealth.org). The concept was developed by and is a trademark of the Wildlife Conservation Society. It was adopted as the basis for a strategic framework in October 2008 to reduce the risks of infectious diseases at the interface of animal–human–ecosystems by a group of international agencies—which included FAO, the World Organisation for Animal Health (OIE), the World Health Organization (WHO), the United Nations Children's Fund (UNICEF)—and by the World Bank and the UN System Influenza Coordinator (UNSIC) (FAO et al. 2008. https://www.preventionweb.net/files/8627_OWOH14Oct08.pdf).

A need for better understanding of the drivers and causes of the emergence and spread of infectious disease was agreed upon during the New Delhi International Ministerial Conference on Avian and Pandemic Influenza held in December 2007. Here, a broad cooperation among the disciplines and sectors is envisaged with focus on emerging infectious diseases at the interface of animal–human–ecosystems, with potential for epidemics and pandemics resulting in wide ranging impacts at the local, regional, national, and international levels. It aims to establish procedures to lower the risk and global impact of epidemics and pandemics of emerging infectious diseases (EIDs). It mandates for better disease intelligence, surveillance, and emergency response systems for wildlife and livestock at all levels. This requires strong public and animal health services along with effective communication strategies. When human health and veterinary disciplines function in isolation, the lack of communication compromises effective control and prevention of EIDs.

A key role is played by the national authorities in devising, financing, and implementing these strategies framework which has five elements:

- building robust and well-governed public- and animal-health systems compliant with the WHO International Health Regulations and OIE international standards, through the pursuit of long-term interventions,
- preventing regional and international crises through the control of disease outbreaks applying improved national and international emergency response capabilities,

- shifting focus from developed to developing economies and from potential to actual disease problems, besides enhanced focus on the drivers of a broader range of locally important diseases,
- promoting wide-ranging collaboration across sectors and disciplines,
- developing a rational and targeted disease-control programme through the conduct of strategic research.

40.2 The Objective

The strategic framework has an overall objective for an international public good. It does not prioritise diseases to target. It aims to benefit the poor by helping to reduce the risks of infectious diseases of local importance—e.g., tuberculosis, brucellosis, rabies. The One World, One Health (OWOH) paradigm to improve global, national and local public health, food safety and security, besides livelihoods of poor farming communities everywhere apart from protecting fragile ecosystems (FAO 2009).

The cost of human-animal diseases impacted India, Nigeria, and Ethiopia the most (Gilbert 2012). Livestock contributed up to half the income of poor families and 6–35% of their protein intake. Increasing demand and market expanding globally for livestock products provide opportunity for the farmers to come out of poverty. Zoonotic diseases pose major obstacles. The study estimated that one out of eight animals in poor countries is affected by brucellosis, causing reduction in milk and meat production of cattle by 8%. Additionally, a sign of current or past infection with bacterial foodborne disease was shown by 27% of livestock in developing countries. Thirteen zoonoses together caused 2.4 billion human cases of illness and 2.2 million deaths every year. There are 1415 microbes causing human diseases, of which 75% are zoonoses (Brown 2004).

40.3 Definition

'One Health' is defined as a collaborative, international, cross-sectoral, multidisciplinary mechanism to address threats and reduce risks of detrimental infectious diseases at the animal-human-ecosystem interface (http://www.fao.org/ag/againfo/home/en/news_archive/ 2010 one-health.html).

VPH is route to 'One Health'. It is multidimensional and is already connected to veterinary medicine and animal production and has the potential to connect outside with wildlife and global public health (Narayan 2011). *VPH is 'the sum of all contributions to the complete physical, mental and social well-being of humans through an understanding and application of veterinary medical science'.*

Several good reviews of endemic and emerging infectious disease (EIDs) have appeared to define 'drivers' and suggestions. Kilpatrik and Randolph (2012) reviewed the drivers of vector-borne diseases (VBDs). Karesh et al. (2012) discussed the complex nature of the ecology of zoonoses. Extending the theory of natural nidality to the understanding of EIDs has led to the identification of the causes or 'drivers' that challenge a 'balanced ecosystem/landscape' and create bridges between pathogen and susceptible population that need to be understood to plan control measures (Daszak et al. 2001). Chomel et al. (2007) identified 'drivers' and classed them as: (a) micro-genetic changes mutation in pathogen, e.g. HPAI, vector, e.g. *Aedes albopictus* and (b) macro-agricultural practices, modification of habitats, human behaviour [see manuscript VBDs]. Lambin et al. (2010) suggested an integrated analysis at the landscape scale for a better understanding of interactions between changes in ecosystems and climate, land use and human behaviour, and the ecology of vectors and animal hosts of infectious agents.

Constituents of inter-sectoral teams would vary depending upon the 'drivers' and these are diverse. However, health, veterinary, and the affected/concerned human population would be common in all such teams.

40.3.1 Understanding the 'Drivers' and Sectors

The phrase 'emerging infectious diseases' was coined by the American microbiologist Joshua Lederberg. Microbes possess enormous potential mechanisms of genetic diversity unlike human. Their numbers, rapid fluctuations, and amenability to genetic change provide tools to microbes for adaptation that far outpace what human can generate on any short-term basis. Host determinants are immunity, physiology, population, behaviour, travel-transport, societal, commercial, and iatrogenic. Environmental determinants are ecological and climate. Population and their domestic animal movement—into arthropod habitat cause emergence, e.g. emergence of yellow fever is linked to entry of human into the jungles of Central America to construct the Panama Canal leading to deforestation and creation of new tropical forest and farm margins thereby exposing the free and domestic livestock to new arthropods and the viruses they harboured. Viral infections of Brazilian woodcutters who cleared Amazon Forest, with Mayaro and Oropouche viruses as examples.

40.4 Ecology and Evolution

Interaction between populations of two species, pathogens and hosts, creates conditions favouring the evolution of a pathogen. The interaction of waterfowl, domestic poultry, and then human beings is considered to have led to the emergence of H5N1 (Guan and Smith 2013).

Culling of infected poultry has so far not allowed the mutation of H5N1 to cause epidemic in human population. Inter-sectoral collaboration such as the departments of health and animal husbandry, administration, poultry farmers, and traders in a country, and hooking the efforts to international organisations such as OIE and WHO has brought this result.

40.4.1 Land Use Change, Extractive Industries and Zoonoses

Humans venturing into forest may get exposed and infected with pathogens naturally maintained, e.g. Ebola, Lyme disease. Humans, thus, act as sentinel. Entry into forests may be for hunting, recreation, search of foods, extractives such as coal, iron, etc. (mining), oil and gas followed by deforestation for agriculture and commercial agri-farming. Lyme disease—burden and spatial distribution in the USA was an outcome of historical deforestation and reforestation and habitat fragmentation; human alveolar echinococcosis in Tibet caused by *Echinococcus multilocularis* has been correlated with overgrazing and degradation of pastures resulting to the increase in small mammal (intermediate hosts) densities. Similar alteration may also be natural. Rinderpest depopulated cattle population in Africa forcing tsetse flies to feed upon human beings causing sleeping sickness.

Sectors that need to be integrated to control/prevent such infectious diseases are the departments of Forest, Mining, Oil & Natural Gas, Agriculture.

40.4.2 Increasing Demand of Animal Produce for the Expanding Global Population

The increased demand for high quality animal products has substantially increased the risk of foodborne zoonoses that are part of the production chain from agriculture/ livestock and poultry and their produce—brucellosis, tuberculosis, salmonella, campylobacter, etc. There is an additional demand for wildlife meat.

It is estimated that central African countries alone consumed 1.0 billion kg meat of wild animal. Wildlife meat—rearing of deer, wild boar, or forest restaurants as in China, etc. for delicacies may lead to new zoonotic infections, e.g. Corona, SARS.

Sectors that need to be integrated are the departments of Foods, Food Industry, Dairying, Livestock, Poultry & Egg and Meat Industry, Agriculture Marketing, and Food Quality Control.

40.4.3 Increasing Demand for Food and Antimicrobial Resistance (AMR)

The following are based on FAO (2020) report, Chap. 2 on climate change:

To meet the demand of a growing population, the agricultural production has to be increased across the globe. Agricultural intensification has increased the dependence on the use of fertilisers, pesticides, and antimicrobials. The microbial resistance against these agents is emerging and the effectiveness of these agents is reducing. Antibiotics used against human pathogens are sprayed on plants; nearly 73% of global use is in meat production. Antibiotics therapy failed by >50% in pigs and 40% in chickens. Horizontal transfer of plasmids mediated resistance genes in microbes may be facilitated by warmer temperatures This has serious public health implications, leading to an estimated death of 700,000 people every year due to drug-resistant diseases (including non-foodborne diseases).

According to CDC, antibiotic-resistant foodborne pathogens caused 430,000 cases every year in the United States of America., e.g. *S. Infantis* in 2019 through raw chicken products, *S. Urbana* in 2017 through papayas, besides many others (FAO 2020). Recently, in the Democratic Republic of Congo, there was isolation of extensively drug resistant *S. typhimurium* ST313.

The prevalence of fungal infections is likely to increase in climate change-led warmer temperatures. *Candida auris* (currently a great health threat) may be grown at 37 °C—adapted to grow in climate-change led warmer conditions. Azoles, as fungicides, are extensively used in crop protection and as antifungal drugs in human and animal healthcare. Rapid emergence of resistance has led to nearly 100% patient mortality. Azole-resistant *Aspergillus* was found in agricultural soils of Colombia where vegetable crops are grown.

Rapid mitigative response required a One Health approach. International Food Safety Authorities Network (INFOSAN) provides a channel for the rapid information exchange of imminent threats of foodborne diseases among members. Cross-sectoral and integrated surveillance, monitoring, and transparent data sharing form key aspects.

40.4.4 Import of Wildlife and Other Products

It brings in pathogens endemic in the exporting country, e.g. *Y. pestis* with rodents, *Francisella tularensis* with prairie dog. Import may be legal or illegal. Agents of wildlife origin are H5N1, Nipah, and Corona-SARSV. Simian retroviruses—simian foamy virus (SFV), simian immunodeficiency virus (SIV), simian human-T-lymphotropic virus (HTLV), human immunodeficiency virus (HIV) [HIV-1 and HIV-2 emerged because of a number of spill over events of SIV from non-human primates (NHPs), chimpanzees, and mangabeys, respectively, which were likely hunted for bush meat in central and western Africa. Azad (2004) highlighted human health risks of the unregulated trade of wild-caught animals. Export and import of animals alter the composition of native flora and fauna, and the translocation of animals facilitate pathogens to jump species and get established in population of native animals.

Sectors that need to be integrated—Wildlife trade, Laboratories using animals, Import-Export Control agencies, Animal Quarantine centres.

40.4.5 Climate Change

The El Niño events of 1991–92 and 1997–98 led to human Hantavirus cases in the south-western USA via an ecological cascade. Increased vegetation consequential to El Niño led to precipitation that caused increased rodent population and mild or subclinical infection with Hantavirus. Human exposure increased.

The number of cholera cases increased during 2000 and 2014 during El Niño events by 50,000 in East Africa (Moore et al. 2017).

Climate-induced changes in the environment will cause an increased net burden of food- and waterborne diseases, varying with pathogens, geographic distribution, persistence of pathogens in environment, and rate of transmission. Animals under heat stress shed enteric pathogens. Some may replicate faster. Pathogens with low infective dose will be more likely to cause food poisoning. Morbidity burden due to Salmonella, Campylobacter, and rotavirus is likely to increase. An increase of temperature by 1 °C (beyond the ambient) caused increase in cases of salmonellosis by 5–10% in several European countries, of *C. jejuni* by 16.1%, of *C. coli* by 18.8% in Israel (ambient temperature of 27 °C), and rota viral diarrhoea by 40.2% for each 1 °C rise in threshold temperature of 29 °C (FAO 2020).

Sectors/institutions/professional to combine are—Environment and Environmentalist, Epidemiology and Predictive Epidemiologist, Microbiology and related Research institutions.

40.4.6 Natural Disaster: The Plague Epidemic in India (1994)

The plague occurred between mid-August to first week of October 1994. There were 234 deaths. The epidemiological investigation in Mamla, district Beed, Maharashtra linked this epidemic with the 1993 earthquake in Latur. Mamla village had the first warning—'rat fall' in mid-August (Tysmans 1994). The survivors of earthquake in September 1993 had converted the old, damaged homes into granaries and used them. The rodent and flea population grew exponentially; the intensity of flea infestation was 1.8 between October 1993 and July 1994 in these granaries (Saxena and Verghese 1996). An admirable relief and rehabilitation operation during and after earthquake had been carried out. Possibly it was beyond imagination that these sites would become a natural nidus of *Y. pestis,* and epidemic would be caused after a year. Disaster management system needs to be more holistic.

40.5 How to Make This Concept Workable?

Let us go back to the '"recommendations of the strategic framework" to make a robust and well-governed public- and animal-health system compliant with the WHO International Health Regulations and international standards of OIE'. This requires a 'national authority and funding'. Considering the diverse nature of the 'drivers', the nation needs to be empowered to select the most relevant authority, for the 'inter-sectoral team'. The United Kingdom made a comprehensive ministry—Department of Environment, Food and Rural Affairs (DEFRA). Reviewing the state of Public Health in India, John et al. (2011) suggest India 'to rethink. . .revise health policy, broaden the agenda of disease control. . . make it comprehensive, redesign health system'.

Responding to the challenges of the modern society requires a holistic approach encompassing a comprehensive multi-sectoral and multidisciplinary approach. Here, the One Health approach fits best, which has also been advocated by the WHO, FAO, and OIE (Bhatia 2019). However, it faces major challenges on various accounts such as fragmented governance of medical, veterinary, and environmental sectors marred with host of disagreements among these sectors. There is also lack of a clear understanding among the stake holders about the application and benefits of One Health concept.

It is with this background that an effective application of One Health approach needs apart from the scientific understanding of the issues, a strong political commitment to have a sustained financial and administrative support for the policy formulation, inter-institutional collaboration, information sharing, and implementation. Although a simple concept, it has a highly complex process for its implementation (Bhatia 2019).

40.5.1 Horizontal Integration of Sectors may be a Solution (Explained Below; Fig. 40.1)

Ministries/departments generally function like '"Vertical" organisations'. The institutions (e.g., health, veterinary sectors) operate independent of one another, restricting to their respective disciplines or sectors. The system is beset with certain gaps and sometimes overlaps.

The priority of health sector in most countries (particularly resource-poor countries) is primary health care and diseases causing the highest burden, such as mortality in child and mother, and control of HIV/AIDS, malaria, and tuberculosis. The highest priority in veterinary services is 'diseases of trade', e.g. FMD, PPR, classical swine fever.

Both sectors fail to afford working on zoonoses (Fig. 40.1). Wildlife agencies are concerned with deaths of monkeys due to KFD. Zoonotic infections, as seen in the

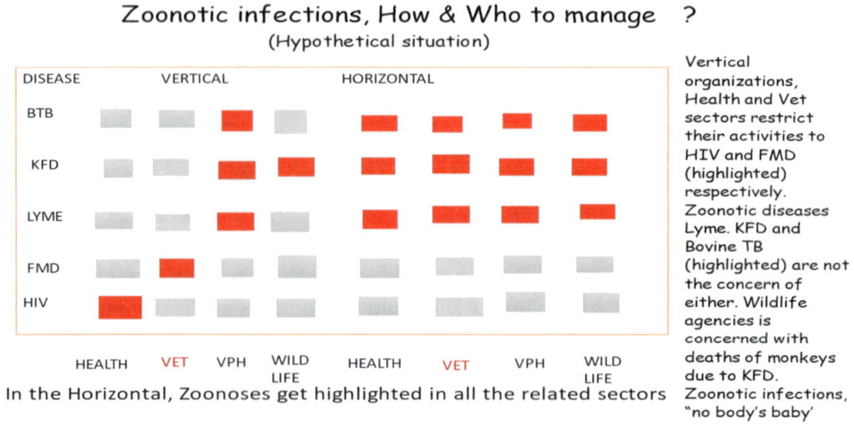

Fig. 40.1 Horizontal integration of sectors

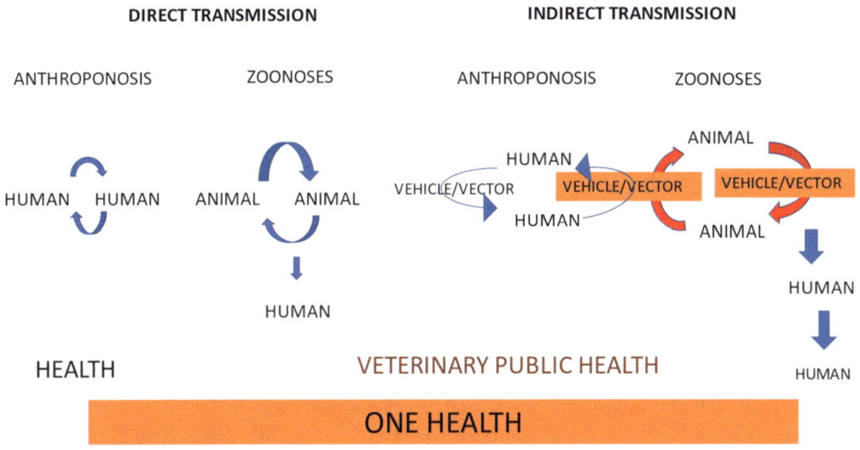

Fig. 40.2 VPH as core of One Health

figure remain 'nobody's baby'. VPH working at domestic & pet animal-human interface should be working at wildlife-human interface, expanding to environmental and wildlife health. This would reduce the burden on health sector.

What is the remedy? Creating another vertical or integrated approach as has been suggested (World Bank 2010). See horizontal in the figure above.

The integrated approach reorients thinking along the horizontal line. The thought process 'What is my responsibility?' *'It is not my job'* in a vertical sector is oriented to *'the work needs to be done'*. The problem is addressed 'additively' through effective communication between each and relaying the efforts made by one to the other for further action like in a relay race.

In the absence of horizontal integration, communication gap (see below Q fever) and dispute are likely to happen.

Bovine TB nearing eradication in England met a barrier in the form of Badger TB (reservoir). The dispute between the two vertical sectors, veterinary and wildlife, was settled, and cull was allowed. A single cull was effective for 6.5 years. Tackling BTB benefited both domestic and wildlife in Australia.

Operationally, this horizontal integration may be limited to/begin with surveillance and monitoring, extendable to areas when needed.

Creating 'One Health' organisation as an option has a merit of inherent 'authority to decide and act on time' which is diluted in horizontal system. Action related to saving life/stopping transmission cannot wait for a debate (among sharers of responsibility) or command to trickle. VPH concept is older to One Health. VPH neither take off even after decades nor One Health after its birth in 2008. A VPH organisation covers most of the human infectious diseases (Fig. 40.2). A functional VPH organisation would have certainly prevented epidemics of diseases such as West Nile fever, Rift Valley fever, and Swine fever, and contributed to reducing disease burden due to bird flu and SARS. Building over it an organisation like One Health would have been easy. VPH has acceptance everywhere, but implementation is limited to some advanced countries. It is sad that highly populated countries with problems where VPH may have answers and could contribute significantly, an organisation of VPH is non-existent.

Where to find a professional man for One Health? It requires engagement of multiple sectors and community education. Rift Valley Fever (RVF) as example illustrates that knowledge of veterinary medicine is essential to control disease in animals. VPH for stopping RVF spread to human and human medicine for attending the ill humans. Combination of veterinary and health professionals, viz. One Health is essential. Veterinarian needs additional knowledge about human medicine and a physician needs to know zoonoses. Veterinary education and practice have inherently strong base of 'preventive medicine'. Further, a veterinarian is a 'comparative pathologist, medicine...' professional. A bridge course for both and orientation on public health (preventive medicine) will make them a One Health professional.

The University of Florida, University of North Carolina in the US and Centre for One Health Education, Advocacy, Research and Training, Kerala Veterinary and Animal Sciences University are some institutions offering courses on One Health.

A vertical One Health organisation with career opportunities and employment appears necessary for the translation of the concept into a functional structure.

One must not undermine 'individual care/case-oriented medicine (clinical medicine)'. There is a huge burden of saving life in the face of the pandemic, say Ebola.

Strong disease intelligence, monitoring, surveillance, scanning and risk assessment, and effective communication systems are essential for the management of epidemic/pandemic.

Reporting diseases, especially Public Health Emergency of International Concern (PHEIC):

It needs to be compliant to the International Health Regulations (IHR) that legally binds countries to report a disease constituting PHEIC. Often, reporting of animal disease has major trade implications. Therefore, OIE member countries have accepted the legal obligation to notify the organisation of an emerging animal disease under Terrestrial Animal Health Code of OIE.

Common reporting procedures and communication channels in the event of an outbreak is important. The *communication channels* to bridge professional and institutional divisions, public and animal health agencies need to be defined. Some Global Disease Information Systems (World Bank 2010) are:

1. Global Public Health Information Network (GPHIN) WHO—Influenza, Polio, SARS and Smallpox + any emergency of Public Health concern.
2. Global Outbreak Alert and Response Network (WHO)—follows up GPHIN identified problem.
3. Programme for Monitoring Emerging Diseases (ProMED) is a reporting system of the International Society for Infectious Diseases.
4. Global Early Warning System for Major Animal diseases (GLEWS)—tracks diseases in high-risk areas. Principal source of data is FAO, OIE, WHO and ProMED, and GPHIN.

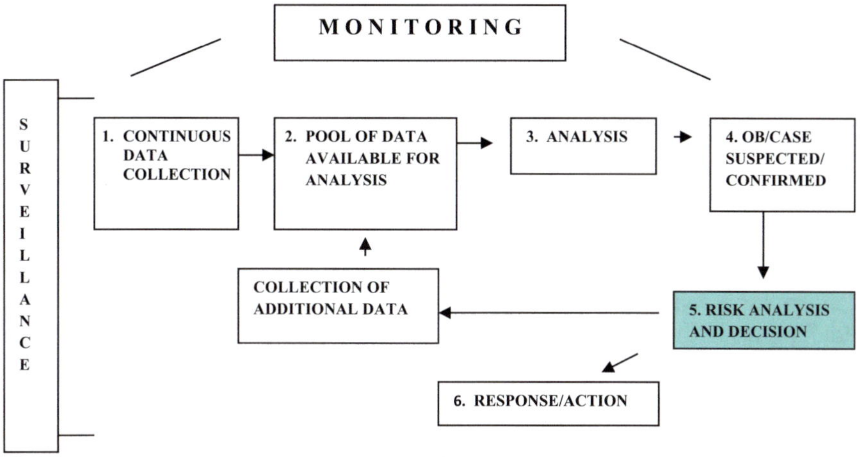

Fig. 40.3 Surveillance system

5. World Animal Health Information Database (WAHID) of disease reported to OIE.
6. Med-Vet-Net—European database on zoonoses and foodborne for prevention and control.

   The important US systems are

7. Global Emergency Infections Surveillance and Response System (GEIS) for infections potential health risk for US military personnel.
8. Emerging Infectious disease Network (EIN) – of US CDC.

Monitoring (1–4 in the Fig. 40.3) is data collection and detection of a case or an outbreak. Risk analysis and decisions (5 in Fig. 40.3) and response actions (6 in Fig. 40.3) makes the system a surveillance system (Vrbova et al. 2010). Actions 1–6 need to be fast, faster than the cycle of spread.

Surveillance is an on-going systematic collection, collation, and analysis of data with timely dissemination of information to the concerned so that action can be taken. *Monitoring* is continuous and on-going or intermittent or episodic with no response.

Scanning

Websites on disease information and digitalisation of data allow opportunity to scan these and analyse. In the UK, Horizon scanners include Health Protection Agency (HPA), Veterinary Laboratory Agency (VLA), DEFRA, UKZG (UK Zoonoses group), Department of Health (DH), Food Safety Agency (FSA), Advisory Committee on Dangerous Pathogens (ACDP), Chief Medical officer (MO) and CVO (Chief Veterinary Officer). They consult global information system sites (vide supra and more).

They prepare a document and circulate to members of (a) National Expert Panel on New and Emerging Infections (NEPNEI), (b) Department of Health, and

(c) others working in the protection of Human and animal health (Walsh and Morgan 2005).

This facilitates the integration of human and animal health surveillance data, experts, and officials.

Example 40.1 From mainland Asia, Ebola virus infection in wildlife has been detected. A total of 276 bats of different genus tested for antibodies to Ebola Zaire (ZEBOV), a highly lethal *Filovirus*. 5/141 (3.5%) *Rousettus leschenaultia* bats were seropositive. This and other fruit bat species visited palm trees ten times more than *Pteropus* spp. found associated with human Nipah infection and disease caused by drinking date palm sap which was contaminated with bat excreta in Bangladesh (Olival et al. 2013). Nipah has been reported in India too.

The scanners have to examine 'the risk' this finding poses to India.

In the UK, scanners refer to expert group. Once confirmed as 'potential risk'—a statement is issued to DH, HPA, UKZG, ACDP, CMO, CVO, and others for action. If the risk is negligible, a statement to this effect is issued and 'monitoring' is continued.

Bio-surveillance is the detection of disease outbreaks in real-time. Collection, collating, and analysis of data from various places and different sources are done. This is the approach to fight bioterrorism. The United States has developed Real-time Outbreak Diseases Surveillance (RODS) and is able to detect a probable bioterrorism within a shortest possible time. The Global Emerging Infections Surveillance and Response system of the USA is used for worldwide bio-surveillance.

Communication channels have to open, and communication made fast.

The Dutch government was faulted in a massive Q fever outbreak and delayed in responding because the issue was being handled by two ministries—of Agriculture and Health that did not communicate well (Martin Enserink, 24th November 2010, 2:19 PM Science Insider http://news.sciencemag.org/scienceinsider/2010/11/dutch-government-faulted.html#more). More than 4000 people fell ill since the outbreak of Q fever that started in 2007, and 14 died. Robust control programme was launched, including compulsory vaccination of goats and sheep and the culling of 62,500 pregnant animals from infected farms. So far, only 382 persons have fallen ill with Q fever in 2010, as compared to over 2300 in 2009.

Example 40.2 Identification of Developing 'Driver'-Anthropogenic and Socio-Economic Changes The earlier system of Government Pig Breeding farms cum Bacon factories in India had built-in arrangement to assure freedom from diseases, identification of sick/infected pigs, and traceability. This failed to meet the increasing demand and was replaced by a cluster of private small farmers but lost the three important ingredients of ensuring safety to pig farmers and pork consumers. Pig farming is remunerative, attracted many who have adopted it as a business. Rural market and consumers have sprung. Pigs are reared in small holdings. However, all in the chain from rearing pigs through slaughter, marketing and consumers are not aware of the associated biohazards—zoonoses such as *Salmonella*, Hepatitis E virus (oral/environmentally spread), and mosquito-borne Japanese encephalitis and bat associated Nipah virus. Similarly, the butchers and processors are ignorant. Meat inspection is absent. *Salmonella*, Hepatitis E virus, Nipah virus, *Taenia solium* (cysticercosis), Trichinellosis, and Toxoplasma occur. Narayan (2012a, b) explained the application of the concept of One Health and suggested the monitoring of these infections and meat inspection with harmonised epidemiological indicator.

Example 40.3 Illustrates the Effectiveness of One Health Approach in Control of a Pandemic In February 2003, SARS was first reported in China. By the time the WHO declared the outbreak over on 5 July 2003, more than 8000 cases were reported in 32 countries across the world with over 800 fatalities. The rapidity of spread, international intervention and emergency response, the speed with which the authorities in different nations responded, and peoples' cooperation that led to its control are appreciated.

Lessons learnt are:

1. Select weapons that have speed faster than the speed of transmission of infectious agent.
2. Understand the drivers of emergence—this knowledge enables 'prevention of recurrence of similar events'.
   It is complex and difficult to understand the 'drivers' of emergence of infection. SARS-CoV was identified in palm civet (*Pagumala varta*) and other species in wet markets of mainland China. Palm civet was consumed in winter as substitute for fresh fruit often not available in winter. It was believed that eating the animal (colloquially known as 'fruit fox' or 'flower fox' because of its dietary preferences) provided the same health benefits as eating fruit, and they are healthier (with better taste) compared with the grain-fed farmed counterparts. In August 2003, a causal model was developed by a mission of the WHO to China with (a) interacting natural, (b) market, (c) human, and (d) peri-human animal components to conceptualise the likely complexity of the market system and to identify possible control points for transmission. For example, the regulation (or elimination) of the trade in wild-caught wildlife might help in the control of transmission to market and farm populations, and thereby to humans, and elimination of infection in the farmed wildlife population. Transmission within this group might be controlled by on-going monitoring, thus, to wildlife markets and humans.
3. Immediate control measures—this required intelligence, planning, pooling of resources, mustering authoritative support, and funds for action.
4. SARS was controlled by following the 'traditional intervention' methods (Bell and World Health Organization Working Group on Prevention of International and Community Transmission of SARS 2004). Connecting with the WHO for advice and action. Control at airports—use of thermal scanning to detect patients among the arrivals; identify and isolate infected persons and contacts; monitor and quarantine, infection control in healthcare settings were useful.

Example 40.4 Illustrates the One Health Approach in Efforts To Control Hendra Viral Infection A case study was conducted by Landford and Nunn (2012)—the management of incidents of Hendra virus in Australia using One Health approach. Seventy cases in horses and seven in human with four deaths were reported in Queensland and New South Wales (NSW) in Australia since it was recognised in 1994. The virus spilled from bats and shedding increased significantly as revealed in 2011. In June and July 2011, a cluster of cases were reported leading to the formation of an intergovernmental Hendra task force by the Premier of Queensland and the Premier of NSW comprised of senior managers. This required the arrangement of specialised skills with broad collaboration across a wide range of disciplines to understand the ecology of bat and epidemiology of Hendra viral infection and to develop mitigation strategies.

Drivers for spill over of virus, transmission identified:

- seasonal translocation of bats to areas providing food sources (during 1994–2010 dry season),
- clearing of natural vegetation led to bats' translocation to vegetation in urban and peri-urban areas,

Transmission and mitigating strategies:

- horses shed virus even before appearance of symptoms and are infectious,
- the candidate vaccine antigen is identified and tested, and found to provide excellent protection against clinical disease in horses and reduce viral shedding.
- convey the key messages to veterinarians and horse owners about appropriate biosecurity and personal protective.

The Singapore experience

Often, the Public Health department is caught unaware when an epidemic appears, especially so when it is due to EID. The situation is like managing a crisis. Singapore experienced SARS epidemic. The first case was detected on 6 March 6 and the last on 11 May 2003; by 30 July, the epidemic ended as a result of rapid action. According to Quah and Hin-Peng (2004), Singaporeans had faith in the public health and environmental regulations, government's efficiency and readiness to control the epidemic. The public was educated through campaign—symptoms of SARS, the need to wash hands, especially after coughing, sneezing and nose cleaning, and accepted quarantine and other restrictive measures with discipline. Subsequent to successful control of the new disease, SARS, a continuous scrutiny on all fronts—people entering the country, people at home and laboratory—was desired.

40.6 Advantage of One Health and Advocacy

One Health epidemiological studies are aimed at improved animal, human, and ecosystem health, and expected to reveal relationship that are bi- and/or multi-directional between animal and human health and their relation to their ecosystems (healthy or otherwise). Inter-sectoral collaboration is made easy. It implies that study, data, analysis, and interpretation are integrated. This is advantageous compared to silo-type studies limited to animal/human/ecosystem in many ways. The time of detection is reduced, access to care improved, intervention accelerated, cost is shared, and the intervention at source and food security are made possible. The results are satisfying as human and animal lives are saved, their suffering minimised, and the ecosystem services are improved such as reforestation, safe water, and clean pasture.

Advocacy is required. It is *'a process through which groups of stakeholders can be influenced to gain support for and reduce barriers to specific initiatives or programmes'.* Six advocacies were identified by the WHO (2009), namely (a) Social, (b) Administrative, (c) Legislative, (d) Regulatory (e) Legal, and (f) Media. Strategic advocacy plan includes one or more of these.

Community education and awareness is of prime importance. The drive against vaccination in general led to the reversion of measles epidemic in countries from where it had been eliminated. Microbes have enormous mechanisms, number, replication rate, amenability to genetic change, etc. for adaptation to what human activities create.

40.7 Methods of Disease Control and Prevention

The disease control and prevention methods are traditional, useful, and have not changed. These are isolation, quarantine, increasing 'social distance', personal protective measures (masks, gloves, etc.), culling, host population control, mass vaccination, chemotherapy and chemoprophylaxis, and environmental control such as sanitation, disinfection, vector-control, and mass education.

One uses weapons after the presence of a pathogen inside a territory or in the neighbourhood has been reported. Therefore, making strong disease intelligence and response system is important as outlined above.

Few examples on the use of these weapons are as follows:

Culling of bird flu infected poultry has succeeded in preventing the mutation of H5N1 to a pandemic strain. In the USA, a campaign followed by accelerated vaccination of pet dogs succeeded in pushing rabies to its natural wildlife habitat. However, the status of protection at the dog population level and immunisation schedule needs to be monitored. Watanabe et al. (2013) observed that the schedule of vaccination followed in Japan provided adequate protection, but the registration system and vaccination need to be improved to ensure that more number of dogs are vaccinated against rabies. Combined sterilisation and vaccination of street dogs is currently the accepted method of rabies control. In Bhutan, the 2008 outbreak appeared to follow the road networks, towns, and areas of high human density associated with large, free-roaming dog population. Culling of such dogs was necessary and controlled the outbreak (Tenzin et al. 2010). Effective media reporting increases the demand for Rabies Post Exposure Prophylaxis. The US Centers for Disease Control and Prevention (CDC) customarily issues instructions to the stake holders after a disease is identified—e.g., once poultry-associated *Salmonella* is detected, poultry breeders, traders, processing plants, consumers and others are posted with relevant information on preventive measures. Randolph et al. (2010) observed that the campaign protected people from Tick Borne Encephalitis in Latvia. Zoonoses such as SARS, Swine flu, plague, Marburg, and Nipah spread fast by human-to-human transmission once it has spilled over to human. Making clinicians aware and hospitals equipped have helped controlling these.

Health is an individual's concern and property. There are numerous health issues that cannot be solved by any one individual. Public Health and Veterinary Public Health are therefore required. The PH and VPH are like a 'team sport' and not an 'individual sport' such as a 100 m race. Good performance of the team requires a synchronised and harmonised orchestrated performance of each dedicated player. Even healthcare in a hospital requires stitching together responsibilities and activities of doctors, nurses, sanitary workers, etc. Nosocomial infections and bacterial drug resistance develop in hospital setting. Animal food production chain is another setting where bacterial drug resistance develops. The extension of the concept of One Health often becomes necessary to control/prevent these. Anybody can report a disease but action is initiated only after 'notification'. Notification is done only by an 'authority'. This is the beginning of 'One Health' activities. Thus "One health' is inherently 'inter-sectoral'. Narayan (2012a) appealed to the professionals of different disciplines/sectors to demolish 'barriers-whatsoever' and implement health programmes. Citing Swami Swatmanandan, President and Acharya, Chinmaya Mission, Mumbai (www. transformingindians.org) he reiterated—'implement the great vision of "one health" and do not let it remain an "imagination"'. Success with SARS and bird flu has proven that we are a peaceful, strong global family.

Abbas et al. (2011) assessed 'rabies control initiative in Tamil Nadu' to conclude that it is possible to implement a successful 'One Health' programme in an environment of strong political will, evidence-based policy innovations, clearly defined roles and responsibilities of agencies, coordination mechanisms at all levels, and a culture of open information exchange.

40.8 Conclusion

One Health is a unifying concept. It is based on spiritual philosophy. 'Oneness' is important for a harmonious family, strong nation, and a peaceful global family... The implementation and application of knowledge is required for 'transformation'... Transformation brings permanent change, *transform attitude and mindset... for world redemption that is saving from sin, error, and evil*" –

Swami Swatmanandan, President and Acharya, Chinmaya Mission, Mumbai (www.transformingindians.org).

The management of zoonoses requires the transformation of attitude and mindset, developing vision of 'One Health', striving for a strong public health for world redemption (from pandemics).

References

Abbas SS, Venkataramanan V, Pathak G, Kakkar M (2011) Rabies control initiative in Tamil Nadu, India: a test case for the 'one health' approach. Int Health 3(4):231–239

Azad AF (2004) Prairie dog: cuddly pet or Trojan horse? Emerg Infect Dis 10(3):542–543

Bell DM, World Health Organization Working Group on Prevention of International and Community Transmission of SARS (2004) Public health interventions and SARS spread, 2003. Emerg Infect Dis 10(11):1900–1906

Bhatia R (2019) Implementation framework for one health approach. Indian J Med Res 149:329–331

Brown C (2004) Emerging zoonoses and pathogens of public health significance – an overview. Rev Sci Tech 23(2):435–442

Chomel BB, Belotto A, Meslin FX (2007) Wildlife, exotic pets, and emerging zoonoses. Emerg Infect Dis 13(1):6–11

Daszak P, Cunningham A, Hyatt A (2001) Anthropogenic environmental change and the emergence of infectious diseases in wildlife. Acta Trop 78:103–116

FAO (2009) The state of food and agriculture. https://www.fao.org/3/i0680e/i0680e.pdf

FAO (2020) Climate change: unpacking the burden on food safety. Food safety and quality series No. 8. Rome. https://doi.org/10.4060/ca8185en

FAO, OIE, WHO, UNSIC, UNICEF, The World Bank (2008) Contributing to One World, One Health. A strategic framework for reducing risks of infectious diseases at the animal–human–ecosystems interface https://www.preventionweb.net/files/8627_OWOH14Oct08.pdf

Gilbert N (2012) Cost of human-animal disease greatest for world's poor. Nature

Guan Y, Smith GJ (2013) The emergence and diversification of panzootic H5N1 influenza viruses. Virus Res 178(1):35–43. https://doi.org/10.1016/j.virusres.2013.05.012. Epub 2013 Jun 2. PMID: 23735533; PMCID: PMC4017639

John JT, Dandona L, Sharma VP, Kakkar M (2011) Continuing challenge of infectious diseases in India. Lancet 377(9761):252–269

Karesh WB, Dobson A, Lloyd-Smith JO, Lubroth J, Dixon MA et al (2012) Ecology of zoonoses: natural and unnatural histories. Lancet 380:1936–1945

Kilpatrik AM, Randolph SE (2012) Drivers, dynamics and control of vector borne emerging zoonoses. Lancet 380:1946–1955

Lambin EF, Tran A, Vanwambeke SO et al (2010) Pathogenic landscapes: interactions between land, people, disease vectors, and their animal hosts. Int J Health Geogr 9:54. https://doi.org/10.1186/1476-072X-9-54

Landford J, Nunn M (2012) Good governance in 'one health' approaches. Rev Sci Tech 31(2):561–575

Moore SM, Azman AS, Zaitchik BF, Mintz ED, Brunkard J et al (2017) El Niño and the shifting geography of cholera in Africa. Proc Natl Acad Sci U S A 114(17):4436–4441

Narayan KG (2011) Veterinary Public Health – a route to 'One health'. Dr. M. R. Dhanda oration. IXth All India Conference of Association of Public Health Veterinarians and National symposium on "Challenges and strategies for Veterinary Public Health in India" Feb. 18–19, 2011

Narayan KG (2012a) One Health Initiative in addressing Food Safety Challenges. National seminar organised by Kerala Veterinary and Animal Science University, Department of Veterinary

Public Health, College of Veterinary and Animal Sciences, Mannuthy and Indian Association of Veterinary Public Health Specialists, Feb. 16-17, 2012, Thrissur, Kerala

Narayan KG (2012b) Key note address -the national symposium and Xth all India conference of the Association of Public Health Veterinarians, West Bengal University of Animal & Fishery Sciences, Kolkata-700037. 14–15th Dec 2012

Olival KJ, Islam A, Yu M, Anthony SJ, Epstein JH et al (2013) Ebola virus antibodies in fruit bats, Bangladesh. Emerg Infect Dis 19(2):270–273

Quah SR, Hin-Peng L (2004) Crisis prevention and management during SARS outbreak, Singapore. Emerg Infect Dis 10(2):364–368

Randolph SE on behalf of the EDEN-TBD sub-project team (2010) Human activities predominate in determining changing incidence of tick-borne encephalitis in Europe. Euro Surveill 15(27): 19606

Saxena VK, Verghese T (1996) Ecology of flea transmitted zoonotic infection in village Mamla, district Beed. Curr Sci 71:800–802

Tenzin, Sharma B, Dhand NK, Timsina N, Ward MP (2010) Re-emergence of rabies in Chhkha District, Bhutan, 2008. Emerg Infect Dis 16(12):1925–1930

Tysmans JB (1994) Plague in India –1994 conditions, containment and goals. http://www.wastetohealth.com/plague_in_india_1994.html

Vrbova L, Stephen C, Kasman C, Boehnke NR, Doyle-Waters M et al (2010) Systematic review of surveillance systems for emerging zoonoses. Transbound Emerg Dis 57(3):154–161

Walsh AL, Morgan D (2005) Identifying hazards, assessing risk. Vet Rec 157:684–687

Watanabe I, Yamada K, Aso A, Suda O, Matsumoto T et al (2013) Relationship between virus-neutralizing antibody levels and the number of rabies vaccinations: a prospective study of dogs in Japan. Jpn J Infect Dis 66:17–21

WHO Dengue (2009) Guidelines for diagnosis, treatment, prevention and control. A Joint Publication of the World Health Organization (WHO) and the Special Programme for Research and Training in Tropical Diseases (TDR) New edition. 2009.9789241547871_eng-Dengue.pdf

World Bank (2010) People, Pathogens and Our Planet. Vol. 1: Towards a One Health Approach for Controlling Zoonotic Diseases. Report No. 50833-GLB. The World Bank, Agriculture and Rural Development Health, Nutrition and Population, Washington, DC

Appendix A

Specific Information Depending Upon the Questions and Demanded by Students Should Be Provided from Farm Records (Tables A.1, A.2, A.3, A.4, A.5, A.6, A.7, and A.8)

Table A.1 Total number of animals

Age group	Holstein Friesian	Cross bred	Total
Neonates	300 (240 F+ 60 M)	250 (210 F +40 M)	550
1–3 months	100 (80 F+ 20 M)	50 (30 F+ 20 M)	150
4–12 months	150 (120 F + 30 M)	100 (75 F+25 M)	250
1–2 years (females)	125	75	200
2–3 years (females)	550	400	950[a]
>3 years (females)	25	75	100
Total	1250	950	2200

Number of females pregnant = 1000
Number of pregnant animals which parturated = 956
[a]Mother cows of calves 0–12 months old

Table A.2 Number of animals, morbidity, and mortality

	Total		Number Sick		Deaths		Total	
Age	HF	CB	HF	CB	HF	CB	Sick	Deaths
0–7 days	100	80	12	10	04	02	12 + 10 = 22	04 + 02 = 06
8–14 days	90	80	15	10	05	02	15 + 10 = 25	05 + 02 = 07
15–21 days	60	60	10	05	06	03	10 + 05 = 15	06 + 03 = 09
22–30 days	50	30	08	02	05	01	08 + 02 = 10	05 + 01 = 06
1–3 months	75	50	20	10	02	02	20 + 10 = 30	02 + 02 = 04
4–6 months	75	50	05	02	0	0	05 + 02 = 07	0
7–9 months	50	25	01	0	0	0	01 + 00 = 01	0
10–12 months	50	25	02	0	0	0	02 + 0 = 02	0
1–2 years	125	75	25	10	05	02	25 + 10 = 35	05+02=07
2–3 years	550	400	75	50	25	10	75 + 50 = 125	25+10=35
>3 years	25	75	10	10	05	05	10 + 10 = 20	05+05=10

K. G. Narayan et al., *Veterinary Public Health & Epidemiology*,
https://doi.org/10.1007/978-981-19-7800-5

Table A.3 Distribution of diseases and deaths in neonates according to breed

	Holstein Friesian			Cross bred		
Neonates	Naval ill	Scour	Pneumonia	Naval ill	Scour	Pneumonia
0–7 days	02/08	01	02/03	02/07	02	01
8–14 days	05/12	02	01	02/06	02	02
15–21 days	02/04	02/03	02/03	½	01/01	01/02
22–30 days	0/0	03/05	02/03	0	½	0
Total	09/24	05/11	06/10	05/15	02/07	01/05

Numerator is the number of deaths and denominator the number of sick neonates

Table A.4 Distribution of diseases according to breed and age

				Age in months			
Diseases (total)	Breed	Neonates 0–4 weeks	Weaned 1–3 month	4–12	13–24	25–36	>36
Naval ill (09/24)	HF	09/24					
(05/15)	CB	05/15					
Calf scour (05/11)	HF	05/11					
(02/07)	CB	02/07					
Pneumonia (14/40)	HF	06/10	15		02/04	05/10	01/01
(02/16)	CB	01/05	01/06			05	
Mastitis (13)	HF					10	03
(05)	CB					05	
Abortion (05)	HF				03		02
(01)	CB						01
Milk fever (01/06)	HF					05	01/01
(02)	CB						02
Stomach worm (13)	HF			08	05		
(01/07)	CB			02	01/05		
Septicaemia (22/36)	HF		02/05		02/03	15/25	03/03
(08/11)	CB		¼			05/05	02/02
Johne's disease (05/10)	HF					05/10	
(09/29)	CB				01/04	05/20	03/05
Ephemeral fever (25)	HF				10	15	
(16)	CB				01	15	
Total (57/183)	HF	20/45	02/20	08	05/25	25/75	05/10
(27/109)	CB	08/27	02/10	02	02/10	10/50	05/10

Table A.5 Ephemeral fever—dates on which cases were first recorded and dates of recovery

Dates cases recorded	Number	Dates—recovered	Duration of illness	Incubation period
25.2.2000	2 CB	29.2.2000		
26.2.2000	3 HF	01.3.2000		
05.03.2000	4 CB	09.03.2000		
07.03.2000	5 HF	10.03.2000		
08.03.2000	4 CB	11.03.2000		
08.03.2000	6 HF	12.03.2000		
10.03.2000	4 CB	13.03.2000		
11.03.2000	2 CB	14.03.2000		
11.03.2000	6 HF	14.03.2000		
12.03.2000	5 HF	15.03.2000		

Table A.6 Months of introduction of cows of Holstein Friesian (HF) and Cross Bred (CB) in the age group of 25–36 months

Months of introduction	Number introduced HF/CB
01.02.2000	100/40
01.03.2000	100/40
01.04.2000	90/30
01.05.2000	80/30
01.06.2000	90/30
01.07.2000	70/25
01.08.2000	20/45
01.09.2000	0/30
01.10.2000	0/40
01.11.2000	0/30
01.12.2000	0/40
01.01.2001	0/20
Total	550/400

Note that the population of the rest of the categories, *i.e.*, age groups is assumed to be the same as shown in Table A.1. The data in this table alters the month-wise number of animals and hence necessitates calculation of denominator as 'animal-months-of-risk'

Table A.7 Distribution of sickness and deaths according to population, breed, and sex

	Holstein Friesian			Cross bred			
Age	Male	Female	Total	Male	Female	Total	Total
0–30 days P	60	240	300	40	210	250	550
S	20	25	45	12	17	29	64
D	12	8	20	4	4	8	28
1–3 months P	20	80	100	20	30	50	150
S	6	14	20	4	6	10	30
D	–	2	2	2	–	2	4
4–12 months P	30	120	150	25	75	100	250
S	4	4	8	1	1	2	10
D	–	–	–	–	–	–	–
1–2 years P	–	125	125	–	75	75	200
S	–	25	–	–	10	–	35
D	–	5	–	–	7	–	12
2–3 years P	–	550	550	–	400	400	950
S	–	75	75	–	50	50	125
D	–	25	25	–	10	10	35
>3 years P	–	25	25	–	75	75	100
S	–	10	10	–	10	10	20
D	–	5	5	–	5	5	10

Note: The distribution of cases of each of the diseases according to the date of onset and the date-wise cumulative numbers has been dictated to students so as to enable them to calculate the prevalence (cumulative) and incidence rates

Table A.8 Result

Date	New cases	Cumulative No.	Remarks
1.2.00	4		Point prevalence on 1.3.00 will have 14 cases Incidence on this date will have 5 new cases Duration of illness not being considered
15.2.00	5	9	
1.3.00	5	14	

Appendix B

Websites, Software, and Apps Useful for Disease Surveillance and Intervention

Major international agencies which are playing an important role in disease surveillance, prevalence, and control are WHO-OIE-FAO collectively known as International Technical Agencies along with WTO (World Trade Organization) supported by disease tracking initiatives as ProMED-mail, GIDEON, EMPRES, EHTF, AHEAD, Fsnet, Agnet, etc. WHO, OIE, and FAO have developed various programmes and initiatives to generate authentic and reliable information on animal health and productivity and publish jointly Animal Health Yearbook. They have long-standing experience in direct collaboration regarding disease control and surveillance. These are integrated, holistic, and transdisciplinary joint initiative called 'One Health'. Veterinary occupies the central position.

WHO continues to track the evolving infectious disease situation, sound the alarm when needed, share expertise, and mount the kind of response needed to protect populations from the consequences of epidemics, whatever and wherever might be their origin

1. *Global Disease Alert, Warning, Risk assessment, Report and Action system* (https://www.who.int/csr/alertresponse/en/) Disease outbreak news; Informa tion resources; Strategic Health Operations Centre (SHOC).
2. *CORDS (Connecting Organizations for Regional Disease Surveillance)* https:// www. cordsnetwork.org/strategic-objectives/):
   It was established in 2012 as an informal governance cooperative of six regional disease surveillance networks (EAIDSNet, SACIDS, SEEHN, APEIR, MECIDS, and MBDS) working across national borders to tackle emerging infectious diseases. The main purpose is to speed up the capabilities of all CORDS members by combining the strengths of all networks of the area in order to boost up the global surveillance against various infectious diseases of humans and animals. It further supports the mandate of FAO, WHO, and OIE to improve global health security vision. Its vision is a world united against infectious diseases.

K. G. Narayan et al., *Veterinary Public Health & Epidemiology*,
https://doi.org/10.1007/978-981-19-7800-5

3. *ProMED* (Programme for Monitoring Emerging Diseases)–mail (http://www.promedmail.org)
   It is one of the first online disease reporting systems since 1994, currently used in at least 185 countries with the main intent to assist local, national, and international organisations as well as scientists, physicians, epidemiologists, public health professionals, and others interested in infectious diseases on a global scale.
4. *ECDC* (European Centre for Disease Prevention and Control; https://www.ecdc.europa.eu/en):
   The mission of ECDC is to strengthen Europe's defences against infectious diseases. The Centre was established in 2004 with its headquarter in Solna, Sweden. The core activities are surveillance, epidemic intelligence, response, scientific advice, microbiology, preparedness, public health training, international relations, health communication, and the scientific journal *Eurosurveillance*.
5. *WOAH* (World Organization for Animal Health; http://www.oie.int/en/):
   WAHIS: This interface provides access to all data held within OIE's new World Animal Health Information System (WAHIS). A comprehensive range of information is available from:
   (a) Immediate notifications and follow-up reports submitted by Country/Territory Members notifying exceptional epidemiological events current in their territory
   (b) Six-monthly reports stating the health status of OIE-listed diseases in each Country/Territory
   (c) Annual reports providing health information and information on the veterinary staff, laboratories, vaccines, etc.
6. *INFOSAN* (International Food Safety Authorities Network; http://www.who.int/foodsafety /areas_work/infosan/en/):
   It is a global network of 186 national food safety authorities, managed jointly by FAO and WHO with the secretariat in Geneva, WHO headquarter. It assists member states in managing food safety risks, ensuring rapid sharing of information during food safety emergencies to stop the spread of contaminated food from one country to another.
7. *GLEWS+* (Global Early Warning System for Major Animal Diseases including Zoonoses; https://www.who.int/zoonoses/outbreaks/glews/en/):
   It is a joint system that builds on the added value of combining and coordinating alert mechanisms of FAO, OIE, and WHO. Networks from the international community and stakeholders are linked to assist in early warning, prevention, and control of animal disease threats, including zoonoses. The objective of GLEWS is to improve data sharing and risk assessment for animal disease threats of the three sister organisations (FAO, OIE, and WHO) for the benefit of the international community.
8. *EMPRESS Food Safety* (Emergency Prevention System for Food safety; http://www.fao.org/food-safety/food-control-systems/empres-food-safety/en/):

It was established in 2009 with aims to contribute towards fulfilling FAO's mandate of ensuring access to a safe and affordable food supply for the world's population, with focus on proactive identification of emerging issues (Foresight, early warning), and Coordination and management of INFOSAN.

9. *MINEADEP* (Middle and Near East Regional Animal Production and Health Project; http://www.fao.org/ag/againfo/programmes/en/empres/gemp/avis/glossary/MINEADEP.html):
   FAO under animal production and health had initiated MINEADEP— Pan African Programme for the Control of Epizootics (PACE), and the Regional Animal Disease and Surveillance Control Network (RADISCON).
10. International Livestock Research Institute (ILRI; https://www.ilri.org/):
   It is an international agricultural research institute based in Nairobi, Kenya, and founded in 1994 by the merging of the International Livestock Centre for Africa and the International Laboratory for Research on Animal Diseases. ILRI works for better lives through livestock in developing countries. ILRI is co-hosted by Kenya and Ethiopia, has 14 offices across Asia and Africa, employs some 700 staff, and has an annual operating budget of about USD80 million.

Organisations in American continent

11. *CDC* (Centers for Disease Control and Prevention; http://www.cdc.gov/):
   It is the leading national public health institute of the USA under the Department of Health and Human Services headquartered in Atlanta, Georgia, with the main objective to protect public health and safety through the control and prevention of disease, injury, and disability in the USA and internationally. It especially focuses its attention on infectious diseases including zoonosis, foodborne pathogens, environmental health, occupational safety and health, health promotion, injury prevention, and educational activities designed to improve the health of US citizens.
12. *CEAH* (Center of Epidemiology and Animal Health; https://www.aphis.usda.gov/aphis/ourfocus/animalhealth/):
   It is one of the science centres within Veterinary Services Science, Technology, and Analysis Services of USDA with a mission to promote and safeguard US agriculture by providing timely and accurate information and analysis about animal health and veterinary public health, which facilitate decision-making in government and industry.
13. *NAHMS* (National Animal Health Monitoring System; https://www.aphis.usda.gov/aphis/ourfocus/animalhealth/monitoring-and-surveillance/nahms):
   It conducts national studies on the health and health management of US domestic livestock and poultry populations.
14. *NAHRS* (National Animal Health Reporting System; https://www.aphis.usda.gov/aphis /ourfocus/animalhealth/monitoring-and-surveillance/sa_disease_reporting/ct_usda_aphis_animal_health):
   It is the only comprehensive reporting system for World Organization for Animal Health (OIE)-reportable diseases in the USA.

15. *Pulse-Net* (https://www.cdc.gov/pulsenet/index.html): It is a nationwide foodborne disease surveillance system under CDC in the USA.
16. *Pan American Health Organization* (*PAHO;* https://www.paho.org/en): It is an international public health agency, established in 1902, works to promote and coordinate efforts of American countries to combat diseases, and supports veterinary public health services concerning zoonoses and sanitary inspection of livestock and fishery products.
17. *Canadian Animal Health Surveillance System* (*CAHSS;* https://www.cahss.ca): It is an initiative of the National Farmed Animal Health and Welfare Council (NFAHWC) with broad-based collaborative support of industry and governments designed to fill the need for strengthened animal health surveillance in Canada.
18. *Caribbean Animal Health Network* (*CaribVET;* https://www.caribvet.net/): It is a collaborative network established in 2006 involving official veterinary services from 34 Caribbean countries/territories as well as research institutes {CIRAD (Guadeloupe) and CENSA (Cuba)}, veterinary faculties {School of Veterinary Medicine of the University of the West Indies (Trinidad and Tobago), University of Guyana, Ross University (Saint-Kitts-et-Nevis), and St. George's University (Grenada)}.

Organisations in Europe

19. *The Pirbright Institute, UK* (https://www.pirbright.ac.uk/our-science): This institute provides the UK with capacity to predict, detect, understand, and respond to the threat and potential attack of serious viral diseases of livestock and viruses that spread from animals to humans. These viral diseases may not be present in the UK (endemic) and only circulating abroad (exotic).
20. *Southern African Centre for Infectious Disease Surveillance* (*SACIDS;* http://www.sacids.org/): It is established to harness innovation in science and technology in order to improve sub-Saharan Africa's capacity to detect, identify, and monitor infectious diseases of humans, animals, and their interactions in order to better manage the risk posed by them. SACIDS Secretariat is in Morogoro, Tanzania.
21. *The East African Integrated Disease Surveillance Network* (*EAIDSNet;* https://www.cordsnetwork.org/networks/eaidsnet/): It is a collaborative, intergovernmental initiative between the National Ministries for human and animal health and the National health research and academic institutions of Burundi, Kenya, Rwanda, Uganda, and Tanzania with a mission to improve the health of the people of East Africa by promoting the exchange and dissemination of appropriate information on emerging diseases, combining disease surveillance systems within the region and ensuring continuous exchange of expertise and best practice on infectious disease so that morbidity and mortality due to common communicable diseases in this region can be reduced.

Organisations in Asia

22. *Mekong Basin Disease Surveillance Network* (*MBDS;* http://www.mbdsnet.org/):
    One of the oldest successful self-organised infectious disease surveillance network comprising six countries (Cambodia, China, Lao PDR, Myanmar, Thailand, and Vietnam) of Mekong Basin Area in Asia, which is considered to be a hot spot for the emergence of new emerging diseases. The secretariat is in Nonthaburi, Thailand.
23. *Middle East Consortium on Infectious Disease Surveillance* (*MECIDS;* https://www.nti.org/about/projects/middle-east-consortium-infectious-disease-surveillance/):
    Initiated in 2003, it comprises Israel, The Palestinian authority, and Jordan. In 2009, it coordinated efforts against the dreaded H1N1 influenza outbreak in these countries.
24. *Asian Partnership on Emerging Infectious Disease Research* (*APEIR;* http://www.apeir.net/):
    It is a research network composed of researchers, practitioners, and senior governments officials from Cambodia, China, Lao PDR, Indonesia, Thailand, and Vietnam. A multi-country, multi-sectoral, multi-disciplinary research partnership launched in 2006 for regional collaboration in influenza research, later expanded its scope to include all emerging infectious diseases.
25. *Asia Pacific Strategy for Emerging Diseases* (*APSED;* https://apps.searo.who.int/):
    APSED was launched in 2005 as a common strategic framework for countries and areas of the region to strengthen their capacity to manage and respond to emerging disease threats, including influenza pandemics. It is a regional strategic framework for prevention and control of zoonoses in the South-East Asia Region with 5 major components, viz. Surveillance warning and rapid response, Laboratory diagnosis, Risk communication, Infection control/biosafety, and Zoonoses

Organisations and Programmes in India

26. *ICMR* (Indian Council of Medical Research; https://www.icmr.gov.in/aboutus.html):
    It is the apex body in India for the formulation, coordination, and promotion of biomedical research with headquarters in New Delhi. It was founded in 1911 and is one of the oldest medical research bodies in the world. It addresses the growing demands of scientific advances in biomedical research as well as finding practical solutions to the health problems of the country.
27. *NCDC* (National Centre for Disease Control; https://www.ncdc.gov.in/):
    It is an institute under the Indian Directorate General of Health Services, Ministry of Health and Family Welfare. It was established in July 1963 for research in epidemiology and control of communicable diseases and to reorganise the activities of the Malaria Institute of India. Previously it is known as National Institute of Communicable Disease (NICD). During the

12th five-year plan, this institute strengthened its laboratories, manpower, and IEC (information, education, and communication) activities for zoonotic diseases.

28. *NIE* (National Institute of Epidemiology; http://www.nie.gov.in/):
It is a research organisation founded in 1999 under Indian Council of Medical Research (ICMR) located in Chennai, Tamil Nadu. NIE conducts research including interventional studies, disease modelling, and health systems and conducts epidemiological investigations and clinical trials of traditional remedies.
29. *NIV* (National Institute of Virology, Pune; http://www.niv.co.in/):
It is a virology research institute under ICMR, previously known as 'Virus Research Center', and was founded in collaboration with the Rockefeller Foundation in 1952 as a part of the global programme of investigations on the arthropod-borne group of viruses. It has been designated as a WHO H5 reference laboratory for SE Asia region. At present it is WHO Collaborating Center for arboviruses and haemorrhagic fever reference and research. It is also the National Monitoring Centre for Influenza, Japanese encephalitis, Rota, Measles, Hepatitis, and Coronavirus.
30. *National Institute of Tuberculosis and Respiratory Diseases* (*NITRD;* http://www.nitrd.nic.in):
LRS Institute of Tuberculosis & Respiratory Diseases is an autonomous institute under the Ministry of Health & Family Welfare, Govt. of India, with the objective to act as an apex institute in the country for the prevention, control, and treatment of Tuberculosis and Allied Diseases under National Tuberculosis Control Programme by providing training, teaching, and research activities.
31. *NISHAD* (*National Institute of High Security Animal Diseases;* http://www.nihsad.nic.in/):
A premier institute of India in Bhopal for research on exotic and emerging pathogens of animals under ICAR. Previously its name was *High Security Animal Disease Laboratory* (HSADL), a regional station of Indian Veterinary Research Institute (IVRI), Izatnagar. Since 8th August 2014, it is known as NIHSAD. Its role in diagnosis of Avian Influenza is highly appreciated.
32. *CADRAD* (Centre for Animal Research and Diagnosis; http://www.ivri.nic.in/DiseaseDiagnosis/default.aspx):
It was established at Indian Veterinary Research Institute, Izatnagar, on 10th March 1986 with a view to provide health care and diagnosis of animal diseases in the country, and is recognised as Central Disease Diagnostic Laboratory (CDDL) by the Department of Animal Husbandry & Dairying, Ministry of Agriculture (Govt. of India).
33. *NIVEDI* (National Institute of Veterinary Epidemiology and Disease Informatics; https://www.nivedi.res.in):
The institute was established in 2013 in Bengaluru under ICAR to cater the needs of surveillance and monitoring of livestock diseases and thereby caring for the country's animal health. It is working towards designing of various

forecasting and forewarning modules in order to predict livestock disease outbreaks.

34. *National Surveillance Programme on Communicable Diseases* (*NSPCD*; https://hetv.org/india/mh/healthstatus/communicable-diseases.htm):
    The programme is initiated during 1997-98 for strengthening the disease surveillance capacity to respond to emerging and reemerging infectious diseases.
35. *Integrated Disease Surveillance Project* (*IDSP;* https://idsp.nic.in/index1):
    It was launched with World Bank assistance in November 2004 to detect and respond to disease outbreaks quickly. The project was extended for 2 years in March 2010, i.e., from April 2010 to March 2012; World Bank funds were available for Central Surveillance Unit (CSU) at NCDC and 9 identified states (Uttarakhand, Rajasthan, Punjab, Maharashtra, Gujarat, Tamil Nadu, Karnataka, Andhra Pradesh, and West Bengal) and the rest 26 states/UTs were funded from domestic budget.
36. *Livestock Health and Disease Control Scheme*:
    The Department of Animal Husbandry, Dairying and Fisheries (DADF), Govt. of India, under this scheme runs a number of control programme of animal diseases like FMD, PPR, Brucellosis, Classical Swine fever besides Assistance to States for Control of Animal Diseases (ASCAD), National Project on Rinderpest Surveillance and Monitoring (NPRSM), National Animal Disease Reporting System (NADRS), Establishment and Strengthening of Existing Veterinary Hospitals and Dispensaries (ESVHD), and Professional Efficiency Development (PED). The NADRS includes about 143 animal diseases scheduled in the Prevention and Control of Infectious and Contagious Diseases in Animals Act, 2009.

Important Epidemiological Software/Websites

1. *Epi Info*: Epi Info™ is a public domain software tool which provides easy data entry form and database construction, a customised data entry experience, and data analyses with epidemiologic statistics, maps, and graphs for public health professionals. Epi Info™ can be used for outbreak investigations; for developing small to mid-sized disease surveillance systems; as analysis, visualisation, and reporting (AVR) components of larger systems; and in the continuing education in the science of epidemiology and public health analytic methods at schools of public health around the world.
   Source: https://www.cdc.gov/epiinfo/index.html
2. *QGIS*: QGIS (previously known as Quantum GIS) is a cross-platform free and open-source desktop geographic information system (GIS) application that supports viewing, editing, and analysis of geospatial data. QGIS functions as geographic information system (GIS) software, allowing users to analyse and edit spatial information, in addition to composing and exporting graphical maps. QGIS supports both raster and vector layers; vector data is stored as either

point, line, or polygon features. Multiple formats of raster images are supported and the software can georeference images.
Source: http://www.qgis.org/en/site/forusers/download.html

3. *Whitebox GAT*: Whitebox GAT was intended to have a broader focus than its predecessor, positioning it as an open-source desktop GIS and remote sensing software package for general applications of geospatial analysis and data visualisation. Whitebox GAT is intended to provide a platform for advanced geospatial data analysis with applications in both environmental research and the geomatics industry more broadly. It was envisioned from the outset as providing an ideal platform for experimenting with novel geospatial analysis methods. Equally important is the project's goal of providing a tool that can be used for geomatics-based education.
   Source: http://www.uoguelph.ca/~hydrogeo/Whitebox/
4. *GRASS GIS*: Geographic Resources Analysis Support System (commonly termed GRASS GIS) is a geographic information system (GIS) software suite used for geospatial data management and analysis, image processing, producing graphics and maps, spatial and temporal modelling, and visualising. It can handle raster, topological vector, image processing, and graphic data.
   Source: https://grass.osgeo.org/
5. *DIVA GIS*: DIVA-GIS is a free geographic information system—software for mapping and geographic data analysis. The software is especially designed for mapping and analysing biodiversity data.
   Source: http://www.diva-gis.org/
6. *Epi Tools*: The site is intended for use by epidemiologists and researchers involved in estimating disease prevalence or demonstrating freedom from disease through structured surveys, or in other epidemiological applications.
   Source: http://epitools.ausvet.com.au/
7. *EpiData*: EpiData Analysis performs basic statistical analysis, graphs, and comprehensive data management, e.g. descriptive statistics, SPC Charts, Recoding data, label values and variables, and defining missing values.
   Source: http://www.epidata.dk/

Certain Customised Apps

Smartphone and GPS technology

1. *'Estimation of street dog population and location'—method is applicable for wildlife also. American crow in West Nile epidemic/migratory birds in avian influenza.*
   Smartphone-GPS technology combines the two methods (Mark-resight surveys applying the Lincoln-Peterson corrected Chapman method and applying the logit-normal mixed model to estimate population size) of estimating dog population more precisely, with less efforts and in the shortest possible time.

Built-in GPS, integrated camera, high-quality Web connectivity, and Android devices displayed 3 superimposed elements: the Google map as background, the perimeter of the areas to survey and the user position—surveyors could use their own phones/tablets to help municipalities, vets, NGOs involved in dog population census and management—is user friendly, average time spent to complete a dog file is 30 s.

Automatically recorded on excel sheet—data, standardised, downloaded, statistical, or descriptive analysis possible.

2. *The Community-Based Rabies Surveillance System (CBRS), GARC,* is a rabies-dedicated software tool launched in the Philippines for comprehensive surveillance of both humans and animals exposed to rabies. Data from active surveillance in a country gathered through an integrated approach including inputs from community health workers, veterinarians, human health professionals, and laboratory professionals (also automated SMS ad e-mail) are stored, analysed, and aggregated in a single system. It is useful for Rabies epidemiological Bulletin. It tracks and links suspect animals and humans that have been potentially exposed to rabies (Overview of the Community-Based Rabies Surveillance software module. Diagram: Dr. Terrence Scott, GARC *Rabies Epidemiological Bulletin administrator).*
3. Contact tracing apps
Tracing the movement of a 'spreader–asymptomatic shedder' and the 'contacts' followed by isolating all of them is the method of arresting the spread of infection. Tracing and monitoring the contacts of infected person works backward from an infected person to identify people who may have been exposed to disease so that they may be tested, isolated, and hospitalised if required.

   Smart Contact tracing was done in South Korea using only a Bluetooth-based app that linked 'contact-tracing codes' to user's phone IP address. India uses similar app *Arogya Setu*. The app is downloaded on a smartphone. Each phone constantly transmits unique code and simultaneously also saves codes from other phones that come within range for several minutes. If one of your 'contacts' tests positive for COVID-19 your app alerts you and provides information about self-quarantining and getting tested.

   By targeting recommendations to only those at risk, epidemic could be controlled without need for mass quarantines that are harmful to society. Control of epidemic may be achieved if used on enough people.

Glossary

Aetiology (Etiology) (The study of) the causes of disease.

Aetiological fraction The reduction in disease when a risk factor is removed.

Absolute risk Risk of a disease is your risk of developing the disease over a time period.

Abiotic factors These are non-living chemical and physical parts of the environment that affect living organisms and the functioning of ecosystems.

Accessory reservoir A reservoir that contributes to the maintenance of a pathogen in nature but is not the primary reservoir for such agent.

Accuracy It is the extent to which a measurement reflects the true value. It is the tendency of test measurement to centre around the true value.

Acquired immunity The inherited potential to resist a disease or infection.

Active immunity Resistance to a disease, developed in response to an antigen (an infecting agent or a vaccine) and usually characterised, or distinguished, by the presence of antibodies produced by the host.

Active surveillance The process in which health departments (or responsible agencies) contact clinicians, laboratories, or other data sources to seek out information about disease cases.

Age-adjustment/Age-standardisation A technique used to compare populations that are quite different in age.

Age-adjusted mortality rate A mortality rate statistically modified to eliminate the effect of different age distributions in the different populations.

Agent A factor, such as a microorganism, chemical substance, or form of radiation, whose presence, excessive presence, or (in deficiency diseases) relative absence is essential for the occurrence of a disease.

Age-specific rate A rate limited to a particular age group. The numerator is the number of occurrences in that age group; the denominator is the number of persons in that age group in the population.

Age-specific mortality rate A mortality rate limited to a particular age group. The numerator is the number of deaths in that age group; the denominator is the number of persons in that age group in the population.

K. G. Narayan et al., *Veterinary Public Health & Epidemiology*,
https://doi.org/10.1007/978-981-19-7800-5

Aggregative fallacy An erroneous application to individuals of a causal relationship observed at the group level. A type of ecological fallacy (sometimes just a synonym).

Airborne transmission The spread of an infection by droplets or dust, with a particle spread of more than three feet through the air. It is considered to be a form of indirect transmission.

Apthisation It is an old method of immunisation to control an outbreak when neither vaccine nor treatment and not even the aetiology was known. It involves deliberately infecting healthy animals with excretions of ill to infect them so as to induce development of natural immunity; example is infecting healthy cattle with salivary discharge from FMD cases.

Analysis of variance (ANOVA) A statistical technique that isolates and assesses the contribution of categorical independent variables to the variance of the mean of a continuous dependent variable. The observations are classified according to their categories for each of the independent variables, and the differences between the categories in their mean values on the dependent variable are estimated and tested.

Analytic epidemiology A focused study of the determinants of disease or reasons for high or low frequency of disease in specific groups. The aspect of epidemiology concerned with the search for health-related causes and effects. Uses comparison groups, which provide baseline data, to quantify the association between exposures and outcomes, and test hypotheses about causal relationships. Analytic epidemiology is search for health-related causes and effects.

Analytical sensitivity It refers to the ability of an assay to detect minimum detectable concentration of a target antibody or antigen.

Analytical specificity It refers to the ability of an assay to measure particular organism or substance rather than others.

Analytic study A comparative study intended to identify and quantify associations, test hypotheses, and identify causes. Two common types are cohort study and case-control study.

Anamorphic map A diagrammatic method of displaying administrative jurisdictions of a country or any other region in two-dimensional 'maps' with areas proportional to any statistic related to the region.

Animal health Animal health is a state of physical, physiological, and behavioural well-being of animals which leads to maximum possible levels of production, draught efficiency, and economic benefit.

Antenatal (Prenatal) The period between conception and birth.

Anthropurgic ecosystem It is the type of ecosystem created by man.

Antibody A protein produced in the blood of vertebrates following exposure to an antigen. The antibody binds specifically to the antigen and thus stimulates its inactivation by other parts of the immune system.

Antigenic drift It is a mechanism for variation in viruses that involves the accumulation of mutations within the genes that code for antibody-binding sites.

Antigenic shift It is the process by which two or more different strains of a virus, or strains of two or more different viruses, combine to form a new subtype having a mixture of the surface antigens of the two or more original strains.

Antiseptics Agents used to keep a check on sepsis, are used on skin, mucosa, wound as mouth wash, vaginal and uterine douche, etc. These are quick in action and are called fungistat, bacteriostat, etc.

Applied epidemiology The application or practice of epidemiology to address public health issues.

Assessment Evaluation or study. For example, a community health assessment would be a study, or evaluation, of the health of a community.

Association Statistical relationship between two or more events, characteristics, or other variables.

Attack rate A variant of an incident rate, applied to a narrowly defined population observed for a limited period of time, such as during an epidemic.

Attenuation It is the process which makes an infectious agent harmless or less virulent.

Attributable fraction It is the proportion of disease in the exposed group that is due to exposure. AF is calculated as the proportion that the attributable risk represents within total disease risk in exposed individuals.

Attributable proportion A measure of the public health impact of a causative factor; proportion of a disease in a group that is exposed to a particular factor which can be attributed to their exposure to that factor.

Attributable risk (rate) It is defined as the increase or decrease in the risk (or rate) of disease in the exposed group that is attributable to exposure.

Autochthonous ecosystem It is the type of ecosystem e coming from land itself.

Average length of stay The average length of stay per discharged patient is computed by dividing the total number of hospital days for a specified group by the total number of discharges for that group.

Bar chart A visual display of the size of the different categories of a variable. Each category or value of the variable is represented by a bar. The lengths of the bars represent frequencies of each group of observations.

Benefit-cost ratio or cost-benefit analysis A ratio between the amount of monetary gain realised by performing a project versus the amount it costs to execute the project.

Bias A flaw in either the study design or data analysis that leads to erroneous results. Bias is the deviation of results or inferences from the truth, or processes leading to such systematic deviation. Any trend in the collection, analysis, interpretation, publication, or review of data that can lead to conclusions that are systematically different from the truth.

Bimodal distribution A distribution that has two distinct modes or peaks.

Biologic transmission The indirect vector-borne transmission of an infectious agent in which the agent undergoes biologic changes within the vector before being transmitted to a new host.

Biome A large naturally occurring community of flora and fauna occupying a major habitat. Major biotic communities are biomes, *e.g.* forest or tundra.

Biosecurity It is the management practice activities that reduce the opportunities for infectious agents to gain access to, or spread within, a food animal production unit.

Biotic community or Biocenosis A collection of living organisms (plants, animals, and the microorganisms) in a biotope.

Biotope An area of uniform environmental conditions providing a living place for a specific collection of plants and animals. Biotope is almost synonymous with the term habitat.

Box plot/Box and whiskers plot A visual display that summarises data using a 'box and whiskers' format to show the minimum and maximum values (ends of the whiskers), interquartile range (length of the box), and median (line through the box).

Carrier Animals/human beings harbouring potentially transmissible infectious agent(s) and are also donors of infection. They are mostly subclinical/inapparent cases. They may be: (a) true carriers, *i.e.* not manifesting any signs and symptoms of infection and shedding the agent or are infectious to others in the population; (b) incubatory carriers are cases between the time of entry to the time of appearance of first sign and symptoms of disease, (c) convalescent carriers are cases during the period of convalescence, *i.e.* disappearance of symptoms and final egress of the infectious agent, (d) transient carriers like the incubatory and convalescent shed the agent for short period, (e) persistent/chronic/lifelong carriers shed infectious agents for long time.

Case In epidemiology, a countable instance in the population or study group of a particular disease, health disorder, or condition under investigation. Sometimes, an individual with the particular disease.

Case-control study A type of observational analytic study. Enrolment into the study is based on presence (case) or absence (control) of disease. Characteristics such as previous exposure are then compared between cases and controls.

Case-crossover study In which a set of cases (subjects) is identified and a period of time before the onset of disease is selected (termed the case window) wherein the exposure to the risk factor of interest is evaluated. For each subject a second, non-overlapping time window (the control window) of the same length as the case window is selected, during which the subject did not experience the disease.

Case definition A set of standard criteria for deciding whether a person has a particular disease or health-related condition, by specifying clinical criteria and limitations on time, place, and person.

Case fatality rate The proportion of persons with a particular condition (cases) who die from that condition. The denominator is the number of incident case and the numerator is the number of cause-specific deaths among those cases.

Case report study A type of descriptive study that consists of a careful, detailed profile of an individual patient.

Case series study A type of descriptive study that describes characteristics of number of patients with a given disease.

Causality The relating of causes to the effects they produce. Some of the criteria for inferring a causal relationship between an implicated food and illness include strength of association, consistency of the observed association, temporal sequence of events biological plausibility of the observed association, effect of removing the exposure, dose-response relationships, and the exclusion of alternate explanations.

Cause of disease A factor (characteristic, behaviour, event etc.) that directly influences the occurrence of disease. A reduction of the factor in the population should lead to a reduction in the occurrence of disease.

Cause-specific mortality rate The mortality rate from a specified cause for a population. The numerator is the number of deaths attributed to a specific cause during a specified time interval and the denominator is the size of the population at the midpoint of the time interval.

Census The enumeration of an entire population, usually with details being recorded on residence, age, sex, occupation, ethnic group, marital status, birth history, and relationship to head of household.

Chance Unexpected, random, or unpredictable.

Chain of infection A process that begins when an agent leaves its reservoir or host through a portal of exit and is conveyed by some mode of transmission, then enters through an appropriate portal of entry to infect a susceptible host.

Chi square test A test of statistical significance. A Chi Square ($\chi 2$) test looks at the difference between what we observe in the data and what we would expect if the exposure was not associated with the illness.

Circular epidemiology Continuation of specific types of epidemiologic studies beyond the point of reasonable doubt of the true existence of an important association or the absence of such an association. It is an extreme example of studies of the consistency of associations.

Class interval A span of values of a continuous variable which are grouped into a single category for a frequency distribution of that variable.

Clinical disease A disease that has been identified by its symptoms and features.

Clinical trial An experimental study with patients as subjects. The goal is to evaluate a potential cure to prevent disease sequelae such as death or disability.

Climate It is the statistics of weather, usually over a 30-year interval of particular location. The weather can change in just a few hours; climate takes hundreds, thousands, even millions of years to change.

Climax It is the eventual balance reached among species in any given area. It is a stable ecological system resulting from the natural succession of plants and animals with eventual dominance of some and subordination or even possible extinction of others.

Cluster An aggregation of cases of a disease or other health-related condition, particularly cancer and birth defects, which are closely grouped in time and place. The number of cases may or may not exceed the expected number; frequently the expected number is not known.

Cohort A well-defined group of people who have had a common experience or exposure, who are then followed up for the incidence of new diseases or events, as in a cohort or prospective study. A group of people born during a particular period or year is called a birth cohort.

Cohort study A type of observational analytic study. It involves comparing disease incidence over time between groups (cohorts) that are found to differ on their exposure to a factor of interest. Cohort studies are either prospective or retrospective. Enrolment into the study is based on exposure characteristics or membership in a group. Disease, death, or other health-related outcomes are then ascertained and compared.

Colonised A carrier state that occurs when a person is not infected with a pathogen, but simply has it on the skin or mucous membrane.

Common source outbreak An outbreak that results from a group of persons being exposed to a common noxious influence, such as an infectious agent or toxin. If the group is exposed over a relatively brief period of time, so that all cases occur within one incubation period, then the common source outbreak is further classified as a point source outbreak. In some common source outbreaks, persons may be exposed over a period of days, weeks, or longer, with the exposure being either intermittent or continuous.

Communicable disease An infectious disease transmitted from an infected person, animal, or reservoir to a susceptible host through an intermediate plant, animal, or the inanimate environment.

Communicable period The period of time during which an infected host (person) remains capable of passing along the infective agent (*e.g.* a virus).

Confidence interval A range of values for a variable of interest, *e.g.* a rate, constructed so that this range has a specified probability of including the true value of the variable. The specified probability is called the confidence level, and the end points of the confidence interval are called the confidence limits. The statistical values described in this factsheet are frequently presented with upper and lower confidence limits. Confidence limits can be used as a guide to assess whether there is a significant difference between samples. The usual degree of confidence presented is 95%, *i.e.* the statistic presented is 95% certain to fall within the upper and lower confidence limits.

Confidence limit The minimum or maximum value of a confidence interval.

Confounding The distortion of the association between an exposure and a health outcome by a third factor that is related to both. This can occur when an association between a risk factor and disease can be explained by a factor associated with both disease and risk factor. For example, an association between smoking, alcohol consumption, and lung cancer is observed.

Consistency Reliability or uniformity of results or events.

Contact Exposure to a source of an infection, or a person so exposed.

Contact transmission The spread of an agent directly (person-to-person), indirectly, or by airborne droplets from less than three feet away.

Contagious Capable of being transmitted from one person to another by contact or close proximity.

Contingency table A two-variable table with cross-tabulated data.

Control A comparison group of people in a case-control study who do not have the disease or condition being studied. In a case-control study, comparison group of persons without disease.

Correlation The degree to which two or more measurements show a tendency to vary together. A measurement of the association or relationship between variables.

Cross-sectional study/Horizontal study A type of descriptive study in which a set of individuals are studied at a single point in time (or over a defined period of time) for the prevalence of disease. Both risk factors and disease status are ascertained at the same time. Cross-sectional studies commonly involve surveys to collect data.

Crude rate The rate calculated for an entire population.

Crude mortality rate The mortality rate from all causes of death for a population.

Cumulative frequency In a frequency distribution, the number or proportion of cases or events with a particular value or in a particular class interval, plus the total number or proportion of cases or events with smaller values of the variable.

Cumulative frequency curve A plot of the cumulative frequency rather than the actual frequency for each class interval of a variable. This type of graph is useful for identifying medians, quartiles, and other percentiles.

Cumulative incidence The risk of new disease occurrence is quantified using cumulative incidence, also called incidence risk. It is defined as the proportion of disease-free individuals developing a given disease over a specified time, conditional on that individuals not dying from any other disease during the period.

Data Numerical information. Data is a plural term; the singular is datum.

Death-to-case ratio The number of deaths attributed to a particular disease during a specified time period divided by the number of new cases of that disease identified during the same time period.

Demography/Demographic information The 'person' characteristics—age, sex, race, and occupation—of descriptive epidemiology used to characterise the populations at risk.

Denominator The lower portion of a fraction used to calculate a rate or ratio. In a rate, the denominator is usually the population (or population experience, as in person-years, etc.) at risk.

Dependent variable/predictor A variable that may be predicted by or caused by one or more other variables, called independent variables. In a statistical analysis, the outcome variable(s) or the variable(s) whose values are a function of other variable(s).

Deterministic model A mathematical model in which the parameters and variables are not subject to random fluctuations, so that the system is at any time entirely defined by the initial conditions chosen.

Descriptive epidemiology The aspect of epidemiology concerned with organising and summarising health-related data according to time, place, and person.

Descriptive statistics Quantitative, or numerical, information used to describe a set of observed cases.

Detection bias This type of bias can occur when persons with a risk factor are more likely to have disease detected because of more intense follow-up.

Determinant Any factor, whether event, characteristic, or other definable entity, that brings about change in a health condition, or in other defined characteristics.

Discrete variable It is a variable for which there is a definite distance from one value of the variable to the next possible value.

Direct transmission The immediate transfer of an agent from a reservoir to a susceptible host by direct contact or droplet spread.

Disease burden The effect of a health problem measured by financial cost, death, illness, or other indicators.

Disease-free zone Attempts are made to control a specific disease to bring it to zero level in certain defined administrative/geographic area. Animals reared in such a zone are thus free from the disease against which this concerted effort has been made. For example, FMD-free zones in some southern states of India are attempted.

Disease investigation/Outbreak investigation The investigation of the occurrence of a disease in a specific group of people.

Disinfection It is the process of making places and objects free from vegetative pathogens. The agents used are called disinfectants, *e.g.* bactericides, germicides, fungicides, virucides. These are used on inanimate objects, like equipment, tables, premises, and not on skin or tissues.

Distribution In epidemiology, the frequency and pattern of health-related characteristics and events in a population. In statistics, the observed or theoretical frequency of values of a variable.

Dot plot/dot map A visual display of the actual data points of a non-continuous variable. In other words it is a visual display of the specific data points of a variable that has a finite number of values, such as race or sex.

Droplet nuclei The residue of dried droplets that may remain suspended in the air for long periods, may be blown over great distances, and are easily inhaled into the lungs and exhaled.

Droplet spread The direct transmission of an infectious agent from a reservoir to a susceptible host by spray with relatively large, short-ranged aerosols produced by sneezing, coughing, or talking.

Ecological (or correlational) study A type of descriptive study involving the comparison of disease frequency (incidence or prevalence) between populations that are different with respect to one or more risk factors of interest. The risk factor information is not known for individual subjects, but rather as a total population characteristic.

Ecological epidemiology A branch of epidemiology which views disease as a result of the ecological interactions between populations of hosts and parasites.

Ecological fallacy With an ecological study, the risk factor information is not known for individual subjects, but rather as a total population characteristic. For example, an ecological study may find that Japanese people have a high rate of stomach cancer and also a high rate of rice consumption. However, with an ecological study, it is not known if the same individuals who eat rice are the same as those who have stomach cancer.

Ecological interfaces An ecological interface is a junction of two ecosystems. Infectious diseases can be transmitted across these interfaces.

Ecological mosaics An ecological mosaic is a modified patch of vegetation, created by man, within a biome that has reached a climax.

Ecosystem A combination of biotic community and its environment.

Effect modification This refers to variation in the magnitude of a measure of exposure effect across levels of another variable.

Effectiveness The degree to which an intervention or programme produces the intended or expected results under real-world conditions.

Efficacy The degree to which an intervention or programme produces the intended or expected results under ideal conditions.

Endemic fadeout Parasite extinction occurring because endemic levels are so low that it is possible for small stochastic fluctuations to remove all parasites.

Endemic disease The constant presence of a disease or infectious agent within a given geographic area or population group; may also refer to the usual prevalence of a given disease within such area or group.

Environment The third part of the epidemiological triangle, which brings the other two parts of the triangle—the host (or, person) and the agent (or, virus)—together so that a disease occurs.

Environmental factor An extrinsic factor (geology, climate, insects, sanitation, health services, etc.) which affects the agent and the opportunity for exposure.

Epidemic The occurrence of more cases of disease than expected in a given area or among a specific group of people over a particular period of time.

Epidemic curve A histogram or graph that shows the course of a disease outbreak or epidemic by plotting the number of cases by time of onset.

Epidemic fadeout Parasite extinction occurring because numbers are so low immediately following an epidemic that it is possible for small stochastic fluctuations to remove all parasites.

Epidemic period A time period when the number of cases of disease reported is greater than expected.

Epidemiologic triad/Epidemiological triangle The traditional model of infectious disease causation. It includes three components: an external agent, a susceptible host, and an environment that brings the host and agent together, so that disease occurs.

Epidemiology The study of distribution and determinants of health-related states or events in specified populations, and the application of this study to the control of health problems.

Epiphytotic An epidemic in a plant host population.

Epizootiology It is the study of disease in animal populations and of factors that determine its occurrence.

Equilibrium A state in which a system is not changing. A population size might be at a static equilibrium at which nothing is happening (there are no births or deaths) or a dynamic equilibrium at which different processes are balanced (there are the same numbers of births and deaths). More generally, the state to which a system eventually evolves, for example sustained periodic oscillations, might be called an equilibrium.

Equivalent Average Death rate (EADR) In this method of adjustment each age-specific rate is weighted with the corresponding interval length rather than the number of people for which the rate is computed. It is a measure of mortality in a dynamic population. It is calculated by number of animals died divided by total number of animal days multiplied by 1000. It is usually expressed as EADR per 1000 animal days.

Equivalent Average Morbidity rate (EAMR) In this method of adjustment each age-specific rate is weighted with the corresponding interval length rather than the number of people for which the rate is computed. It is a measure of morbidity in a dynamic population. It is calculated by number of animals morbid divided by total number of animal days multiplied by 1000. It is usually expressed as EADR per 1000 animal days.

Evaluation A process that attempts to determine as systematically and objectively as possible the relevance, effectiveness, and impact of activities in the light of their objectives.

Exotic disease Disease which is of foreign origin for a country. For example, Blue tongue in India was recorded in sheep in 1984. It is supposed to have been imported with exotic breeds of sheep. Exotic disease is imported also with animal feed or other products of animal origin.

Exzootic disease A disease that has been stamped out or eradicated from a country. For example Rabies, Bovine tuberculosis, brucellosis in many countries.

Experimental study A study in which the investigator specifies the exposure category for each individual (clinical trial) or community (community trial), then follows the individuals or community to detect the effects of the exposure.

Exposed (group) A group whose members have been exposed to a supposed cause of disease or health state of interest, or possess a characteristic that is a determinant of the health outcome of interest.

Exponential growth An increase in which the rate of growth is always proportional to the amount of material remaining; the constant of proportionality is the rate constant.

False-negative A negative test result for a person who actually has the condition.

False-positive A positive test result for a person who actually does not have the condition.

Feedback It involves deliberately infecting pigs with infected intestine so that the herd develops natural protective antibodies. The method is long, complex, needs strict follow-up till virus is considered eliminated; many pigs die in the process; and not applicable to pigs with suppressed immunity because of co-infection of porcine respiratory and reproductive syndrome virus. In case of Porcine Epidemic Diarrhoea in absence of vaccine the alternate option may be feedback.

Foodborne transmission A type of disease transmission in which the infectious agent (which can be bacteria, parasites, viruses, fungi, and their products, or toxic substances not of microbial origin) is passed on through food.

Fomite An inanimate object that can be used to transmit an infectious agent. This may be contaminated transfusion products or injections, towels or bedding, surgical instruments, or contaminated food, water, or air.

Frequency distribution A complete summary of the frequencies of the values or categories of a variable; often displayed in a two-column table: the left column lists the individual values or categories and the right column indicates the number of observations in each category.

Frequency polygon A graph of a frequency distribution with values of the variable on the x-axis and the number of observations on the y-axis; data points are plotted at the midpoints of the intervals and are connected with a straight line.

Graph A way to show quantitative data visually, using a system of coordinates.

Habitat Food area

Health A state of complete physical, mental, and social well-being and not merely the absence of disease or infirmity.

Health indicator A measure that reflects, or indicates, the state of health of persons in a defined population, *e.g.* the infant mortality rate.

Health information system A combination of health statistics from various sources, used to derive information about health status, health care, provision and use of services, and impact on health.

Herd immunity The resistance of a group to an infectious agent. This group resistance exists because a high proportion of people in the group are immune to the agent. Herd immunity is based on having a substantial number of people who are immune, which reduces the probability that they will come into contact with an infected person. By vaccinating large numbers of people in a population to protect them from smallpox, for example, health officials used herd immunity to control and eradicate the disease.

High-risk group A group in the community with an elevated risk of disease.

Histogram A graphic representation of the frequency distribution of a continuous variable. Rectangles are drawn in such a way that their bases lie on a linear scale representing different intervals, and their heights are proportional to the frequencies of the values within each of the intervals.

Holoendemic When essentially every individual in a population is infected.

Holoendemic Transmission occurs all year long.

Horizontal survey A study of a community perhaps stratified by age, sex, ethnicity, etc., but at one point in time or over a short time interval. Although a snapshot, horizontal surveys of prevalence and intensity within different age classes of a community can nevertheless provide valuable information on the rate at which hosts acquire infection through time, provided that the host and parasite populations have sufficiently low, therfore thre population has limited or no immunity to it.

Horizontal transmission Transmission occurring generally within a population, but not including vertical transmission.

Host A person or other living organism that can be infected by an infectious agent under natural conditions.

Host factor An intrinsic factor (age, race, sex, behaviours, etc.) which influences an individual's exposure, susceptibility, or response to a causative agent.

Hygiene It deals with principles and procedures employed for promoting health. Veterinary hygiene is concerned with health problems and specific diseases of domestic animals, poultry, and wildlife with a view to ensure their health and/or socio-economic utility.

Hyperendemic When a disease is continuously present to a high level, affecting all age groups equally.

Hypoendemic Denoting a population or area in which a disease incidence is sufficiently low that the population has limited or no immunity to it.

Hypothesis A supposition arrived at from observation or reflection, which leads to refutable predictions. Any conjecture cast in a form that will allow it to be tested and refuted.

Hypothesis, alternative The hypothesis, to be adopted if the null hypothesis proves implausible, in which exposure is associated with disease.

Hypothesis, null The first step in testing for statistical significance in which it is assumed that the exposure is not related to disease.

Informatics It is the supply of information through the medium of the computer.

Immunity, active Resistance developed in response to stimulus by an antigen (infecting agent or vaccine) and usually characterised by the presence of antibody produced by the host.

Immunity, herd The resistance of a group to invasion and spread of an infectious agent, based on the resistance to infection of a high proportion of individual members of the group. The resistance is a product of the number susceptible and the probability that those who are susceptible will come into contact with an infected person.

Immunity, passive Immunity conferred by an antibody produced in another host and acquired naturally by an infant from its mother or artificially by administration of an antibody-containing preparation (antiserum or immune globulin).

Immunisation Introducing weakened or killed germs or toxins into the body so that the immune system will make protective antibodies that will destroy the disease-causing agent (for example, a virus) if it enters the body at a later time.

Immunogenicity The ability of a vaccine to stimulate the immune system, as measured by the proportion of individuals who produce specific antibody or T cells, or the amount of antibody produced.

Incidence density Incidence density (also called true incidence rate, hazard rate, force of morbidity or mortality) is defined as the instantaneous potential for change in disease status per unit of time at time t, relative to the size of the disease-free population at time t.

Incidence rate A measure of the frequency with which an event, such as a new case of illness, occurs in a population over a period of time. The denominator is the population at risk; the numerator is the number of new cases occurring during a given time period. Incidence is the number of new cases occurring in a specified period of time and in a defined population.

Incubation period A period of subclinical or inapparent pathologic changes following exposure, ending with the onset of symptoms of infectious disease.

Independent variable An exposure, risk factor, or other characteristic being observed or measured that is hypothesised to influence an event or manifestation (the dependent variable).

Index case The first case of a disease or health condition that is known to investigators. Identifying the index case can be helpful in determining the origin of a disease outbreak.

Indicator species A dominant organism for a particular climax.

Indirect transmission The transmission of an agent carried from a reservoir to a susceptible host by suspended air particles or by animate (vector) or inanimate (vehicle) intermediaries.

Individual data Data that have not been put into a frequency distribution or rank ordered.

Infection It is invasion of body of a living organism with living agent and often without any evidence of disease.

Infectious period The time period during which infected are able to transmit an infection to any susceptible host or vector they contact. Note that the infectious period may not necessarily be associated with symptoms of the disease.

Infectivity It is an attribute of infectious agent and indicates the ability to invade, lodge, and multiple in a host. In case of contact-borne infection, secondary attack rate measures the infectivity.

Inference, statistical In statistics, the development of generalisations from sample data, usually with calculated degrees of uncertainty.

Information bias The type of bias can occur when interviewers who are aware of the identity of subjects or factors of interest (*e.g.* case or control) and collect information unevenly between subjects.

Isolation/Segregation In order to check the spread of disease from the cases to the healthy, method of segregation/isolation is used. The diseased, *i.e.* cases are kept isolated/segregated from the healthy ones. Depending upon the contagiousness of disease, immediate, strict/less stringent, and complete/incomplete isolation is organised. In case of highly contagious disease, it has to be immediate and complete. In the case of complete isolation, sick animals and all that come in contact with it, like bedding, leftover feed, etc., must also be removed and the latter terminally disinfected. The premises have to be thoroughly cleaned and sanitised. Separate set of attendants is required to look after the sick animals. Examples of such diseases are FMD, HS, and Anthrax. In the cases of mastitis, injuries, fractures, nutritional diseases less stringent and incomplete isolation can do. However, farm hygiene should never be compromised. Animal attendants should be asked to look after the healthy animals first and then the sick ones. The waste of the farm should be safely disposed. Premises should be kept clean and sanitised.

Interaction Two or more component causes acting in the same sufficient cause.

Interquartile range The central portion of a distribution, calculated as the difference between the third quartile and the first quartile; this range includes about one-half of the observations in the set, leaving one-quarter of the observations on each side.

Isolation Limiting movement of or separating people who are ill with a contagious disease.

Landscape epidemiology The study of diseases in relation to the ecosystems in which they are found.

Latency period A period of subclinical or inapparent pathologic changes following exposure, ending with the onset of symptoms of chronic disease.

Life expectancy Life expectancy is the average number of years of life remaining to a person at a particular age and is based on a given set of age-specific death rates, generally the mortality conditions existing in the period mentioned. Life expectancy may be determined by race, sex, or other characteristics using age-specific death rates for the population with that characteristic.

Live birth A live birth is the complete expulsion or extraction from its mother of a product of conception, irrespective of the duration of the pregnancy, which, after such separation, breathes or shows any other evidence of life such as heartbeat, umbilical cord pulsation, or definite movement of voluntary muscles, whether the umbilical cord has been cut or the placenta is attached. Each product of such a birth is considered live born.

Line listing A list, or spreadsheet, of cases containing demographic characteristics and other key descriptions.

Mass screening Large-scale screening of whole, unselected population groups.

Measure of association A quantified relationship between exposure and a particular health problem.

Mean, arithmetic The measure of central location commonly called the average. It is calculated by adding together all the individual values in a group of measurements and dividing by the number of values in the group.

Mean, geometric The mean or average of a set of data measured on a logarithmic scale.

Measure of association A quantified relationship between exposure and disease; includes relative risk, rate ratio, odds ratio.

Measure of central location A central value that best represents a distribution of data. Measures of central location include the mean, median, and mode. Also called the measure of central tendency.

Measure of dispersion A measure of the spread of a distribution out from its central value. Measures of dispersion used in epidemiology include the interquartile range, variance, and the standard deviation.

Median The measure of central location which divides a set of data into two equal parts.

Medical surveillance The monitoring of potentially exposed individuals to detect early symptoms of disease.

Mesoendemic It is an endemic disease that affects a moderate proportion of the population at risk.

Mesoendemic Regular seasonal transmission.

Metaphylaxis It is the prevention of symptoms. Disease is present in metaphylaxis. As an example, if you are deworming your dog every 4 weeks, that is a metaphylactic treatment in that it does not prevent parasitic infection, but it prevents the dog from shedding eggs and developing symptoms as a result of that infection. However, dictionary defined it as the timely mass medication of group of animals (drove/flock/herd) to eliminate or minimise an expected outbreak of disease, *e.g.* the routine administration of antibiotics in livestock.

Midrange The halfway point or midpoint in a set of observations. For most types of data, it is calculated as the sum of the smallest observation and the largest observation, divided by two. For age data, one is added to the numerator. The midrange is usually calculated as an intermediate step in determining other measures.

Misclassification This type of bias can occur when there is error in classifying subjects by disease or risk factor that tends to distort associations between disease and risk factors. The effect of misclassification with respect to exposure or disease is dependent on the individual's disease or exposure status. When the misclassification is random or non-differential, the proportions of subjects erroneously classified in the study groups are approximately equal. With differential misclassification, the proportions of subjects classified incorrectly differ between groups.

Mode A measure of central location, the most frequently occurring value in a set of observations.

Mode of transmission The way or ways in which a disease is transmitted. The transmission can be direct (person-to-person) or indirect.

Molecular epidemiology A kind of epidemiologic investigation that uses molecular laboratory techniques to detect outbreaks.

Morbidity Any departure, subjective or objective, from a state of physiological or psychological well-being.

Mortality/mortality rate A measure of the frequency of occurrence of death in a defined population during a specified interval of time (or) the number of deaths due to a disease occurring in a specified period of time and in a defined population.

Mortality rate, infant A ratio expressing the number of deaths among children under 1 year of age reported during a given time period divided by the number of births reported during the same time period. The infant mortality rate is usually expressed per 1000 live births.

Mortality rate, neonatal A ratio expressing the number of deaths among children from birth up to but not including 28 days of age divided by the number of live births reported during the same time period. The neonatal mortality rate is usually expressed per 1000 live births.

Mortality rate, postneonatal A ratio expressing the number of deaths among children from 28 days up to but not including 1 year of age during a given time period divided by the number of live births reported during the same time period. The postneonatal mortality rate is usually expressed per 1000 live births.

Natural history of disease The temporal course of disease from onset (inception) to resolution.

Necessary cause A causal factor whose presence is required for the occurrence of the effect (of disease).

Negative predictive value The proportion of those testing negative in a screening test for a disease who truly do not have the disease.

Nested case-control study It is similar to a cohort study with the key difference that a sample of non-cases is selected for analysis (rather than the entire cohort, as in the case of a cohort study).

Niche It is a place or relationship of a particular species with respect to such things as food and its enemies. Biotope is address of the organism; niche is its occupation.

Nidus It is a place where something originates, develops, or is located or it is a place or substance in an animal or plant where bacteria or other organisms lodge and multiply. It is a focus of infection.

Nominal scale Classification into unordered qualitative categories; *e.g.* race, religion, and country of birth as measurements of individual attributes are purely nominal scales, as there is no inherent order to their categories.

Nosoarea A nosoarea is a nosogenic territory in which a particular disease is present.

Nosogenic territory An area that has ecological, social, and environmental conditions that can support a disease outcome.

Normal curve A bell-shaped curve that results when a normal distribution is graphed.

Normal distribution The symmetrical clustering of values around a central location. The properties of a normal distribution include the following: (1) It is a continuous, symmetrical distribution; both tails extend to infinity; (2) the arithmetic mean, mode, and median are identical; and (3) its shape is completely determined by the mean and standard deviation.

Notifiable disease A list of diseases is notifiable in every country. The health administration keeps a constant vigil and reports the occurrence of a notifiable disease. The notification is obligatory. The list of notifiable diseases changes. The notifiable animal diseases in India are: FMD, HS, blackleg, rabies, anthrax, Johne's disease, tuberculosis, glanders, epizootic lymphangitis, clostridial diseases of cattle and sheep and surra.

Numerator The upper portion of a fraction.

Observational study Epidemiological study in situations where nature is allowed to take its course. Changes or differences in one characteristic are studied in relation to changes or differences in others, without the intervention of the investigator.

Odds ratio A measure of association which quantifies the relationship between an exposure and health outcome from a comparative study; also known as the cross-product ratio.

Ordinal scale Classification into ordered qualitative categories; *e.g.* social class (I, II, III, etc.), where the values have a distinct order, but their categories are qualitative in that there is no natural (numerical) distance between their positive values.

Outbreak It is an epidemic of localised nature. The spatial distribution is small, e.g. food poisoning outbreak.

Outbreak investigation The investigation of the occurrence of a disease in a specific group of people.

Outlier In statistics, an observation or value that is significantly different from the rest of the scores.

Oversample A sampling procedure designed to give a demographic or geographic population a larger proportion of representation in the sample than the population's proportion of representation in the overall population.

p-value The probability of obtaining a result at least as extreme as a given data point, assuming the data point was the result of chance alone.

Pathogenicity (or virulence) It is a property of an infectious agent indicating its ability to induce clinical disease in the host invaded. The ratio = infected with disease (divided by) total infected measures the pathogenicity.

Panel study It combines the features of cross-sectional and prospective cohort designs. It can be viewed as a series of cross-sectional studies conducted on the same subjects (the panel) at successive time intervals (sometimes referred to as waves).

Pandemic/panzootic An epidemic occurring over a very wide area (several countries or continents) and usually affecting a large proportion of the population.

Parity Parity is defined as the total number of live births ever had by the woman. This number is distinguished from gravidity, which is the total number of times she has been pregnant. Nulliparous women are those who have had no live births, and parous women are those who have given birth to at least one baby.

Passive immunity Immunity conferred by an antibody produced in another host. This type of immunity can be acquired naturally by an infant from its mother or artificially by administration of an antibody-containing preparation (antiserum or immune globulin).

Passive surveillance A provider-based approach to data collection, in which health departments or the Centers for Disease Control and Prevention (CDC) depend on disease reports to be submitted by laboratories, clinicians, and the public.

Pathogenicity The proportion of persons infected, after exposure to a causative agent, who then develop clinical disease.

Percentile The set of numbers from 0 to 100 that divide a distribution into 100 parts of equal area, or divide a set of ranked data into 100 class intervals with each interval containing 1/100 of the observations. A particular percentile, say the 5th percentile, is a cut point with 5 percent of the observations below it and the remaining 95% of the observations above it.

Period prevalence The amount a particular disease present in a population over a period of time.

Person-years The sum of the lengths of time of experience or exposure of a group of people who have been observed for varying periods of time, in other words, the total amount of time, expressed in years, that the entire group been exposed, observed, or at risk.

Person-time rate A measure of the incidence rate of an event, *e.g.* a disease or death, in a population at risk over an observed period to time, that directly incorporates time into the denominator.

Pie chart A circular chart in which the size of each 'slice' is proportional to the frequency of each category of a variable.

Point prevalence The amount of a particular disease present in a population at a single point in time.

Point source outbreak An outbreak that results from an exposure to the same source.

Population The total number of inhabitants of a given area or country. In sampling, the population may refer to the units from which the sample is drawn, not necessarily the total population of people.

Population attributable risk (rate) It is the increase or decrease in incidence risk (or rate) of disease in the population that is attributable to exposure or it is the impact that a specified exposure may have on the total population with respect to a particular outcome.

Population attributable fraction/aetiologic fraction It is the proportion of disease in the population that is due to the exposure.

Population at risk The total number of inhabitants of a given area who may contract the disease of interest.

Portal of entry A pathway into the host that gives an agent access to tissue that will allow it to multiply or act.

Portal of exit A pathway by which an agent can leave its host.

Positive predictive value A measure of the predictive value of a reported case or epidemic; the proportion of cases reported by a surveillance system or classified by a case definition which are true cases.

Precision 'Precise' means sharply defined or measured. Data can be very precise, but inaccurate.

Prepatent period It refers to the time between infection and when the agent becomes first detectable, and the period of communicability is the time during which the infected host is capable of transmitting the agent.

Prevalence The number or proportion of cases or events or conditions in a given population. Prevalence is the number of people currently living with a disease and provides a useful indication of the number of patients being actively treated for their disease.

Prevalence rate The proportion of persons in a population who have a particular disease or attribute at a specified point in time or over a specified period of time.

Primary case A person who acquires a disease from an exposure, for example, to contaminated food.

Proclimax A biological community held short of its natural climax by man-made factors, such as agriculture.

Programme evaluation The study of the activities and outcomes of a programme or project in order to assess its effectiveness or value.

Propagated outbreak An outbreak that does not have a common source, but instead spreads from person to person.

Prophylaxis It is a case-specific administration of preventative medicine (vaccine, antibiotic, etc.) to an individual patient. There is no disease present in prophylaxis.

Proportion A type of ratio in which the numerator is included in the denominator. The ratio of a part to the whole, expressed as a "decimal fraction" (*e.g.* 0.2), as a fraction (1/5), or, loosely, as a percentage (20%).

Proportionate mortality The proportion of deaths in a specified population over a period of time attributable to different causes. Each cause is expressed as a percentage of all deaths, and the sum of the causes must add to 100%. These proportions are not mortality rates, since the denominator is all deaths, not the population in which the deaths occurred.

Prospective study At the time a study begins, either the exposure or the outcome of interest has not yet occurred.

Public health surveillance The systematic collection, analysis, interpretation, and dissemination of health data on an ongoing basis, to gain knowledge of the pattern of disease occurrence and potential in a community, in order to control and prevent disease in the community.

Quarantine Limiting movement of or separating people who are not sick but are presumed to have been exposed to a contagious disease.

Questionnaire A set of questions used to collect information. Typically questions can be grouped into the following categories: identifying, demographic, clinical, risk, and reported information.

Race-specific mortality rate A mortality rate limited to a specified racial group. Both numerator and denominator are limited to the specified group.

Random sample A sample derived by selecting individuals such that each individual has the same probability of selection.

Randomised clinical trials The randomised clinical trial is the epidemiologic design that most closely resembles a laboratory experiment.

Range In statistics, the difference between the largest and smallest values in a distribution. In common use, the span of values from smallest to largest.

Rate An expression of the frequency with which an event occurs in a defined population.

Rate ratio A comparison of two groups in terms of incidence rates, person-time rates, or mortality rates.

Ratio The value obtained by dividing one quantity by another.

Recall bias This type of bias can occur in retrospective studies when persons with disease tend to report past exposures and events differently from persons without disease.

Relative risk It is ratio of the rate of disease (incidence or mortality) among those exposed to the rate among those not exposed to the factor (supposedly causing disease or death).

Reliability Refers to the consistency of a measurement when repeated on the same subjects.

Repeated survey It is a series of cross-sectional studies performed over time on the same study population, but each is sampled independently.

Representative sample A sample whose characteristics correspond to those of the original population or reference population.

Reservoir They are generally such animals that naturally harbour infective agents. Any human, animal, arthropod, plant, soil, or even inanimate matter in which an infectious agent normally lives and multiplies and on which it depends primarily for its survival reproducing itself in a manner that it can be transmitted to a susceptible host is a reservoir of infectious agent.

Retrospective study At the time a study begins, both the exposure and the outcome of interest have occurred.

Risk The probability that an event will occur, *e.g.* that an individual will become ill or die within a stated period of time or age.

Risk analysis A process consisting of three components: risk assessment, risk management, and risk communication.

Risk assessment A scientifically based process consisting of the following steps: (a) hazard identification, (b) hazard characterisation, (c) exposure assessment, and (d) risk characterisation.

Risk characterisation The process of determining the qualitative and/or quantitative estimation, including attendant uncertainties, of the probability of occurrence and severity of known or potential adverse health effects in a given population based on hazard identification, hazard characterisation, and exposure assessment.

Risk communication The interactive exchange of information and opinions concerning risk and risk management among risk assessors, risk managers, consumers, and other interested parties.

Risk Estimate Output of risk characterisation.

Risk factor An aspect of personal behaviour or lifestyle, an environmental exposure, or an inborn or inherited characteristic that is associated with an increased occurrence of disease or other health-related event or condition.

Risk Management The process of weighing policy alternatives in the light of the results of risk assessment and, if required, selecting and implementing appropriate control options, including regulatory measures.

Risk ratio A comparison of the risk of some health-related event such as disease or death in two groups.

Sample A selected subset of a population. A sample may be random or non-random and it may be representative or non-representative.

Sample size The size of the group being studied. 'N' is used to indicate the sample size; for example, if you have a sample of 34 people, $n = 34$.

Sanitation It refers to public health conditions related to clean drinking water and adequate treatment and disposal of human excreta and sewage. Preventing human contact with faeces is part of sanitation, as is hand washing with soap.

Sanitizer These are substances used to reduce the microbial counts on the surface of objects, *e.g.* operation table. Detergent sanitizers are sanitizers with wetting and emulsifying properties.

Screening The presumptive identification of unrecognised disease or defect by the application of tests, examinations, or other procedures which can be applied rapidly.

Scatter diagram A graph in which each dot represents paired values for two continuous variables, with the x-axis representing one variable and the y-axis representing the other; used to display the relationship between the two variables; also called a scattergram.

Seasonality Change in physiological status or in disease occurrence that conforms to a regular seasonal pattern.

Secondary attack rate A measure of the frequency of new cases of a disease among the contacts of known cases.

Secondary case A person who gets a disease from exposure to a person with the disease, or primary case.

Secular trend Changes over a long period of time, generally years or decades.

Selective screening Screening of selected high-risk groups in the population.

Sensitivity The ability of a system to detect epidemics and other changes in disease occurrence. The proportion of persons with disease who are correctly identified by a screening test or case definition as having disease.

Sentinel surveillance A surveillance system in which a pre-arranged sample of reporting sources agrees to report all cases of one or more notifiable conditions or diseases.

Shifting antigenicity The condition when an infection-causing organism's antibody producing characteristics change greatly, which usually causes immunity to the infection to decrease significantly.

Sex-specific mortality rate A mortality rate among either males or females.

Significance test A test of statistical significance shows how likely one is to get a measure of association as strong as the observed one if there is no difference between the groups.

Skewed A distribution that is asymmetrical.

Specificity The proportion of persons without disease who are correctly identified by a screening test or case definition as not having disease.

Sporadic In this case the diseases appear only rarely or occasionally in individuals of a given population.

Spot map A map that indicates the location of each case of a rare disease or outbreak by a place that is potentially relevant to the health event being investigated, such as where each case lived or worked.

Stamping out It is a concerted effort to 'stamp out' a disease or infection or a foreign vector species from an area, as soon as it is recognised. Action against the recent bird flu in Hong Kong is an example. Bird flu is a direct host density dependent disease. The methods applied are 'early detection, chasing/tracing', and using even coercive or drastic methods like strict isolation/quarantine, slaughter, proper disposal of the carcass, terminal disinfection, thorough disinfection of the premises, etc., mass vaccination for cordoning, etc., depending upon the disease and situation.

Standard deviation The most widely used measure of dispersion of a frequency distribution, equal to the positive square root of the variance.

Standard error (of the mean) The standard deviation of a theoretical distribution of sample means about the true population mean.

Standard population A population used to allow comparisons over time and among different parts of the population. By convention in the USA, the standard population is the US population in the year 2000.

Statistical significance The degree to which a value is greater or smaller than would be expected to occur by chance. Typically, a relationship is considered statistically significant when the probability of obtaining that result by chance is less than five percent if there were, in fact, no relationship in the population being studied.

Study design The methodology that is used to investigate a particular health phenomenon or exposure-disease relationship. Studies can be descriptive or analytical.

Study population The population of specific interest, *e.g.* New Delhi female dog population.

Subclinical/inapparent/latent infection Without apparent symptoms. It is the impact that a specified exposure may have on the total population with respect to a particular outcome.

Sufficient cause A causal factor or collection of factors whose presence is always followed by the occurrence of the effect (of disease).

Superspreader An individual who is much more infective than most other people with the disease.

Surveillance The collection of information on cases of disease or other conditions in a standard way to detect increases or decreases in the disease over time and differences between various geographic areas. Public health officials use the information to detect outbreaks and to plan programmes to help prevent and control disease.

Survival The proportion of individuals diagnosed with a specific disease surviving over a defined period of time.

Survival curve A curve that starts at 100% of the study population and shows the percentage of the population still surviving at successive times for as long as information is available. May be applied not only to survival as such, but also to the persistence of freedom from a disease, or complication or some other endpoint.

Symptom Any indication of disease noticed or felt by a patient

Syndromic surveillance The collection and analysis of pre-diagnosis information that lead to an estimation of the health status of the community. In other words it is monitoring of non-specific health indicators including clinical signs, symptoms, or proxy measures to enable the early identification of the impact (or absence of impact) of potential human or veterinary public health threats.

Synanthropic ecosystem Synanthropic ecosystem is one that is in contact with man. This facilitates transmission of zoonotic infections.

Table A set of data arranged in rows and columns.

Table shell A table that is complete except for the data.

Targeted intervention A programme or activity intended to improve a health condition among a specific group of people.

Theory An explanation accounting for known facts or phenomena, capable of predicting future occurrences or observations of the same kind, and capable of being tested through experiment or proven false through empirical observation.

Threshold host density It is used in wildlife disease ecology. It refers to the minimum concentration of individuals necessary to sustain a given disease within a population. In Direct Host Density Dependent diseases incidence is elevated in high host density conditions, *e.g.* brucellosis, avian influenza, Echinococcus multilocularis. The population may be reduced (not reach extinction) during the course. Reduced population means lower rate of infection, reaching equilibrium. Host Density Independent diseases show no correlation between host population and disease incidence; examples are sexually transmitted diseases in human and animals. Inverse Host Density dependent diseases show increase in incidence of parasitism or disease when host density is low. Vector-borne diseases often exhibit inverse density dependence.

Transmission of infection Any mode or mechanism by which an infectious agent is spread through the environment or to another person.

Trend A long-term movement or change in frequency, usually upwards or downwards.

Type I Errors/alpha error/false-positive Type I errors occur when the null hypothesis is rejected when it is true.

Type II errors/beta error/false-negative Type II errors occur when the null hypothesis is accepted when it is false.

Two-by-two table A table with only two variables, in which each variable has only two categories. Usually one variable represents a health outcome, and one represents an exposure or characteristic.

Universal precautions Recommendations issued by CDC to minimise the risk of transmission of bloodborne pathogens, particularly HIV and HBV, by healthcare and public safety workers. Barrier precautions are to be used to prevent exposure to blood and certain body fluids of all patients.

Vaccine efficacy It stands for the proportion of disease prevented by the vaccine in vaccinated animals. Vaccine efficacy is estimated through subtracting cumulative incidence in vaccinated animals from cumulative incidence in unvaccinated animals, and dividing the resulting value by the cumulative incidence in unvaccinated animals.

Validity The degree to which a measurement actually measures or detects what it is supposed to measure.

Variable Any characteristic or attribute that can be measured.

Variance A measure of the dispersion shown by a set of observations, defined by the sum of the squares of deviations from the mean, divided by the number of degrees of freedom in the set of observations.

Vectors These are generally invertebrates (in some cases vertebrate also) which are responsible for the transmission of an infectious agent from an infected individual or its excreta to a susceptible one to some immediate source such as feed or water.

Vehicle It is any non-living substance or object like dust, milk, food, water, serum, pus, etc. by which or upon which an infectious agent passes from an infected individual to a susceptible one.

Vehicular transmission It refers to transfer of the agent in inanimate substances (fomite).

Virulence It refers to the severity of disease and is dependent upon the agent's ability to leave permanent sequelae, such as death or paralysis or pockmark, etc. Case fatality rate (death is the permanent sequelae) or number of severe cases (define severity, *e.g.* paralysis in Polio) divided by total number of cases measures the virulence of the infectious agent/its serotype/strain. In laboratory animal experiments, LD50 is measured using Reed and Muench technique.

Vital statistics Systematically tabulated information about births, marriages, divorces, and deaths, based on registration of these vital events.

Years of potential life lost A measure of the impact of premature mortality on a population, calculated as the sum of the differences between some predetermined minimum or desired life span and the age of death for individuals who died earlier than that predetermined age.

Zoonoses An infectious disease that is transmissible under normal conditions from animals to humans.

Printed in the United States
by Baker & Taylor Publisher Services